Social Skills Training for Schizophrenia

SOCIAL SKILLS TRAINING FOR SCHIZOPHRENIA

A Step-by-Step Guide

Second Edition

Alan S. Bellack
Kim T. Mueser
Susan Gingerich
Julie Agresta

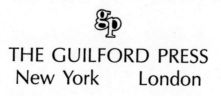

THE GUILFORD PRESS
New York   London

Library of Congress Cataloging-in-Publication Data

Social Skills training for schizophrenia: a step-by-step guide / Alan S. Bellack . . . [et al.].—2nd ed.
   p. ; cm.
Includes bibliographical references and index.
   ISBN 1-57230-846-X (paper: alk. paper)
   1. Schizophrenia—Rehabilitation. 2. Social skills—Study and teaching.
   [DNLM: 1. Schizophrenia—rehabilitation. 2. Behavior Therapy—Methods. 3. Interpersonal
Relations. 4. Psychotherapy, Group—methods. 5. Social Behavior. WM 203 S678 2004]
   I. Bellack, Alan S.
   RC514.S595 2004
   616.89'806—dc22

2003024140

About the Authors

Alan S. Bellack, PhD, ABPP, is Professor of Psychiatry and Director of the Division of Psychology at the University of Maryland School of Medicine and Director of the VA Capitol Health Care Network Mental Illness Research, Education, and Clinical Center (MIRECC). He is a past president of the Association for Advancement of Behavior Therapy and of the Society for a Science of Clinical Psychology; a diplomate of the American Board of Behavior Therapy and the American Board of Professional Psychology; and a fellow of the American Psychological Association, the American Psychological Society, the Association for Clinical Psychosocial Research, and the American Psychopathological Association. He was the first recipient of the American Psychological Foundation Gralnick Foundation Award for his lifetime research on psychosocial aspects of schizophrenia, and the first recipient of the Ireland Investigator Award from the National Alliance for Research on Schizophrenia and Depression (NARSAD). Dr. Bellack is coauthor or coeditor of 31 books, and has published over 150 journal articles and 46 book chapters. He has had continuous funding from the National Institutes of Health since 1974 for his work on schizophrenia, depression, social skills training, and substance abuse. He is a consultant to the United States Justice Department on behavioral treatments and rehabilitation for psychiatric patients. Dr. Bellack is editor and founder of the journals *Behavior Modification* and *Clinical Psychology Review*, and serves on the editorial boards of nine other journals, including *Schizophrenia Bulletin*.

Kim T. Mueser, PhD, is a licensed clinical psychologist and a Professor in the Departments of Psychiatry and Community and Family Medicine at the Dartmouth Medical School in Hanover, New Hampshire. Dr. Mueser was on the faculty of the Psychiatry Department at the Medical College of Pennsylvania in Philadelphia until 1994, at which time he moved to Dartmouth Medical School. His clinical and research interests include the psychosocial treatment of severe mental illnesses, dual diagnosis, and posttraumatic stress disorder. Dr. Mueser has published extensively and given numerous lectures and workshops on psychiatric rehabilitation, and he is the coauthor of several books, including *Social Skills Training for Psychiatric Patients*; *Coping with Schizophrenia: A Guide for Families*; *Behavioral Family Therapy for Psychiatric Disorders, Second Edition*; and *Integrated Treatment for Dual Disorders: A Guide to Effective Practice*.

Susan Gingerich, MSW, is a full-time trainer and consultant based in Narberth, Pennsylvania, who has over 20 years of research and clinical experience with consumers and families. She has conducted workshops for professionals and families throughout the United States, Canada, and Europe. She and Kim Mueser are the co-leaders of the development team for the Illness Management and Recovery toolkit, part of the Evidence-Based Practices Project sponsored by the Substance Abuse and Mental Health Administration and coordinated by Dartmouth College. She is the coauthor of *Coping with Schizophrenia: A Guide for Families, Behavioral Family Therapy: A Workbook*, and several chapters in *Multiple Family Groups in the Treatment of Severe Psychiatric Disorders*. She appears in the videos *I'm Still Here: The Truth about Schizophrenia* and *The Role of Psychosocial Rehabilitation*.

Julie Agresta, MSS, MEd, is a licensed social worker in private practice based in Cheltenham, Pennsylvania. She has over 15 years of clinical and research experience working with consumers and families, and provides consultation services in the Philadelphia area to community-based programs serving adults and children with mental illness and developmental disabilities. Ms. Agresta is currently completing a PhD in school psychology at Temple University in Philadelphia, Pennsylvania. Her clinical and research interests include school-based mental health services, social skills training for children and adolescents with pervasive developmental disorder, and parent and teacher attitudes toward inclusive education.

Preface

We are most gratified that The Guilford Press asked us to do a second edition of this book, as it reflects the excellent response that the first edition received. Although sales of that edition served as an objective marker of success, in many ways the informal, qualitative responses we have received from students and clinicians are more important to us. They indicate that we achieved our goal of writing a *hands-on* volume that both new and experienced clinicians could use to conduct effective skills training groups. We are also pleased to be able to report that the basic strategies and tactics for skills training that we presented in the prior edition are as valid and effective today as they were 7 years ago and, in fact, as they were when they were developed in the 1970s. The field has changed substantially in the intervening years, the public mental health system has gone through cataclysmic changes, and there are new and more effective antipsychotic medications available. Unfortunately, the basic aspects of schizophrenia and the associated disability have not changed. Most people with the illness continue to have significant impairments in social role functioning, are unable to work, and have problems with substances of abuse. Consequently, social skills training continues to be an important component of a comprehensive system of care. In fact, one of the primary recommendations in the 2002 update of the Schizophrenia Patient Outcomes Research Team, a major project sponsored by the National Institutes of Health to develop treatment guidelines for schizophrenia, is that *persons with schizophrenia should be offered skills training, the key elements of which include behaviorally based instruction, modeling, corrective feedback, contingent social reinforcements, and homework assignments.*

As suggested above, there are no changes in the basic teaching approach presented in this edition, and much of *what* is taught remains the same. However, there are a number of significant changes in the content of the book. We have added an overview of empirical support for social skills training (Chapter 2) and an entirely new chapter (Chapter 9) on skills training for clients with substance abuse problems. A number of new skills sheets have been added to Part II. Chapter 3, on assessment, has been substantially revised, and new, practical instruments have been added. Chapters 3 and 4 from the first edition have been combined in an updated chapter on teaching social skills (Chapter 4), and the former Chapters 8 and 9 on working with clients who present special problems have been combined into a new and updated chapter on troubleshooting (Chapter 8). Some material that was difficult to find in the appendices of the first edition has also been moved to make the current volume more reader friendly. We are confident that readers of the first edition will find this update worth purchasing, and that the book will continue to be helpful to new readers.

Contents

Part II

Steps for Teaching Specific Social Skills: Curricular Skill Sheets

Social Skills Training for Schizophrenia

Part I

PRINCIPLES, FORMAT, AND TECHNIQUES FOR SOCIAL SKILLS TRAINING OF CLIENTS WITH SCHIZOPHRENIA

1

Schizophrenia and Social Skills

If asked to define schizophrenia or explain it, you would probably refer to hallucinations and delusions, the prototypical symptoms. But stop and form an image of a typical patient with schizophrenia. In imagining specific clients and what they are like, you likely think about their appearance and behavior. Even when florid symptomatology is controlled by medication, most individuals with schizophrenia seem a little different or "off center."

It may be difficult to follow their train of thought in a conversation. They may even say some things that sound slightly odd or unrelated to the topic. The person's face and voice may be unusually inexpressive, and he or she may avoid looking at you during the conversation. In fact, you may feel that the person is not really listening to you. Overall, you are apt to feel a little uncomfortable.

Critical factors that lead to your unease can be subsumed under the rubric of *social skills deficits*. Social skills are interpersonal behaviors that are normative and/or socially sanctioned. They include such things as dress and behavior codes, rules about what to say and not to say, and stylistic guidelines about the expression of affect, social reinforcement, interpersonal distance, and so forth. Whether they have never learned social skills or have lost them, most people with schizophrenia have marked skill deficits. These deficits make it difficult for many clients to establish and maintain social relationships, to fulfill social roles (e.g., worker, spouse), or to have their needs met.

In this chapter, we present an overview of the behavioral model of social skills and how the model applies to schizophrenia. We describe the specific behaviors that constitute social skills and then discuss other factors that interfere with social behavior in schizophrenia, especially information-processing deficits. We then describe some social situations that are especially difficult for clients with schizophrenia.

3

THE BEHAVIORAL MODEL OF SOCIAL SKILLS

Definition of Social Skills

Many definitions of social skills have been developed, but most specific definitions fail to account for the broad array of social behaviors.

> Rather than providing a single, global definition of social skill, we prefer a situation-specific conception of social skills. The overriding factor is effectiveness of behavior in social interactions. However, determination of effectiveness depends on the context of the interaction (e.g., returning a faulty appliance, introducing oneself to a prospective date, expressing appreciation to a friend) and, given any context, the parameters of the specific situation (e.g., expression of anger to a spouse, to an employer, or to a stranger). (Hersen & Bellack, 1976, p. 562)

More specifically, social skills involve the

> ability to express both positive and negative feelings in the interpersonal context without suffering consequent loss of social reinforcement. Such skill is demonstrated in a large variety of interpersonal contexts . . and it involves the coordinated delivery of appropriate verbal and nonverbal responses. In addition, the socially skilled individual is attuned to realities of the situation and is aware when he is likely to be reinforced for his efforts. (Hersen & Bellack, 1976, p. 562)

Two aspects of this definition warrant special mention. First, socially skilled behavior is situationally specific. Few, if any, aspects of interpersonal behavior are universally or invariably appropriate (or inappropriate). Both cultural and situational factors determine social norms. For example, in U.S. society, kissing is sanctioned within families and between lovers, but not between casual acquaintances or in the office. Direct expression of anger is more acceptable within families and toward referees at sporting events than toward an employer. The socially skilled individual must know when, where, and in what form different behaviors are sanctioned. Thus, social skill involves the ability to perceive and analyze subtle cues that define the situation as well as the presence of a repertoire of appropriate responses.

Second, social competence involves the maximization of reinforcement. Marriage, friendship, sexual gratification, employment, service (e.g., in stores, restaurants), and personal rights are all powerful sources of reinforcement that hinge on social skills. The unskilled individual is apt to fail in most or all of these spheres and, consequently, experience anxiety, frustration, and isolation, all of which are especially problematic for people with schizophrenia. Thus, social skills deficits may increase the risk of relapse, whereas enhanced social competence may decrease that risk.

Social Skills and Social Behavior

The following discussion elaborates the elements of the social skills model depicted in Table 1.1. First, interpersonal behavior is based on a distinct set of *skills*. The term *skill* is used to emphasize that social competence is based on a set of *learned* performance abilities, rather than traits, needs, or other intrapsychic processes. Conversely, poor social behavior is often the result of social skills deficits. Basic aspects of social behavior are learned in

TABLE 1.1. Social Skills Model

1. Social competence is based on a set of component response skills.
2. These skills are learned or learnable.
3. Social dysfunction results when:
   a. The requisite behaviors are not in the person's behavioral repertoire.
   b. The requisite behaviors are not used at the appropriate time.
   c. The person performs socially inappropriate behaviors.
4. Social dysfunction can be rectified by skills training.

childhood, while more complex behavioral repertoires, such as dating and job interview skills, are acquired in adolescence and young adulthood. It appears as if some elements of social competence, such as the facial expression of affect, are not learned, but are genetically "hard wired" at birth. Nevertheless, research suggests that virtually all social behaviors are *learnable;* that is, they can be modified by experience or training.

As indicated in Table 1.1, social dysfunction results from three circumstances: when the individual does not know how to perform appropriately, when he or she does not use skills in his or her repertoire when they are called for, or when appropriate behavior is undermined by socially inappropriate behavior. The first of these circumstances is especially common in schizophrenia. Individuals with schizophrenia fail to learn appropriate social behaviors for three reasons. First, children who otherwise seem normal but who later develop schizophrenia in adulthood seem to have subtle attention deficits in childhood. These deficits interfere with the development of appropriate social relationships and the acquisition of social skills. Second, schizophrenia often strikes first in late adolescence or young adulthood, a critical period for mastery of adult social roles and skills, such as dating and sexual behaviors, work-related skills, and the ability to form and maintain adult relationships.

Many individuals with schizophrenia gradually develop isolated lives, punctuated by lengthy periods in psychiatric hospitals or in community residences. Such events remove clients from their normal peer group, provide few opportunities to engage in age-appropriate social roles, and limit social contacts to mental health staff and other severely ill clients. Under such circumstances, clients do not have an opportunity to acquire and practice appropriate adult roles. Moreover, skills mastered earlier in life may be lost because of disuse or lack of reinforcement by the environment.

Other Factors That Affect Social Functioning

Why might a person not use behaviors that are still in his or her repertoire, as suggested by item 3b in Table 1.1? As indicated in Table 1.2, a number of factors can be expected to influence social behavior in schizophrenia in addition to social skills per se (Bellack & Mueser, 1993).

Psychotic Symptoms

It should not be surprising that an individual hearing highly intrusive voices, or feeling jeopardized by malevolent forces, would be unable to focus on social interactions. Clients

TABLE 1.2. Factors Affecting Social Performance

1. Psychotic symptoms
2. Motivational factors
     Goals
     Expectancies for success and failure
3. Affective states
     Anxiety
     Depression
4. Environmental factors
     Lack of reinforcement for efforts
     Lack of resources
     Social isolation
5. Neurobiological factors
     Information-processing deficits
     Negative symptoms
     Medication side effects

can be expected to have difficulty fulfilling social roles and behaving in a socially appropriate manner at the height of acute exacerbations.

However, research indicates that clients with schizophrenia have marked deficits in social competence even when psychotic symptoms are under control; conversely, many clients can learn more effective ways of interacting even when they have persistent symptoms. Psychotic symptoms may have a limiting effect on social performance, but they do not explain the bulk of social disability in this population.

Motivational Factors

Many individuals with schizophrenia actively avoid social interactions and appear to have little motivation to develop social relationships. Several factors seem to be involved in this pattern. First, most chronic clients have a history of social failure, rejection, and criticism. As a result, they learn that it may be safer to minimize social interactions than to risk further failure or censure. Second, most clients are engaged in a lifelong struggle to find an equilibrium in which they can control their symptoms, limit their experience of negative affect, and maintain the best possible quality of life. Although at one level they may desire to have improved social relationships and undertake more demanding social roles, venturing out into the social environment may pose an unmanageable threat.

Affective States

As indicated earlier, social interaction is often very anxiety provoking to individuals with schizophrenia which leads to avoidance. Moreover, clients frequently seek to escape from social interactions initiated by others. Research from our laboratory has shown that clients are particularly sensitive to conflict and criticism and will withdraw from potential conflict situations even when they are being taken advantage of or unjustly accused of things they have not done (Bellack, Mueser, Wade, Sayers, & Morrison, 1992).

Environmental Factors

Three aspects of the environment often make it difficult for clients with schizophrenia to use their social skills effectively. First, as their skills tend to be limited, their performance is often odd or imperfect in some way. Unfortunately, many people are not tolerant of idiosyncrasies or social errors and tend to be unsympathetic, impatient, or overtly critical. As a result, clients are not reinforced for their efforts and, in some circumstances, may receive a critical or hostile response. Hence, they tend to become wary of engaging in social interactions.

Second, many clients are unemployed and live in harsh economic circumstances. They do not have the resources to participate in social recreational activities that they might otherwise be able to succeed in and enjoy. Finally, many clients are isolated and do not have good social networks. The illness is stigmatizing, leading others to avoid them. In addition, repeated exacerbations and periods in the hospital disrupt relationships and gradually remove clients from the social environment. Friendships generally develop from the workplace or school, hobbies, volunteer activities, child rearing, and other activities that individuals with schizophrenia often do not participate in. As a result, social contacts for many clients are limited to other clients, mental health staff, and/or family members.

Neurobiological Factors

Several significant neurobiological factors affect social behavior in schizophrenia. The illness is characterized by significant deficits in information processing: the multiple abilities necessary for thinking, learning, and remembering (Green, Kern, Braff, & Mintz, 2000). People with schizophrenia tend to have a variety of problems with attention. They cannot process information as rapidly as others. They have difficulty discriminating important from unimportant stimuli, such as what the interpersonal partner is saying versus voices coming from another conversation or the TV. They have problems with concentrating, focusing attention, sustaining attention over time, or focusing in difficult conditions such as when under stress or when presented with a highly complex task. Thus, they may have great difficulty in attending to what someone is saying if the person speaks rapidly or presents a lot of complex information, if there are distractions (e.g., other conversations going on in the background), if the other person is angry and increasing their level of stress or anxiety, or if the person is providing confusing cues (e.g., subtlety or sarcasm).

Clients with schizophrenia also frequently have problems with memory, especially with short-term verbal memory (e.g., what someone said or told them to do) (Mueser, Bellack, Douglas, & Wade, 1991) and working memory (e.g., ability to retain information *on line* while making a decision or solving a problem). The problem does not seem to be one of forgetting as much as difficulty in initial learning or accessing information that has been learned (e.g., as when you cannot remember a name). Individuals with schizophrenia often seem forgetful or distracted, and they may be accused of not paying attention or not caring about important things. In fact, the real problem may be that the information is not presented in a way that adjusts for their attention problems (e.g., slowly, clearly, and with repetition) or that they simply cannot remember what they did hear unless they are provided with reminders or prompts.

A third important information-processing deficit involves higher-level or complex information processing. People with schizophrenia have trouble in problem solving, in part because they have difficulty in drawing abstractions or deducing relationships between events. A related problem involves the ability to draw connections between current and past experience. Whether it is because they cannot recall past experience, cannot determine when past experience is relevant, or because they simply cannot integrate the diverse processes of memory, attention, and analysis of multiple pieces of information, these individuals have difficulty in learning from experience. They also are unable to effectively organize mental efforts, such as initiating and maintaining a plan of action. As a result, their reasoning and problem solving often seem to be disorganized or even random.

These various problems are not extreme, such as the memory impairment in Alzheimer's disease, but they can nevertheless disrupt social behavior and the ability to fulfill social roles. The fact that these deficits cause significant problems without their being very noticeable to other people sometimes adds to their negative effects, as family members and others in contact with such clients often get frustrated and angry with them when they fail to respond or do things that they appeared to understand (e.g., requests for favors, directions for taking medications). As indicated earlier, disability is often mistaken for laziness, disrespect, and other undesirable personal attributes.

Another significant neurobiological constraint is negative symptoms (Andreasen, 1982). *Positive symptoms*, such as hallucination and delusions, are things that clients experience that normal individuals do not. *Negative symptoms* are things that are deficient as compared with normal levels of functioning. Many persons with schizophrenia suffer from a variety of such deficits, including avolition and anergia, a generalized lack of motivation, energy, and initiative; anhedonia, an inability to experience pleasure and positive emotions; and alogia, a relative inability to generate conversation.

Negative symptoms may result from significant depression or social isolation or from excessive doses of antipsychotic medication. In other cases, they reflect a symptom constellation referred to as the *deficit state*, which appears to be a fundamental biological component of the illness. In either case, these symptoms deprive the patient of the motivation and energy to participate in social activity or to enjoy interactions with others. This symptom constellation is one of the most pernicious aspects of the illness and is also the least responsive to medication.

Components of Social Skills

As specified earlier, social competence is based on a distinct set of component skills (Morrison, 1990). These components can be roughly divided into two broad sets: expressive skills and receptive skills. Table 1.3 provides a list of the most important skills for schizophrenia, including some additional skills that reflect the reciprocal nature of social interaction.

Expressive Skills

There are three groups or categories of expressive behaviors that contribute to the quality of social performance: verbal behaviors, paralinguistic behaviors, and nonverbal behaviors. *Verbal behavior* refers to what we say: the form, structure, content, and amount of words we

TABLE 1.3. Components of Social Skills

Expressive behaviors
  Speech content
  Paralinguistic features
    Voice volume
    Speech rate
    Pitch
    Intonation
  Nonverbal behaviors
    Eye contact (gaze)
    Posture
    Facial expression
    Proximics
    Kinesics

Receptive behaviors (social perception)
  Attention to and interpretation of relevant cues
  Emotion recognition

Interactive behaviors
  Response timing
  Use of social reinforcers
  Turn taking

Situational factors
  Social "intelligence" (knowledge of social mores
    and demands of the specific situation)

emit. Socially skilled individuals are easy to understand. They use vocabulary and sentence structure that are sensible to their audience. Conversely, many clients with schizophrenia are difficult to follow, in part because they use language in an odd or confusing manner. They may use common words to mean something very idiosyncratic, use neologisms (words that are not real words), or use sentence structure that omits key elements (e.g., conjunctions), making it difficult for the listener to discern the meaning of what is being said. Moreover, many persons with schizophrenia have a paucity of relevant and interesting things to say. They often do not work or go to school, they do not read newspapers or attend to current events, and they live relatively restricted lives. Hence, even if they have the desire to converse, they may not have a repertoire of things to talk about. Their conversation may also be dominated by their personal concerns, such as bizarre physical symptoms or delusions.

The manner in which one speaks and presents oneself may be as important as what one says. The term *paralinguistic* refers to characteristics of the voice during speech, including volume, pace, and intonation and pitch. Speech that is very fast is difficult to understand; speech that is very soft may be difficult to hear; speech that is very slow, very loud, or monotonic (as in monotonous) is unpleasant to listen to. High-pitched (e.g., shrill) voices may also be annoying, especially as the volume increases. Speech dysfluencies (e.g., "uh" or "um," stutters) and lengthy pauses may also make it difficult or unpleasant for the listener. These voice and speech characteristics are important for interpreting meaning, as well as for the listener's interest and enjoyment. For example, pace, volume, and intonation are especially important in communicating affect or emotion. Flattened tone, slow pace, and low volume often reflect boredom, depression, or fatigue, but they may also signal a romantic intention (e.g., a slow, deep, sultry voice quality). Loud volume (e.g., raising one's voice) is associated with anger. Rapid pace and high pitch can reflect excitement or fear. Changes in these characteristics are also important in signaling meaning and feelings. For example, increasing loudness can be used to emphasize a point. Schizophrenia, especially the deficit syndrome, is frequently marked by a relatively monotonic voice quality and slow rate of speech that are unpleasant for the listener and hard to interpret. Conversely, excited states can result in pressured, high-pitched speech that is very difficult to follow.

Nonverbal behavior also affects one's interpersonal impact. Facial expression is, perhaps, the primary cue to emotional state: smiling, frowning, grimacing, glowering, and other expressions are substantially reflexive correlates of our mood and feelings. Subtle changes in the muscles around the mouth and eyes signal annoyance, curiosity, surprise, pleasure, or any number of other emotional reactions to what the speaker is saying or doing. The eyes have often been regarded as the primary "window to the soul." Good eye contact is associated with strength, authority, anger, and truthfulness. Lovers will look deeply into each other's eyes. Conversely, "shifty" eyes or avoidance of eye contact is thought to reflect anxiety, discomfort, or dishonesty. Wide-open eyes and dilated pupils can signal heightened interest or fear, whereas narrowed eyes and contracted pupils are associated with suspiciousness, annoyance, or anger. The eyes also play an important role in the flow of conversation. Typically, the speaker looks directly toward the listener's eyes, and the listener moves his or her gaze around the speaker's face. When the speaker is ready to pause and shift the floor to the listener, he or she breaks off eye contact; similarly, the listener wanting to speak tries to catch the speaker's eye to signal the desire for a floor shift. Individuals with schizophrenia tend to be gaze-avoidant. They are uncomfortable in social situations and seem to be especially sensitive to maintaining eye contact. Of course, clients with paranoia may exhibit an unblinking stare that makes the listener uncomfortable or even fearful.

Posture may denote feelings, interest, and authority. A relaxed posture signals comfort, whereas muscular tension (e.g., balled fist, pursed lips, forward lean) signifies arousal or tension. Similarly, leaning forward while speaking or listening is associated with interest and attention, whereas leaning away may reflect fear or distaste. The latter stance is characteristic of many clients with schizophrenia, who are uncomfortable in social interactions.

Proximics, a related behavioral category, refers to the distance between people during their interactions. There are fairly clear, albeit unwritten, cultural rules for the comfortable and appropriate distance between two people during conversations. The acceptable distances vary according to the nature of the relationship and gender, as well as across cultures. For example, familial and romantic relationships allow closer contact than is permitted between employer and employee, especially when they are of opposite sex.

Strangers or casual acquaintances are expected to remain farther apart than friends, although the acceptable distances shorten in crowded subway cars or elevators. A male patient who got as close to a female staff member in an office or on the ward as in a crowded elevator would be perceived as threatening and displaying inappropriate behavior; conversely, if the same staff member approached him to take his blood pressure, the interaction would be entirely acceptable. As previously indicated, many clients with schizophrenia are uncomfortable in close interpersonal situations and maintain inappropriately large interpersonal distances. Some clients with paranoia may be sufficiently threatened as to act out when their "personal space" is violated.

These diverse behavioral elements identified here are each important by themselves, but their impact and interpretation are generally a function of their relationship to one another. When the different components are consistent with one another, they serve to reinforce the speaker's message, as when someone says, "I am angry," in a loud and slow voice, makes direct eye contact with the listener, and has a tense posture with balled fist, clenched teeth, and a forward lean. Conversely, when someone says, "I'm not afraid of you," in a rapid and tremulous voice, avoids eye contact, trembles, and leans backward, the verbal content must be interpreted in light of these inconsistent paralinguistic and nonverbal cues.

Receptive Skills

Regardless of an individual's ability to emit socially skillful responses, he or she cannot be effective without accurate perception of the social situation. The socially skillful individual attends to the interpersonal partner, analyzes the situation, and knows when, where, and how to structure his or her response. This combination of attention, analysis, and knowledge is generally referred to as *social perception*. Not surprisingly, individuals with schizophrenia are thought to have particular difficulty in this area. First, as previously discussed, they have significant difficulties with attention. Effective social perception requires the person to detect a rapidly changing series of facial expressions, verbal content with shifting intonation, and subtle gestural and postural changes. Individuals with schizophrenia may not be able to pick up all of the relevant cues provided by a partner. In addition, accurate interpretation of these various cues requires the individual to integrate the diverse pieces of information, remember them, be able to integrate current information with previous experience (e.g., does Susan express anger directly, or does she do it indirectly by talking more slowly, looking slightly tense, and calling you "John" instead of "Johnny"?), and abstract the crux of the communication by differentiating important and unimportant details. These are all capacities that are limited in schizophrenia.

In addition, it has been suggested that clients with schizophrenia have a specific deficit in the ability to perceive emotions, especially negative emotions such as anger and sadness (Bellack, Blanchard, & Mueser, 1996). This difficulty is thought to be the result of a specific neurological impairment, akin to receptive aphasia for language or agnosia that prevents the interpretation of visual images. The data on this point are somewhat inconsistent, but the clinician should be attuned to the possibility that an individual client who has difficulty interpreting other people's feelings may have a specific, inherited deficit that interferes with the decoding of affect cues.

Social skills depend on the effective use of the constellation of specific elements discussed earlier, but they are not the simple sum of these molecular behaviors. Rather, the ability to communicate and interact effectively is the result of the smooth integration of these behaviors over time, along with ancillary characteristics such as grooming and hygiene. In essence, the whole is greater than the sum of the parts. Moreover, as discussed in the context of our definition of social skill, social behavior is situationally specific. Each situation presents special demands and constraints, and many situations have specific rules that must be mastered. For example, dealing with a high-pressure car salesman may require a false bravado and less candor than is desirable in most other situations. Similarly, effective performance on a job interview demands a style of behavior that would be very difficult to maintain in everyday interactions and would not be appropriate in informal interactions with peers. We refer to these discrete areas of skill as *behavioral repertoires*.

Skills training programs involve development of curricula to teach one or more of these repertoires, depending on the needs of the specific group of clients and the amount of time available. This issue is elaborated in subsequent chapters; Part II provides an extensive set of such curricula. For illustrative purposes, in the rest of this chapter we highlight a few repertoires that we have found to be particularly important for clients with schizophrenia: (1) conversational skills, (2) social perception skills, and (3) skills relevant to special problem situations. Remediation strategies for these repertoires are discussed in subsequent chapters.

Conversational Skills

The ability to initiate, maintain, and terminate a conversation is central to almost every social interaction. Conversational skill is not simply the ability to engage in repartee at cocktail parties, but the basic medium of communication for interactions as simple as asking directions, ordering in a restaurant, and saying "Thank you" for a simple favor. Conversational skills involve verbal and nonverbal responses employed in (1) starting conversations, (2) maintaining conversations, and (3) ending conversations.

A relatively circumscribed repertoire of specific verbal responses can be sufficient for starting and ending most conversations. Responses for initiation include (1) simple greetings, such as "Hi" and "Good morning"; (2) facilitating remarks and open-ended questions, such as "How are you today?" "I haven't seen you in a while, what's new?" "Isn't today a beautiful [miserable] day?" and "Did you listen to the ball game yesterday?" and (3) remarks for entering ongoing conversations, such as "Mind if I join you?" and "Are you talking about the game [show, etc.] last night?" Ending a conversation or leaving a group is frequently an awkward process, and many clients with schizophrenia either leave abruptly or continue ad infinitum. Concluding statements include "I have to go; see you later," "What time is it? I have to meet someone," and "It was nice talking with you. See you tomorrow." Of course, social perception skills (see the next section) are required to ensure that entry and exit are smooth and appropriately timed.

A somewhat more complex set of skills is required to maintain a conversation effectively and to promote satisfactory and reinforcing relationships. A basic requirement is the ability to ask appropriate questions that facilitate a response by the interpersonal partner and/or secure relevant information. The socially skilled individual generally has two types of questioning strategies at his or her disposal. Open-ended questions serve primarily as response facilitators. Examples include "How are you doing?" "What's new?" "What did you think of the game [show, meeting, etc.] yesterday?" and "Do you really think so?" Frequently, the questioner is less interested in the specific answer to such questions than in the general conversation that follows. Specific information is more effectively secured by closed-ended questions, such as: "What was the score of the game yesterday?" "What did you eat last night?" and "Would you like to go downstairs for lunch now?" The individual must also be able to differentiate these two types of questions when they are directed at him or her so as to make an appropriate response. Consider the following reply to the greeting "Hi, what have you been doing?": "Well, I bought a pack of cigarettes this morning, then I went to my group, then I had a hamburger for lunch, and I just went to the bathroom." Although this response might ordinarily be ascribed to a schizophrenia patient's concreteness, it could more profitably be viewed as a manifestation of social skill deficit.

Another factor that is critical for maintaining interactions is periodic reinforcement of the interpersonal partner. Brief interactions can be effectively enacted with an exchange of greetings and/or information, but these minimal responses are not sufficient to maintain longer interactions or to facilitate the development of continuing relationships. Conversational reinforcers include statements of agreement (e.g., "Yeah, you're right," "I agree with you"), approval ("That's a good idea," "I never thought of that, you re right"). Simple verbal facilitators such as "Yeh," "Uh-huh," and "Mm-hmm" have also been shown to have significant reinforcing value. The quality of social interactions is also improved by the appropriate use of social amenities such as "Please," "Thank you," and "Excuse me." The experienced clinician will likely be aware of both the relative infrequency with which most clients with schizophrenia emit either reinforcement of amenities and the rather sterile nature of their conversational style.

There are a number of nonverbal response elements that substantially contribute to socially skillful behavior:

1. Eye contact should be maintained intermittently, interspersed by gazing in the direction of the partner. Both constant eye contact (i.e., staring) and the absence of eye contact are generally inappropriate.
2. Voice volume should approximate a "conversational" level, neither too loud nor too low.
3. Voice tone should not be monotonic, but should include inflection to communicate emphasis, affect, and so on.
4. Response latency to input from the interpersonal partner should generally be brief (see also the discussion of timing in the next section). Mediators such as "Let me think about that" and "Hmm" can be employed when a response must be contemplated.
5. Speech rate should coincide with normative conversational style.
6. Speech dysfluencies should be at a minimum.
7. Physical gestures such as head nods, hand movements (for emphasis), and forward leaning all add to the qualitative impact of the communication.
8. Smiles, frowns, and other facial gestures should be employed in conjunction with verbal content.
9. Physical distance should be maintained according to preferred social norms.
10. Posture should be relaxed, rather than wooden.

These response elements undoubtedly have differential importance in different situations. At present, there are no clear data on their comparative contributions to social effectiveness or on the relative importance of the nonverbal and verbal response components. However, it seems likely that they combine to create a gestalt impression and that anomalous performance of any of the nonverbal elements (e.g., staring, extremely low voice volume) would have deleterious effects on social interactions.

Social Perception Skills

Good conversational behavior also requires effective social perception skills. The most relevant social perception skills for clients with schizophrenia fall into five general categories: (1) listening, (2) getting clarification, (3) relevance, (4) timing, and (5) identifying emotions.

Listening or attending to the interpersonal partner is the most fundamental requirement for accurate social perception. Many clients with schizophrenia exhibit poor interpersonal behavior precisely because their focus of attention is primarily internal and only intermittently and selectively directed outward. Consequently, they fail to secure sufficient accurate information to make an appropriate response and they cannot emit social facilitators or reinforcers.

Even if the individual is an adept listener, he or she will periodically tune out for brief periods and/or occasionally be confused or uncertain about the message being communicated. The skillful individual can identify this confusion and will seek *clarification*. Failure either to perceive confusion or to resolve it frequently results in a breakdown of the subsequent communication process and the emission of inappropriate responses. Clarification can be secured with such statements as "Excuse me, but I didn't hear that," "I don't understand, and I'm not sure what you mean (what you're asking, etc.)." A related and somewhat more subtle skill is perception of confusion on the part of the interpersonal partner. Confusion is often communicated by quizzical or vacant looks, which may include cocking the head to the side, furrowing of forehead and eyebrows, contraction of the pupils, and cessation of social reinforcers (e.g., head nods and "mm-hmms"). By perceiving the partner's confusion, the skillful individual can avoid noncommunicative rambling.

In order to be appropriate, a response must be *relevant* to the conversation as a whole, as well as to the immediately preceding communication. Persons with schizophrenia are frequently seen to be irrelevant in their persistent references to personal problems and family members. Determining relevance is primarily a function of listening to and analysis of the communications. However, relevance can also be increased by self-censoring, such that certain content areas or discrete responses are not emitted in certain types of interactions (or conversely, are allowed only in certain interactions). For example, complaints about ill health, references to idiosyncratic experiences (e.g., hallucinations), and discussion of toileting and sexual behavior are customarily inappropriate other than in conversations with health service providers, family, and close friends.

Timing involves performance of responses at appropriate points in an interaction, as well as with appropriate latency. Effective social interaction involves ebb and flow, including both rapid exchanges and silences. Certain activities and emotional states (e.g., grief) also affect social appropriateness.

The content of the conversation and social norms are the primary determinants of appropriate timing, and thus knowledge of social rules is essential for proper timing. Poor timing is exemplified by interruptions, long latencies to simple closed-ended questions, or leaving an interaction before some resolution is reached (e.g., ignoring requests for delay such as "Let me finish this first" or "Let me think about that").

The final aspect of social perception involves accurate *perception of emotion.* Emotion is frequently communicated by a subtle combination of verbal and nonverbal cues (most people are not sufficiently assertive to communicate their emotions with clear, direct statements). Given that the emotional status of the interpersonal partner is a critical factor in determining an appropriate response, the socially skilled individual must be able to read emotional cues. Minimally, this entails perceiving changes in the nature of the partner's behavior; however, discrimination of emotional states is also necessary. In addition, the skillful individual is able to identify his or her own emotional states, transmit them accurately, and analyze their cause. Such personal perception and analysis enhance accurate communication and are necessary for effective resolution of conflict and distress.

Additional Problem Situations

An individual possessing the full range of conversational and perceptual skills described earlier will be effective in most social situations. However, some interactions are especially difficult to complete because they are anxiety provoking or stressful, because they require great subtlety and nuance, or because they are infrequently encountered. Although an exhaustive list of such situations cannot be supplied, there are a number of situations that we have found to be problematic for a great proportion of clients with schizophrenia.

Assertiveness Skills

One of the most frequently encountered deficits is lack of skill in appropriate assertion. There are generally considered to be two forms of assertion. Hostile or negative assertion involves the expression of negative feelings, standing up for one's rights, and refusing unreasonable demands. Examples of appropriate negative assertion include returning food (in a restaurant) or merchandise that is unsatisfactory or damaged, standing up to an authority figure (police officer, employer, teacher) who is treating you unfairly or inappropriately, requesting an intruder to get to the back of a line or wait his or her turn at a store counter, and expressing justified anger or annoyance to a repairman who has done faulty work or caused unreasonable delay. Commendatory or positive assertion consists of expression of positive emotions: affection, approval, appreciation, and agreement. This includes, for example, warmly thanking a friend for doing a favor, kissing a spouse and verbalizing affectionate feelings, telling a friend (or employee, child, etc.) that he or she has done a really good job, and complimenting someone on his or her appearance or improvement, and so on.

Individuals with schizophrenia tend to avoid or escape from situations in which they may be criticized or in which there may be conflict. The result is that they are frequently taken advantage of. In addition, they often face increased criticism from frustrated family members or mental health staff for failing to deal directly with difficult issues. Appropriate assertiveness is one of the most critical skills for clients with schizophrenia to learn in order to avoid and reduce distress and avoid mistreatment. Positive assertion is similarly important for them to be able to develop and sustain friendships. Assertiveness skills, along with conversational skills, are the most common focus of skill training programs.

Heterosocial Skills

In addition to the general conversational and perceptual skills described earlier, there are a variety of special demands and social norms that pertain to dating, romantic, or sexual interactions. Comparable skills are needed by clients who wish to develop same-sex romantic and sexual relationships.

Grooming, cleanliness, social amenities, social reinforcement, and positive assertion are of special importance. Age-appropriate, as well as culturally appropriate, dating etiquette (e.g., telephone calls, planning, and engaging in social activities) must be observed. Finally, the individual must have information about sexual functioning, be somewhat sophisticated about how to make and respond to sexual overtures, and know how to perform sexually to maximize pleasure and minimize discomfort. In addition, all clients need to learn about safe-sex practices, including the use of condoms and how to avoid or resist unwanted or dangerous sexual encounters.

Assertion skills targeted on condom use and saying "No" are especially important for female clients, who are particularly vulnerable to manipulation and abuse by male acquaintances. Education about HIV and AIDS should be a standard part of any skills curriculum with clients who are sexually active or may otherwise be at risk.

Independent Living Skills

Although many clients are unable to compete for employment or even to hold jobs in sheltered workshop settings, *job interview skills* are needed by those who are able to look for work. These skills include how to present oneself positively; how to answer questions about experience and abilities; how to ask questions about salary, working conditions, and so forth; and such associated behaviors as grooming, punctuality, and the like. Dealing with one's psychiatric history and long periods of unemployment is particularly important.

Clients need to be taught what information *not* to disclose about their history and symptoms, as well as what should be disclosed and how to disclose this information in the most positive light possible. Many clients experience difficulty in making *satisfactory living arrangements*. Issues here include how to find an apartment, how to speak with a landlord (e.g., what to ask, how to discuss rent), how to make arrangements with a roommate (e.g., sharing rent and chores, visitors), and how to interact with neighbors. A related set of topics, which may or may not be appropriate for social skills training, involves activities of daily living (ADLs), including cooking and grocery shopping, managing money, and using public transportation. Although such training is often covered in vocational rehabilitation, the social skills training technology is particularly effective for teaching these nonsocial skills.

Medication Management

A critical factor in poor posthospitalization adjustment and relapse is failure to follow the prescribed medication regimen. It is our contention that an important factor in this regard is faulty communication between the client and the health service provider. Thus, the client may not effectively communicate about side effects and inconsistent usage or may fail to comprehend the physician's treatment plan or the need to continue with medication.

We believe that interacting with health service personnel is a specific social skill and that treatment compliance can be increased if clients are able to communicate their concerns, reactions, expectations, and desires effectively.

These various behaviors, referred to as *medication management skills*, include education about medication, its importance, side effects, and so forth, as well as specific conversational and assertiveness skills needed to discuss questions and concerns effectively with physicians and nursing staff (Eckman et al., 1992).

SUMMARY

This chapter has provided an introduction and overview of the social skills model. We defined social skills and gave a detailed description of the elements of social behavior. Expressive skills include verbal behavior, paralinguistic behavior, and nonverbal behavior. Receptive skills, referred to as social perception, refer to the ability to attend to and interpret the cues provided by an interpersonal partner. We also discussed factors that interfere with appropriate social behavior and prevent clients from using skills in their repertoires, including significant deficits in information processing, positive and negative symptoms, motivation and affect, and environmental constraints. Finally, we described some of the basic repertoires that constitute effective social performance, including conversational skills, assertiveness, and skills needed in special situations, such as sexual skills and job interview skills. This material was designed to provide an orientation to the rest of the book, which discusses the assessment and treatment of social skill deficits. As the reader will see, the basic building blocks and constraints to effective performance introduced in this chapter are referred to in every subsequent chapter in the volume.

2

Social Skills Training as an Evidence-Based Practice

How effective is social skills training in the rehabilitation of people with schizophrenia and other severe mental illnesses? What areas of functioning has skills training been shown to improve? Which clients with schizophrenia are most likely to benefit from skills training? This chapter addresses these questions and others concerning the effectiveness of social skills training for clients with schizophrenia and other severe mental illnesses.

We begin with a discussion of *evidence-based practices*, including a description of the criteria used to evaluate the effectiveness of interventions and examples of evidence-based practices for severe mental illnesses. We next review research on social skills training for clients with schizophrenia and summarize the results of key reviews of the research literature. We then describe recent research on social skills training and conclude with a brief discussion of future directions for research in this area.

EVIDENCE-BASED PRACTICES

Most people who visit a doctor expect to be provided with information and access to treatments that have been shown to be effective through the use of objective and scientific methods. Even in the absence of cures for certain ailments or diseases, people expect and demand access to effective interventions that decrease the severity of their problems and the associated suffering. The terms *evidence-based practices* and *evidence-based medicine* refer to the preferred use of interventions that have been shown to be effective for improving an illness in rigorously conducted, scientifically objective research studies.

Clinicians, supervisors, mental health program directors, administrators, and policy makers, as well as clients and family members, benefit from knowing which rehabilitation strategies are most effective for schizophrenia. Such knowledge can help in the selection of interventions most likely to improve functioning. Understanding the limitations of interven-

18

tions can also help people set realistic expectations for what specific treatments can and cannot do. To determine whether an intervention is an evidence-based practice, scientists evaluate research studies according to specific criteria that reflect the objectivity and rigor involved in the research.

These criteria include impact on important outcomes, standardization, controlled research, and replication of research findings. First and foremost, an intervention must show that it *improves important outcomes* of mental illness, such as symptoms, social functioning, vocational functioning, self-care, independent living skills, or quality and enjoyment of life. The *standardization* of an intervention in the form of a book or manual (such as this book), including information about assessment, evaluation of ongoing progress, and treatment procedures, is critical for clinicians to deliver the same intervention that has been found to be effective in the research studies. The most objective way to determine whether an intervention is effective is to conduct *controlled research*, including either randomized controlled trials (RCTs), in which clients are randomly assigned to receive different interventions and then followed over time, or rigorous single case studies in which individuals are carefully studied over extended periods of time before and after an intervention is provided. Finding that an intervention is effective in a single study is not compelling evidence; rather, the *replication* of research findings across multiple studies and investigators is necessary to show that a treatment is effective in the hands of many clinicians and is not just the product of chance or a few exceptional clinicians.

There is broad consensus that several different interventions for persons with schizophrenia are supported by research and may be considered evidenced-based practices (Lehman & Steinwachs, 1998; Mueser, Torrey, Lynde, Singer, & Drake, 2003). These interventions include family psychoeducation (Dixon et al., 2001), supported employment (Bond et al., 2001), assertive community treatment (Bond, Drake, Mueser, & Latimer, 2001), integrated treatment for substance abuse in severe mental illness (dual disorders) (Drake et al., 2001), and cognitive-behavior therapy for psychosis (Gould, Mueser, Bolton, Mays, & Goff, 2001). In the next section we review the evidence supporting social skills training as an evidence-based treatment.

RESEARCH ON THE EFFECTIVENESS OF SOCIAL SKILLS TRAINING

Since development of social skills training procedures in the 1960s and 1970s, the effects of skills training on individuals with schizophrenia and other severe mental illnesses have been extensively studied. Early research during the first two decades of work on social skills training emphasized the application of rigorous single-case-study designs to evaluate the effects of skills training on skill acquisition and functioning (Bellack & Hersen, 1979). Subsequent research has emphasized experimental group designs, including randomized controlled trials (RCTs).

Single-Case-Study Research

A wide variety of rigorous single-case-study designs have been developed and employed in evaluating the effects of social skills training. One of the most common designs is the multiple-baseline approach. With this approach, a person's social skills (and possibly other areas of functioning as well) are assessed several times before treatment (e.g., social skills training) is initiated, and the same areas continue to be assessed periodically as different components of the intervention are systematically taught (e.g., different skills or skill components, such as nonverbal and paralinguistic skills and verbal content). Demonstrating that specific social skills improve when they are targeted by skills training, but not otherwise, provides strong evidence for the effectiveness of skills training in teaching those skills. Similarly, showing that other areas of functioning (e.g., social relationships) fail to improve spontaneously, but improve following the initiation of skills training, can provide compelling evidence for the clinical effects of social skills training.

For example, Hersen and Bellack (1976) conducted a multiple-baseline study of 4–5 weeks of skills training for assertiveness skills in two symptomatic inpatients with schizophrenia. The results showed that the clients were able to learn more appropriate assertiveness skills (e.g., making requests of others, responding to requests) and that these skills were maintained at a 2-month follow-up. In another example, Mueser, Foy, and Carter (1986) used a multiple-baseline approach to evaluate the effects of social skills training on job performance for a psychiatric client who was competitively employed but was having interpersonal difficulties on the job, such as in socializing with coworkers, controlling his temper when faced with unexpected problems, and appropriately asserting himself with his supervisor. A total of 16 skills training sessions were conducted over a 4-month period, targeting the following skills: voice volume, eye contact, affect, responsiveness (for socialization), eliciting suggestions (for problem situations), requesting clarification (for supervisor situations), and self-assertion (for supervisor situations). The multiple-baseline analysis demonstrated that skills training was effective at improving the client's social skills, and the gains were maintained at a 3-month follow-up. Furthermore, independent ratings of the client's work performance indicated improvements over treatment and follow-up as well, including improved interactions with customers, coworkers, and his supervisor and the cessation of complaints from customers.

Numerous single case studies conducted mainly in the 1970s and 1980s were pivotal in both establishing the feasibility of social skills training with clients with schizophrenia and evaluating its effects. However, such studies are limited by publication bias (unsuccessful case reports are less likely to be published), the intensive assessment procedures required, and the emphasis on individual skills training as opposed to group skills training. For these reasons, controlled group studies of skills training have predominated in recent years.

Reviews of Research on Social Skills Training

Over the past several decades, numerous studies of social skills training have been conducted, often with mixed samples of clients with different psychiatric disorders, but who share common impairments in their social functioning. In fact, so many studies have been conducted on social skills training that it is possible to conduct a selected review of the reviews to summarize what has been learned from research.

Table 2.1 summarizes eight reviews of research on the effects of social skills training for clients with schizophrenia and other severe mental illnesses, published between 1988

TABLE 2.1. Reviews of Research on Social Skills Training (SST) for Schizophrenia

Reviewer	Method of review	Number of studies	Focus of review	Conclusions
Donahoe & Driesenga (1988)	Narrative	39	Chronic mental patients	• Clients learn new social skills, retain them over time, and generalize them to other situations • Unclear effects on stress reduction, quality of life, symptoms, hospitalization
Benton & Schroeder (1990)	Meta-analysis	27	Schizophrenia 1972–1988	• Clients learn, maintain, and generalize new skills • SST improves assertiveness, hospital discharge, relapse rate • Marginal benefits of SST on symptoms and functioning
Corrigan (1992)	Meta-analysis	73	Adult psychiatric patients 1970–1988	• Clients can learn and maintain skills • SST reduces symptoms • SST effects stronger in outpatient than inpatient settings
Dilk & Bond (1996)	Meta-analysis	68	Severe mental illness 1970–1992	• SST has moderate efforts on skill acquisition, reduced symptoms, improved personal adjustment • Limited research on effects of SST on role functioning
Smith et al. (1996)	Narrative	9	Controlled studies of schizophrenia 1983–1995	• Clients learn and retain new social skills • Some evidence that skills generalize to improved social functioning
Wallace (1998)	Narrative	6	Recent controlled research on schizophrenia	• Specific and highly structured SST improves social functioning and quality of life
Heinssen et al. (2000)	Narrative	27	Schizophrenia 1994–1999	• Clients learn, retain, and generalize new social skills
Piling et al. (2002)	Meta-analysis	9	Randomized controlled trials for schizophrenia	• No effects of SST on relapse, treatment adherence, global adjustment (2 studies), social functioning (1 study), quality of life (1 study)

and 2002. From this table it can be seen that four reviews employed meta-analysis (a statistical technique in which the effects of each study are estimated and aggregated over multiple studies) (Benton & Schroeder, 1990; Corrigan, 1991; Dilk & Bond, 1996; Pilling et al., 2002) and four reviews provided narrative summaries of the research (Donahoe & Driesenga, 1988; Heinssen, Liberman, & Kopelowicz, 2000; Smith, Bellack, & Liberman, 1996; Wallace, 1998).

Inspection of this table indicates that seven of the eight reviews reached remarkably similar conclusions regarding the effects of social skills training, namely:

- Clients can learn new social skills.
- Clients can retain social skills over time and after the end of training.
- Some degree of spontaneous generalization of skills occurs from training sessions to new situations.
- Social skills training improves social functioning, including the quality and number of social relationships.
- Social skills training has limited effects on the severity of symptoms, relapses, and rehospitalizations.

The eighth review (Pilling et al., 2002) was more negative, but the methods employed and conclusions reached are flawed in several respects (Bellack, in press). First, by limiting the review to RCTs for people with schizophrenia, the greatest amount of research on social skills training was excluded. This led the authors to reach the untenable conclusion that skills training was ineffective at improving social adjustment, quality of life, or general adjustment, based on a mere one or two studies. Second, the authors combined studies comparing skills training to standard care with studies comparing skills training to another effective intervention, leading to the erroneous conclusion that skills training had no impact when the comparison intervention was effective. These and other limitations of this review, combined with the contrasting positive findings of other reviews, cast doubt on the validity of the conclusions reached by the authors. However, they also point to the need for more rigorously controlled research on social skills training.

The reviews raise important issues concerning the generalization of social skills and the (lack of) effects of skills training on psychopathology.

Generalization

One point of agreement across all of the reviews has been the question of the extent of generalization of the effects of skills training from the office into clients' day-to-day interactions. For skills training to be effective, social skills learned in the group (or individual) treatment setting must be transferred to new and different contexts, but serious questions have been raised as to the extent to which such generalization occurs in clients with schizophrenia (Halford & Hayes, 1991), especially considering the cognitive impairments characteristic of the disorder. Although generalization refers to the transfer of skills to new situations, the assessment of generalization varies across studies. Some studies examine generalizability by doing training on one set of role play situations and testing subjects on a parallel set. Most of these studies indicate good levels of generalization (Donahoe & Dresenga, 1988). Other studies examine the generalization of trained skills to spontaneous social interactions, which also suggest moderate levels of generalization (Furman, Gleller, Simon, & Kelly, 1979; Liberman et al., 1984). Still others evaluate the extent to which skills training results in significant improvement in measures of social functioning, such as extent and quality of social relationships and use of leisure time (Marder et al., 1996). Results of these studies are more mixed and may depend, at least partly, on the skills training procedures employed. Studies that incorporate booster sessions and *in vivo* training sessions appear to show better generalization of skills training to social functioning in the community (Kopelowicz, Corrigan, Schade, & Liberman, 1998).

Enhancing the generalization of social skills continues to be an important research priority. A recently developed approach designed to enhance generalization is *in vivo* amplified skills training (IVAST), in which the case manager is formally involved in helping clients complete homework assignments in the community, looking for opportunities to spontaneously prompt and reinforce skills, and developing links with existing or potential support systems (Liberman, Blair, Glynn, Marder, & Wirshing, 2001). Some controlled research supports this approach (Glynn et al., 2002), as reviewed the a following section, "Recent Research on Social Skills Training."

Effects of Skills Training on Psychopathology

From its inception, social skills training was developed as an intervention intended to address social impairments, either related to mental illness or not (Mueser, 1998). Some versions of the stress–vulnerability model of schizophrenia have posited that improved social competence (i.e., social skills) would result in lower levels of psychopathology and susceptibility to relapses (Liberman et al., 1986). However, the available research has not found consistent effects of skills training on psychiatric symptoms. Although some research suggests that skills training may have a modest effect on negative symptoms (e.g., social withdrawal, apathy) in schizophrenia (Matousek, Edwards, Jackson, Rudd, & McMurry, 1992; Patterson et al., 2003), the preponderance of studies indicate few or no effects on other symptoms.

The lack of effect of skills training on psychopathology and relapses should come as no surprise. Social skills training is not a stand-alone intervention, but rather should be one possible component in a comprehensive treatment package that includes pharmacological treatment and other psychosocial treatment or rehabilitation strategies, such as supported employment, family psychoeducation, and cognitive–behavioral therapy for persistent psychotic symptoms, as well as basic services such as housing and access to medical care. The Supplemental Reading List in Appendix A of this book provides references concerning the comprehensive treatment of schizophrenia.

RECENT RESEARCH ON SOCIAL SKILLS TRAINING

Because research on schizophrenia continues to accumulate, with increasingly rigorous research designs, in this section we provide an update on recent controlled research on social skills training. Many of the most recent studies on social skills training focus on the application of the approach to very specific problems, such as those of clients preparing for discharge from the hospital back into the community, clients participating in vocational rehabilitation programs, or elderly clients with schizophrenia. We describe research on social skills training for schizophrenia and severe mental illness published since the publication of the first edition of this book in 1997.

Daniels (1998)

A study by Daniels (1998) evaluated the effectiveness of a group approach that combined social skills training with group process methods, referred to as interactive behavioral-skills

training (IBT). A total of 40 clients with schizophrenia were randomly assigned to participate in a 16-session, twice weekly IBT group or treatment as usual. IBT focused on basic interpersonal skills. Assessments at the end of treatment indicated that clients who had received IBP showed significantly greater improvements in global functioning and marginally
greater improvements in the quality of interpersonal relationships and asociality, but no
differences in overall psychopathology or overall negative symptoms. This study is unique
for its formal incorporation of group process concepts (e.g., universality, altruism, cohesion, self-disclosure) into social skills training procedures. Interpretation of the findings is
limited by the absence of follow-up assessments.

Liberman et al. (1998)

Liberman et al. (1998) examined the effects of 6 months of intensive social skills training
(12 hours weekly) with equally intensive occupational therapy in 84 men with schizophrenia
and persistent symptoms. Skills training focused on basic conversational skills, leisure and
recreational skills, skills for medication management, and symptom management skills. A
2-year follow-up showed that the clients who received social skills training had better independent living skills and lower levels of distress than the clients who received occupational
therapy. This study was important because it showed very positive effects of social skills
training on the long-term outcomes of clients with severe symptoms, with treatment effects
still present 18 months after the end of the program.

Kopelowicz, Wallace, and Zarate (1998)

A study by Kopelowicz, Wallace, and Zarate (1998) examined 59 recently admitted inpatients with schizophrenia or schizoaffective disorder who were assigned to eight sessions of
social skills training or occupational therapy provided over approximately 4 days. Skills
training focused on "community re-entry skills," which included providing basic information about schizophrenia and its treatment, developing an after-care plan, dealing with
stress, and avoiding drug and alcohol abuse. Assessments conducted at the end of treatment indicated that clients who received social skills training learned more of the targeted
information and social skills than clients who received occupational therapy. In addition,
clients who received skills training were more likely to attend their first aftercare appointment than clients who received occupational therapy.

   This study made two important contributions. First, it demonstrated the feasibility of
conducting intensive social skills training with recently admitted inpatients. Despite the
acuteness of their symptoms, clients were able to learn the targeted skills. Second, the study
showed that teaching clients basic principles about the management of their mental illness
was associated with better attendance at their first aftercare appointment in the community. This finding is important because clients with schizophrenia often fail to follow
through on outpatient treatment recommendations, including medication monitoring and
management, and are therefore at increased risk for relapse when living in the community.
The study suggests that there is an important place for brief inpatient social skills training
oriented toward teaching clients practical strategies for the management of their mental illness and to support their active participation in aftercare treatment.

Tsang (2001); Tsang and Pearson (2001)

Improving vocational outcomes is an important goal for many people with schizophrenia. A study reported by both Tsang (2001) and Tsang and Pearson (2001) evaluated the effects of a 10-week social skills training program on work outcomes in 97 people with schizophrenia. Skills training covered basic social skills (e.g., conversational skills), grooming and hygiene, skills for obtaining and keeping a job, and problem-solving skills. Clients were randomly assigned to one of three groups: skills training with monthly follow-up contacts, skills training without follow-up contacts, and no skills training. Work outcomes were tracked for 3 months following the end of intervention. The results indicated that clients who received skills training plus follow-ups had the best work outcomes, followed by those who received skills training alone, followed by clients who received usual care. This study showed that skills training can be effective at helping clients achieve their vocational goals and that relatively modest follow-up efforts to help clients maintain their skills conferred an additional benefit in improving outcomes.

Tauber, Wallace, and Lecomte (2000)

Tauber, Wallace, and Lecomte (2000) examined the effects of involving support persons for clients in social skills training in order to help them learn and practice new social skills in their own natural day-to-day encounters. The study involved 85 clients who were randomized to either social skills training alone or social skills training combined with regular meetings with a support person. These regular meetings focused on informing the support person about the nature of the targeted skills, appropriate situations for using these skills, and making plans for how the client could practice the skills. Biweekly meetings were held between skills training staff and support persons such as the client's family members or friends. Training, provided over a 6-month period of time, included skills for basic conversations, medication management, leisure and recreation, and symptom management.

The results showed that at 6- and 12-month assessments, clients who had received skills training plus the help from a support person had better interpersonal functioning than clients who received only social skills training. This study contributed to understanding how social skills training works and underscores the importance of planning for the generalization of skills in clients' natural settings. Specifically, clients who had a support person who was involved and informed about the nature and goals of social skills training showed more improvements in their interpersonal functioning than clients who received the same skills training package but whose natural supporters were not involved in skills training. Although the involvement of significant others in helping clients learn and generalize social skills in their natural environments has long been recognized to be a vital component of social skills training, this study was the first to rigorously demonstrate the importance of involving these support people in improving social functioning.

Glynn et al. (2002)

Although practicing social skills in the community is considered to be an important component of social skills training, Glynn and colleagues (2002) conducted the first study to formally evaluate the effects of such *in vivo* skills training sessions. Sixty-three clients with schizophrenia were randomized to either social skills training alone or social skills training and *in vivo* amplified skills training (IVAST). The IVAST component involved individual based *in vivo* training sessions conducted in the community, such as a trip to a pharmacy or attending a social gathering. Social skills training was provided over 60 weeks, and included medication symptom management, social problem solving, and living skills. Clients in the IVAST group also participated in biweekly *in vivo* community trips to practice their skills.

The results at 2 years indicated that both groups had improved in social functioning, but the clients who received IVAST had improved significantly more. This study is important because it demonstrates that providing community trips in which clients have an opportunity to practice the skills they have learned yields stronger effects for social skills training than just involving clients in clinic-based training sessions. The findings are consistent with the observations of practitioners of social skills training (and the methods outlined in this book), that training is most likely to generalize to clients' personal lives when it is conducted across multiple settings rather than in a single setting.

Patterson et al. (2003)

The population of older adults in the United States is expected to grow significantly over the next few decades, and, because of advances in medical and psychiatric care, it is anticipated that the number of older individuals with schizophrenia and other severe mental illnesses will grow disproportionately greater (Jeste et al., 1999). Despite this projected growth, there is a paucity of research aimed at evaluating the effects of psychiatric rehabilitation in this population. Patterson and colleagues (2003) conducted a study to examine the effects of a skills training intervention on middle-aged and older persons with schizophrenia.

A total of 32 clients with chronic psychotic disorders were randomized to either group-based functional adaptive skills training (FAST) or treatment as usual and completed pretreatment, posttreatment, and follow-up assessments. FAST included 24 sessions conducted twice weekly and focused on medication management, social skills, communication skills, organization and planning, transportation, and financial management. Results showed that clients who participated in FAST showed significantly greater improvements at follow-up on daily living skills and negative symptoms than the clients who received treatment as usual, but did not differ in positive or other symptoms. This study, the first controlled trial of social skills training with older individuals with schizophrenia, suggests that these clients may benefit from skills training in ways similar to those of younger clients.

Wallace (2003)

People with schizophrenia and other severe mental illnesses often encounter interpersonal problems on the job, such as in interacting with coworkers, customers, and supervisors, which often lead to unsuccessful job endings (Becker et al., 1998). Social skills training has long been used to try to improve job-related interpersonal skills (Mueser et al., 1986), but there have been few systematic evaluations of the effects of skills training on work outcomes. Wallace (2003) conducted a study to evaluate whether social skills training was successful in improving the vocational outcomes of clients participating in a supported employment program. Supported employment is an approach to vocational rehabilitation in which a premium is placed on helping clients find jobs in their areas of interest, with minimal prevocational assessment or skills training, and providing supports (either on the job or off the job) to help them succeed on the job (Becker & Drake, 2003).

A total of 42 clients with severe mental illness participated in the study. All clients were participating in a supported employment program. Half of the clients were randomized to also participate in the Workplace Fundamentals Module, a social skills training program designed to improve interpersonal skills at the workplace (Wallace, Tauber, & Wilde, 1999). The group met twice weekly for 2-hour sessions for 3 months. Assessments were conducted at 6, 12, and 18 months postenrollment. The results provided support for the skills training program. Although the total number of hours worked and the total wages earned between the two groups were the same, clients who participated in the Workplace Fundamentals Module had fewer jobs (indicating less job turnover, presumably due to better skills at the workplace) and high satisfaction with work. In addition, the Workplace Fundamentals group demonstrated better acquisition of the targeted skills than the clients who participated only in the supported employment program. This study provides support for the effect of a focused skills training program on improving job-related skills for clients who are receiving vocational supports and are working at competitive jobs in the community.

FUTURE DIRECTIONS FOR SOCIAL SKILLS TRAINING

Research on social skills training has made advances in demonstrating long-term improvements in social functioning and the importance of programming the generalization of social skills from the clinic to clients' natural community settings. Research has also begun to examine specific applications of skills training, such as preparing briefly hospitalized clients for managing their psychiatric illness in collaboration with others after they leave the hospital, assisting elderly clients, and helping clients improve their social skills for obtaining and keeping jobs. This research demonstrates that skills training has broad applicability for improving social functioning in persons with schizophrenia and other severe mental illnesses.

Whereas there have been great gains in research on social skills training, many important questions remain. An area deserving of more research is how to help clients develop closer and more intimate relationships with other people. Many people with schizophrenia want to have more friends, including intimate relationships with members of the opposite sex (Davidson, 2003). Although social skills training has been shown to improve social functioning in people with schizophrenia, research has not examined the effects of skills training on improving the ability of people to establish these types of close relationships.

Another area worthy of research concerns the leisure and recreational activities of persons with schizophrenia. Because of the early age at the onset of schizophrenia, many clients lack well-developed leisure and recreational activities. The absence of such activities may make these people's lives seem emptier and less rewarding and increase their vulnerability to using drugs and alcohol to fill this void. Although specific social skills have been identified as useful in improving the ability of clients to establish new leisure and recreational activities, the effects of skills training in these areas on increasing the quality of clients' free time has not been established.

Yet another area in need of research concerns the parenting skills of people with schizophrenia who have children. Significant numbers of people with schizophrenia, especially women, have children. Parenting problems among these individuals are common. An unfortunate result is that many mothers with schizophrenia lose custody of their children because of their poor parenting skills. Although teaching parents more effective child-rearing skills is a common application of social skills training in the general population, and among mothers with problems of child neglect, the use of skills training to address this problem in parents with schizophrenia has not been investigated. Successful application of skills training to parents with schizophrenia may decrease the need for child welfare agencies to seek alternative custodial arrangements for their children.

Another area in need of research concerns the application of social skills training to the management of anger problems in people with severe mental illness. People with schizophrenia are at increased risk for violence as compared with people in the general population, and difficulties with the management of anger may be partly responsible for this problem. Social skills training has been applied to improving anger management and the problem of violence in the general population, but systematic applications of skills training to address the problem of anger and violence in people with schizophrenia and other severe mental illnesses have not been evaluated. Social skills training focused on anger management skills may have the potential of decreasing both violence and incarceration, which are common problems in this population.

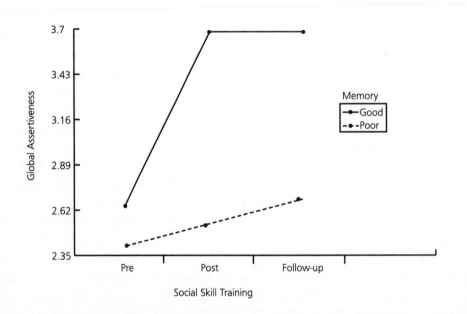

FIGURE 2.1. Improvement in global assertiveness. Improvement was measured from pretreatment assessment to posttreatment and 1-month follow-up assessments for patients with schizophrenia and schizoaffective disorder with good memory versus poor memory (based on a median split of the Weschler Memory Quotient) (N = 30). Adapted from Mueser, Bellack, Douglas, and Wade (1991). Copyright 1991 by Elsevier Ireland, Ltd. Adapted by permission.

Aside from specific applications of social skills training, there are other research questions concerning how to improve the effectiveness of skills training when working with certain clients. For example, it has been found that clients with more severe cognitive impairments tend to learn social skills more slowly (Mueser, Bellack, Douglas, & Wade, 1991; Smith, Hull, Romanelli, Fertuck, & Weiss, 1999). The results of one study demonstrating this effect are summarized in Figure 2.1. This raises the question of how best to help clients with cognitive impairments acquire the targeted skills. Can skills training be just as effective for these clients if intervention is provided over a longer period of time? Do clients with cognitive impairments require additional opportunities and prompts to learn how to use such skills in their natural environments? Can strategies be taught to clients with cognitive impairments to help them compensate for these impairments? Research on these questions may help skills trainers to be even more effective in teaching social skills to clients with cognitive impairments.

SUMMARY AND CONCLUSIONS

Social skills training has been shown to improve social functioning in numerous controlled research studies. These gains can be maintained over time and are especially strong if efforts have been made to systematically program the generalization of skills to clients' natural environments. Examples of programmed generalization include routine community trips with trainers in which clients are given the opportunity to practice their skills in naturally occurring situations, and the involvement of significant others in skills training who can help clients remember to practice their skills in appropriate situations. Social skills training does not appear to improve the positive symptoms of schizophrenia (e.g., hallucination, delusions) or prevent relapses, and the effects on negative symptoms are more mixed. In summary, research indicates that social skills training is an evidence- based practice for improving social functioning in people with schizophrenia and other severe mental illnesses. Further research in social skills training is warranted in order to evaluate the application of this approach to specific problems, such as the development of intimate relationships, parenting skills, and anger management.

Considering that social skills training is the only intervention that has consistently been shown to improve social functioning in schizophrenia, the broad availability of this rehabilitation approach for persons with schizophrenia is an important priority.

3

Assessment of Social Skills

As described in Chapter 1, people with schizophrenia often experience significant problems in social skills and social role functioning. However, there is considerable variability in the precise nature and the severity of these problems. For example, people who have severe forms of schizophrenia and have experienced persistent symptoms over the course of many years may have broad-based, serious social skill problems that are observable even in a brief conversation. Individuals with less severe forms of the illness may have relatively effective social skills in general, but may have difficulties in some specific social skills areas. It is therefore important to conduct an individual, systematic skills assessment before beginning social skills training. Reassessment should be conducted periodically throughout treatment in order to determine the effectiveness of the training and to evaluate the need for continued treatment and/or modification of the training program. It is important to include the person's point of view in planning and assessing all aspects of the training.

The process of assessment can be conceptualized as first gathering general information (Does the person have a problem in social role functioning? In what situations? Does it result from a social skills deficit or a problem in another area?) and then gathering progressively more specific information in order to develop a detailed picture of the person's specific strengths and problem areas. The more general questions can be addressed by interviewing the person and significant others in his or her environment and by informal observation. The more detailed evaluation depends on structured assessments and systematic observation. This chapter discusses general assessment issues, interviewing techniques, and methods for systematic observation using role-play tests. It also provides suggestions for assessing people's progress while participating in social skills training

To help clinicians in a mental health agency conduct systematic assessments, the following tools are described in the text of this chapter and are included as ready-to-use forms in Appendix B.

- Social Functioning Interview
- Social Adaptive Functioning Evaluation (SAFE)

- Social Skills Checklist
- Social Skills Goals Self-Rating Scale
- Social Skills Goals Clinician Rating Scale
- Social Skills Training Group Progress Note
- Social Skills Homework Record
- Social Skills Effectiveness Self-Rating Scale

The following assessment tools, primarily used in research settings but adaptable for mental health agencies, are also described.

- Observation of Role-Play Tests
- Maryland Assessment of Social Competence

GENERAL ISSUES

In assessing a person's social skills, the clinician must start with four questions (Belllack & Morrison, 1982):

1. Does the person manifest one or more problems in interpersonal behavior?
2. What are the specific circumstances in which the interpersonal problem occurs?
3. What is the probable source of the problem (i.e., does it result from a social skills deficit or a problem in another area)?
4. If the problem results from a social skills deficit, what specific deficit does the person have?

These questions are ordered from the most general to the most specific. The answers to each of the first three questions determine whether the subsequent questions need to be answered, and if so, what specific information needs to be pursued. For example, if the person has a problem such as getting into loud arguments when someone disagrees with him or her, what are the circumstance in which this problem occurs? If it is determined that the person usually gets into loud arguments with his or her coworkers but rarely with family members, is this the result of a social skills deficit or of stress experienced on the job? If the loud arguments are the result of a social skills deficit, what is the specific deficit? For example, the person may lack skills in one of the following areas: disagreeing with another's opinion without arguing, making or refusing a request, responding to criticism.

Of course, in the clinical setting, two or more questions may be answered simultaneously, as when a male client reports wanting to meet and talk with women but not knowing how.

- *Question 1: Does the person manifest one or more problems in interpersonal behavior?* The answer to this question can often be determined by the customary clinical evaluation and general observation conducted in most psychiatric settings. For example, a clinician may observe during an intake interview that the person looks down and responds to questions with an extremely soft voice. Or the clinician may notice that while group members are sitting in the waiting room prior to a session, the person is often seen arguing with others, with raised voice and threatening stance. The more severe and generalized the interpersonal problem, the easier it will be to answer this first question. People with less severe problems, however, may not experience difficulties in casual and low-stress interactions, but may have problems in specific situations in the community (e.g., in a store or at work) or their skills may break down in stressful or demanding situations (e.g., refusing requests for money or responding to critical comments from an employer).

• *Question 2: What are the specific circumstances in which the problem occurs?* As with all other behavior, social skills are situationally specific. For example, individuals may be more or less assertive depending on whether the situation involves women or men, acquaintances or strangers, hostile remarks or polite suggestions (Hersen, Bellack, & Turner, 1978). The particular situations in which problems occur will naturally differ across individuals. A social situation that is difficult for one person may be easy for another. Moreover, specific social skills deficits will vary not only across individuals, but across situations for any one individual.

• *Question 3: What is the probable source of the problem?* For many people with schizophrenia, the source of interpersonal difficulties is often specific social skills deficits, but it is important to remember that there are other possible sources as well. For example, even when people have adequate social skills, interpersonal anxiety can inhibit social functioning, depression can reduce the amount and quality of interaction in social situations, and a history of social failure may serve as a disincentive to engage in anything more than minimal interactions. Given that the purpose of assessment is to plan treatment, it must be ascertained whether there is some skill deficit in order to determine whether social skills training or some other intervention is the most appropriate method for helping the person.

It should be emphasized that social skills deficits and factors such as anxiety, depression, and disinterest are not mutually exclusive. For example, Figure 3.1 shows four possible combinations of social anxiety and social skills deficits that an individual may have, with different treatment implications.

An individual represented in box A would have a low level of social skill and low level of anxiety, and therefore social skills training would be the treatment of choice. Box B represents an individual having a low level of anxiety and a high level of social skill (i.e., no dysfunction), and no treatment would be necessary. Box C depicts an individual with a high level of anxiety and low level of social skill. Social skills training would be needed in order to remediate the skills deficit. However, although skills training generally helps reduce anx-

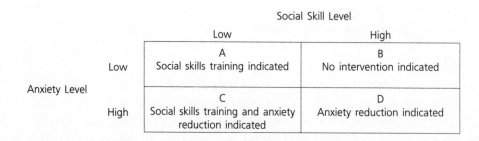

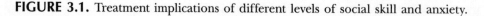

FIGURE 3.1. Treatment implications of different levels of social skill and anxiety.

iety by increasing feelings of self-efficacy about social competence, it is often not sufficient. A supplemental anxiety-reduction strategy would be required if the person is too anxious to try out his or her new social skills. Box D represents a person with a high level of anxiety and high level of social skill. An individual with this profile would require an anxiety-reduction intervention. Social skills training may be a useful adjunct to increase the person's feelings of self-efficacy, but skills development would not be the primary focus of treatment.

• *Question 4: What specific social skills deficit(s) does the person have?* If (a) an interpersonal problem is observed, (b) the situational determinants are identified, and (c) the problem seems to be associated with a social skills deficit, then (d) the specific parameters of the deficit must be isolated. These parameters include the verbal and nonverbal response elements described in detail in Chapter 1, including expressive behaviors (speech content, paralinguistic features, nonverbal behaviors), receptive behaviors (attention to and interpretation of relevant cues, emotion recognition), interactive behaviors (response timing, use of social reinforcers, turn taking), and situational factors (knowledge of social mores and demands of specific situations). The parameters of the deficit also include whether the person has difficulty in one or more of the basic repertoires of skills used in effective social performance, including conversation skill, assertiveness, friendship and dating, conflict management, and so forth. As may be apparent, this is the most difficult aspect of social skills assessment and requires the most detailed analysis of behavior. Whereas the first three questions can often be answered by interview and informal observation techniques, this question usually requires some systematic observation of the person engaging in a relevant social interaction either *in vivo* or in a role-play test.

ASSESSING SOCIAL SKILLS AND SOCIAL FUNCTIONING

Interviewing

Interviewing is among the most useful and cost-efficient assessment techniques. It can provide the clinician with a quick "snapshot" of the person, offer an opportunity to ask questions that reveal a fuller picture of the person's overall social functioning, and help to differentiate the reasons for poor social performance. Three general categories of information can be secured by interview: (1) interpersonal history, (2) informal observational data, and (3) the perspective of significant others in the person's environment, such as family members or staff members at a community residence.

Gathering an Interpersonal History

The interpersonal history is a retrospective picture of the person's current and past levels of social competence, satisfaction, interests, and motivations. It is essential to look for strengths as well as weaknesses. Of special importance is the person's report of situational factors affecting interpersonal competence: where, when, with whom, and under what circumstances do difficulties arise? In addition, the interview can reveal whether the person has ever been able to do something he or she no longer does. For example, the person may have had friends in the past or may have held a part-time job. Interviewing for interpersonal history can be structured around the clinician's specific knowledge about the individual and his or her difficulties.

The preferred interview style consists of asking somewhat general questions, followed by successively more specific questions, and ending with specific examples. For instance, after a general question about managing conflicts and avoiding arguments, the following two sets of questions are likely to yield useful answers:

1. "Can you remember the last time you had an argument with someone at home/where you live?"
   - "When was that?"
   - "Can you describe the situation for me?"
   - "What exactly did you say?"
   - "Is that usually what happens when you argue with him?"

2. "Can you remember an argument you had recently with someone *away* from home/where you live?"
   - "When was that?"
   - "What were you arguing about?"
   - "What exactly did you say?"
   - "Is that what usually happens?"

Social Functioning Interview

The Social Functioning Interview, printed in Appendix B, is designed to help clinicians record information gained from the interviewing process described here. It contains the following general categories:

- Role functioning, past and present
- Social situations that are problematic for the person
- Personal goals
- Social skills strengths and weaknesses identified by the clinician during the interview

Each category of the Social Functioning Interview includes subcategories and may also include a series of questions that prompt further discussion. For example, under the subcategory "Education and work activities" (included in the "Role Functioning" category), the questions include the following:"

- "Are you taking classes or studying subjects on your own?"
- "Do you work part-time or full-time?"
- "Do you volunteer?"
- "Are you participating in a vocational program?"
- "What kinds of jobs did you have in the past? Which did you enjoy most?"
- "What kinds of careers interest you now? What careers interested you in the past?"

As with any self-report data, information gathered in interviews is potentially incomplete and inaccurate. In addition to such factors as incomplete observation of the original event and distorted recall, people with schizophrenia often have difficulties with social perception, which can obscure important data. For example, if the person cannot identify angry feelings, he or she cannot report accurately on the occurrence and handling of this emotion. The person with schizophrenia may also have difficulty recognizing his or her own inappropriate behavior in a situation. However, data secured through interviews are still helpful for generating initial hypotheses about the nature of the person's problems in interpersonal situations.

Structured Social Functioning Interviews

Structured assessments can provide a more systematic index of a person's social functioning than an informal interview and can be used to plan a social skills intervention and to measure progress while the person is participating in social skills training. There are several standardized instruments that are helpful in doing a structured assessment of a person's social functioning, including the following:

- Social Behavior Schedule (Wykes & Sturt, 1986)
- Katz Adjustment Scale (Katz & Lyerly, 1963)
- Social Adjustment Scale—II, client and family versions (Schooler, Hogarty, & Weissman, 1979)
- Life Skills Profile (Rosen, Hazi-Pavlovic, & Parker, 1989)
- Social Functioning Scale (Birchwood, Smith, Cochrane, Wetton, & Copestake, 1990)
- Independent Living Skills Survey (Wallace, Liberman, Tauber, & Wallace, 2000)
- Social Adaptive Functioning Evaluation (SAFE) (Harvey et al., 1997).

The choice of instrument should be based on which particular aspects of functioning are of interest and the extent to which the resulting data will be used in treatment planning and assessment. Practical issues such as cost, time, and available staff are also critical in determining which structured social functioning assessment is feasible (Scott & Lehman, 1998).

The Social Adaptive Functioning Evaluation (SAFE), contained in Appendix B, was originally developed to use with geriatric psychiatric clients (Harvey et al., 1997). The SAFE scale has been adapted for use with people of all ages who have experienced severe functioning problems related to schizophrenia. It is especially helpful in inpatient and long-term residential settings. The scale contains 19 different items, such as "bathing and grooming," "clothing and dressing," "money management," and "conversational skill." The clinician is asked to rate people's functioning in the past month for each item, using a 5-point scale, from "0" (no impairment) to "4" (extreme impairment.) Each of the 5 points on the scale has a behaviorally defined description to make it easier for clinicians to rate the items reliably. For example, in the item "clothing and dressing," a rating of "0" (no impairment) is defined as "The person is able to dress him- or herself without help; he or she chooses to wear clothes appropriate for the season, and if given funds or the opportunity, is able to select and purchase appropriate clothing."

It is recommended that clinicians complete the SAFE at baseline and at 3-month intervals to measure progress in social functioning. To rate some of the items, such as "money management," it may be necessary to ask for additional information from the person, staff members, or family members.

Informal Observation

Interviews with clinicians are a form of informal observation that can be a valuable source of data about how people interact with others. For example, during an interview, the person may look down and speak in a whisper or he or she may speak in a tangential way that makes comprehension difficult. On a general level, the interviewer can appraise his or her own subjective reaction to the person. How easy is the person to talk with? How comfortable/uncomfortable does he or she make the interviewer feel? Can rapport be established, and with how much difficulty? Does the person generate a positive response? The interview also provides a sample of the person's level of verbal and nonverbal skills and interpersonal sensitivity. How well does the person maintain eye contact? Does he or she provide social reinforcers (such as smiling)? Does he or she maintain appropriate interpersonal distance? How is his or her conversational timing (e.g., pauses and taking turns during a conversation)?

As emphasized in Chapter 1, social skills are situationally specific. The generalizability of behavior during an interview may be limited. Similarly, problems in other specific situations (e.g., when strong emotions are expressed or when assertiveness is required) may not be apparent during an interview. However, the more severe the social skills problems, the more likely they are to be manifested across situations. Furthermore, when the clinician observes that the person is able to make appropriate responses in at least one situation (e.g., the interview), it suggests that less training will be required because the social skill problem is circumscribed and not pervasive.

Clinicians can also obtain important data by observing how people interact in the clinic setting, community residence, or hospital. These observations are not like rigorous research assessments, but they provide useful information about people's social skills *in vivo*. The person being observed is usually interacting in a natural fashion, which is likely to reveal specific strengths and weaknesses in social skills. When people live in community residences or in a hospital setting, there is also an opportunity for clinicians to observe what happens at mealtimes, during recreational activities, and during organized trips.

Interviewing Significant Others

Another source of information about the person's social functioning can be utilized by interviewing significant figures in the person's environment, such as family members, spouses, children, roommates, residential staff, and so on. (The clinician will need the person's permission to speak to these individuals if they are not part of the same treatment team.) Significant others often have very helpful information about the person's social skills in real-life situations. In addition, meeting with significant others gives the clinician important information about the person's environment, including areas both of support and conflict. Discussions with these individuals can help answer questions such as, Is the person's environment supportive of change? Does the environment provide positive social reinforcement? Does the environment model appropriate behavior? For example, one community residence may have staff members who are trained to use positive reinforcement, whereas another may encourage staff to use "tough love" or frequent criticism. In gathering information from significant others, the clinician should seek out specific reports and descriptions rather than subjective impressions and general statements.

Direct Observation

Social Skills Checklist

The Social Skills Checklist, printed in Appendix B, is designed as a quick measure of the person's social skills and social functioning over the past month. The checklist is to be completed at baseline and at 3-month intervals during the social skills training intervention. There are 12 skills in the checklist, including "looks at the other person while talking," "maintains appropriate social distance," "initiates conversations," "speaks up for self assertively and politely." The clinician is asked to check off the frequency with which the person uses each skill ("not at all or rarely," "some of the time," "often or most of the time"). Some social skill behaviors occur quite frequently, and it is possible to get a "snapshot" of such behaviors in a brief period of time. For example, by observing a person's behavior in a conversation or during a social skills group, a clinician may have sufficient information to rate the skill of "looking at the other person while talking." For social skill behaviors that occur less often (e.g., "can resolve conflicts without arguments") or that require a knowledge of the person's activities outside the mental health setting (e.g., "maintains at least one close relationship"), it may take longer to develop a picture of the person's skill level. The clinician may need more opportunities to observe the person's behavior or may need to seek additional information from other sources, such as the person him- or herself, staff members, or significant others.

Role-Play Tests

Self-reports and interviews provide *indirect* evidence about social behavior and social skills. Such evidence can provide a good general picture of the person but has limited objectivity and reliability. That is, most individuals do not observe themselves or other people carefully enough or objectively enough to give detailed, accurate reports. The best way to determine what the person does and does not do in specific situations is to collect *direct* evidence by observing the person in the environment. Unfortunately, direct *in vivo* observation is impractical in most settings, especially when the target behavior occurs infrequently (e.g., defending oneself when treated unfairly) or in private (e.g., dating). The optimal strategy for dealing with this constraint is to have the person role play in simulated interactions that mimic the natural environment. Role-play tests are the most commonly used and valid strategy for assessing social skills (Bellack, Morrison, Mueser, Wade, & Sayers, 1990). Although role-play tests are more time-consuming to administer than the other assessment methods described here, they provide a more objective measure of the person's social skills. Role-play tests are most commonly administered in research settings, but they can be simplified and adapted for use in clinical settings.

Many variations have been developed for role playing, but they all essentially follow the same basic plan:

- A standardized, hypothetical social situation is described to the person in a brief and clear manner. For example, a person may be told, "You have broken a vase belonging to your roommate. It was an accident, but you are blamed for breaking it." See Appendix B for examples of a variety of role-play scenes.
- The person is asked to imagine that he or she is actually in the situation and to interact with a staff member, who will play the role of the other person in the hypothetical interaction. For example, the staff member may say, "Did you break my vase?" and ask the person what he or she would say in response. As much as possible, this staff member maintains a neutral manner and avoids guiding the conversation.
- The interaction continues for a time period that may last from 30 seconds to 10 minutes, depending on what is being assessed.
- After the designated time period or a fixed number of responses have been exchanged, additional social situations are presented in the same manner.
- The interactions are audiotaped or videotaped (with the person's written consent) to allow detailed ratings of specific behaviors at a later time.
- A neutral staff member views or listens to the taped interaction to make objective ratings of the person's behaviors. It is important to define target behaviors carefully and to develop rating procedures that accurately and reliably reflect the person's performance. See Appendix B for examples of ratings using a 5-point scale and ratings using a simple "occur/non-occur" designation.

Maryland Assessment of Social Competence (MASC)

The MASC (Bellack & Thomas-Lohrman, 2003) is an example of a fully developed role-play test that can be used in a research setting or modified to use in a mental health agency. This role-play test employs a series of four 3-minute role-played conversations and takes about 20 minutes to administer. The four role-play scenes include one involving initiating conversation with a casual acquaintance, one involving discussion with a health care worker, one involving compromise and negotiation, and one involving standing up for one's rights. The role plays can be altered according to the characteristics of the clients. For example, if a clinician is working with a group of clients who have diabetes, it may be helpful to include a role play involving talking to the doctor about the difficulties of sticking to the recommended diet.

In the MASC, careful attention is paid to ensuring that the person understands clearly what he or she is supposed to do in the role plays. Role-play tests are meant to measure people's behavior in simulated situations; they are not meant to put people under stress or to test their memory or cognitive processing ability. To help facilitate understanding, a description of each role-play scene is typed on a card, which the person is asked to read. The person then hears the description again, either spoken by a staff member or played from a previously recorded audiotape. The person is then asked what he or she will be doing in the role play and what part the staff member will be playing (e.g., a landlord, a new neighbor, a boss, a doctor). If the person's answers show that he or she understands the situation clearly, the staff member then begins the role playing by making an opening statement or asking an opening question. For example, in the role play involving approaching a supervisor, the staff member playing the part of the supervisor may start by looking up and saying, "Yes. May I help you?"

In the role plays, the staff member uses a standardized set of suggested prompts or guidelines for how to interact in response to what the person says. These prompts primarily entail open-ended or minimal responses that put the onus on the person to control the flow of the interchange. The staff member is not restricted to saying the exact words in the prompts, but is advised to limit his or her interactions to general comments and questions. For example, in the role-play scene involving talking to the landlord about fixing the leak in the ceiling, the staff member should avoid making suggestions about how the problem might be solved. Otherwise, the staff member may unintentionally guide the person toward a solution that he or she may not have been able to generate him- or herself.

The interactions are videotaped or audiotaped and rated on verbal skill (the conversational content of the interaction), nonverbal skill (a measure of paralinguistic style, eye contact, and gestures), and overall effectiveness (ability to maintain focus and achieve the goal of the role-play scene). Each item is scored on a 5-point scale from "very poor" to "very good." Table 3.1 presents an example of one role play from the MASC, including the description of the scene and suggested staff member prompts.

TABLE 3.1. A Sample MASC Item

Description of situation: You called your landlord last week about a slow leak in your ceiling. He said that he would be there in the next day or two to fix it. He has not fixed it yet, nor has he called you to let you know when he will be over to fix it. By now, the leak has become much worse. You decide to call your landlord again.

Staff member opening: "Hi, _____. How are you?"

First response: Argue that you haven't had enough time to get over there to fix it.
• "I haven't had enough time."
• "I haven't had enough time to get up there to fix it."
• "I'm a very busy person. I just didn't have enough time."

Second response: Argue that you have other problems that require your attention.
• "There are a lot of other things that require my attention."
• "I have a lot of other tenants with a lot of other problems that are ahead of yours."
• "I have a list and you're on the list, but there are other problems that are more important.

Third response: Argue that you are aware of the problem.
• "You don't need to call any more. I'm aware of the problem."
• "You keep calling, but I'm aware of the problem. I'll be there when I can."
• "I am well aware of your problem."

Fourth response: Argue that the person can do something in the meantime.
• "Do you have a bucket under it?"
• "Can't you just put plastic over your furniture?"

Fifth response: Well, I don't know what I can do about it right now.
• "If the person offers a reasonable solution, question it but don't reject it."

If possible, he or she should talk with the person about each of the topics for approximately the same amount of time (about 45 seconds each). The staff member does not have to use all of the responses. For example, if the person speaks for a long time on the first topic, the staff member may have to skip either the second or the third response in order to have time at the end to generate solutions. The staff member should always leave at least 45 seconds at the end of the interaction for the person to generate solutions.

The MASC is rated on three dimensions: verbal skill, nonverbal skill, and effectiveness. Table 3.2 provides guidelines and sample criteria for conducting the ratings.

IDENTIFYING AND MEASURING PROGRESS TOWARD SOCIAL SKILLS GOALS

Being able to set and pursue personal goals is an essential part of mental health recovery. Social skill assessments should therefore include identifying the person's goals and how they relate to social skills. For example, many people's recovery goals include improving relationships and finding meaningful work. Improving social skills is often an important ingredient to pursuing these goals. As the literature on motivational enhancement has shown (Miller & Rollnick, 2002), the more people see an intervention as contributing to reaching their personal goals, the more actively they participate in the intervention. When people recognize that improving their social skills will lead them closer to achieving something that is important to them, they gain much more from social skills training groups. Chapter 7 provides more detail about how clinicians can select specific social skills to help individuals progress toward their personal goals.

Some people with schizophrenia may find it difficult to identify their goals. Before talking directly about goals, it may be helpful to know more about the person's life. The Social Functioning Interview, described earlier in this chapter and included in Appendix B, provides some questions that help the clinician in this process. For example, the clinician can ask questions such as the following:

- "Where are you living? Do you like it there? Is there anything you would like to change about where you live?"
- "With whom do you spend time? Is there anyone you would like to spend more time with? Would you like to have more close relationships? If so, with whom?"
- "What is a typical day like for you? Is there anything you would rather be doing?"
- "What do you do in the course of a week? Is there anything you would rather be doing during the week?"

It can also be helpful to discuss what the person's goals were before developing schizophrenia, by asking questions such as:

- "When you were younger, what did you imagine yourself doing when you grew up?"
- "What types of things did you used to enjoy doing?"

TABLE 3.2. MASC Rating Categories

<u>Verbal Skill</u>

1	2	3	4	5
Very poor	Poor	Neither good nor poor	Somewhat good	Very good

High Rating for Verbal Skill

The person demonstrates that he or she is able to engage in the interaction by using language that serves to continue or further the conversation (e.g., asking questions, responding appropriately to the staff member's prompts). His or her statements should be clear and reasonable and show that he or she is tracking the content of the scene. Ask yourself, does he or she say things that make sense and show interest in solving the problem? For example, does the person stay on the topic of fixing the leak?

Low Rating for Verbal Skill

The person discourages continuation of the interaction by failing to ask questions, speaking only when prompted, and giving very brief (yes or no) responses. He or she provides inconsistent or unclear responses. The person may make sarcastic comments or be unduly apologetic. He or she may introduce topics only somewhat associated with the role, is vague, or says things that show confusion about what is going on. If you don't understand what the person is trying to say, he or she should get a low rating in this category. For example, if the person starts talking about other apartments he or she has lived in, with little relevance to the leak at hand, the person should get a low rating.

<u>Nonverbal Skill</u>

1	2	3	4	5
Very poor	Poor	Neither good nor poor	Somewhat good	Very good

High Rating for Nonverbal Skill

The person's tone of voice, volume, pace, and inflection are firm, with no hostility. The person should have a confident and self-reliant tone, seem to mean what he or she says, and sound persuasive and insistent. His or her voice should add emphasis to speech content. The person should have good clarity, speak fluently, and maintain a smooth flow in his or her conversation. Speech is clear, well articulated, continuous, and facile. There are few pauses or disruptions within speech units.

Low Rating for Nonverbal Skill

The person's tone may be belligerent, hostile, or angry. You may also hear a dull, monotone, or lifeless tone. It may also be whining, supercilious and/or apologetic. A lower rating should be given for speech that is poorly articulated, pressured, or labored. This would include pauses, mumbling, stammering, and repetitions. Note that true speech impediments are to be disregarded.

<u>Effectiveness</u>

1	2	3	4	5
Very poor	Poor	Neither good nor poor	Somewhat good	Very good

(continued)

TABLE 3.2. *(continued)*

High Rating for Effectiveness

To be effective, the person should be able to stick to the goal of resolving the situation to his or her satisfaction. This should be done firmly, but without being offensive. It may involve compromising, but not "giving in." The person should acknowledge the landlord's point of view and make modifications to his or her suggestions when the landlord does not accept them. The person is able to generate a variety of solutions and compromises in addition to amending those that have not met with approval. He or she should be able to provide the rationale for suggestions made. For example, the person might suggest bringing in a plumber. He or she may then go on to explain how this would minimize damage to the ceiling and free up some of the landlord's time to attend to other tenant problems.

Low Rating for Effectiveness

The person is rigid or unable to generate solutions, compromises, or alternative suggestions. When meeting with resistance, he or she may repeat the same idea over and over, become defensive, or stop the problem-solving process. Alternately, the person may go along with whatever the landlord suggests. For example, when the staff member states that he or she will be unable to fix the leak for several weeks, the person replies, "OK, I'll call back in a month to see if you can fix it then."

- "Did you want to go further in school?"
- "What were your dreams and hopes for your life?"

Depending on the person's answers, the clinician can usually progress to talking about specific goals the person would like to pursue by asking:

- "What kind of changes would you like to make in your life?"
- "What are some goals that you would like to achieve within the next 6 months?"
- "What are some goals that you would like to achieve within the next year?"

Without discouraging ambitious goals, it is important for clinicians to help the person break them down into a series of smaller steps. For example, if the person says he or she wants to get married in the next year, but is not yet dating anyone, the first step toward the goal may be to ask someone to go on a date. If the person is uncomfortable talking to someone that he or she might ask out, the first step may be to become more comfortable in having friendly conversations. The steps leading to this goal, of course, would benefit from several skills from the category "Friendship and Dating."

Examples of common goals related to social skills include:

- Participate in at least one form of recreation.
- Inquire about a job.
- Take a class.
- Refuse requests for money.
- Express angry feelings calmly to roommate.
- Increase the time spent with sibling.
- Find a better apartment.

- Make a new friend.
- Use public transportation confidently.
- Talk to physician about reducing medication.
- Feel more comfortable in a classroom.
- Improve communication with spouse.
- Arrange an enjoyable outing with the whole family.

After the person identifies personal goals that are related to social skills, the clinician can record them on one or both of the following forms provided in Appendix B: the Social Skills Goals Self-Rating Scale and the Social Skills Goals Clinician Rating Scale. Each form provides a space for writing down the person's goals and a scale to rate how much progress has been made on the goals. These forms differ as to whether it is the person or the clinician rating the progress. They can be used at the initial assessment and at 3 months, 6 months, 12 months, and later times to measure the effectiveness of the social skills training and to evaluate the need for continued treatment and/or modification of the training program.

Additional suggestions about how clinicians can help people set realistic goals are provided in Chapter 5 ("Starting a Skills Group").

ASSESSING PROGRESS IN SOCIAL SKILLS TRAINING GROUPS

To evaluate whether social skills are being learned, it is helpful for clinicians to regularly assess the progress made by individuals in the social skills training groups. After each group session, the clinician can complete a progress note, such as the Social Skills Training Group Progress Note provided in Appendix B. This form covers seven group sessions and has blanks for the following information:

- Goal(s) of the person
- Dates of sessions
- Skill taught in each session
- Number of role plays the person performed in each session
- How attentive the person was during the session (on a scale of 1–5)
- Gow well the person cooperated during the session (on a scale of 1–5)
- How well the person performed the skill in the session (on a scale of 1–5)
- Completion of homework assigned at the previous session (on a scale of 1–3)
- Brief description of the specific homework assigned to be completed before the next session

Completing the progress notes gives clinicians a great deal of helpful information. For example, when people cannot perform the steps of a skill in the group session without being prompted, it indicates that they have not adequately learned the skill and require further assistance. When group members are unable to complete their homework, they may require either additional training in the skill or help in overcoming obstacles to generalizing the skill. Chapter 7 ("Tailoring Skills for Individual Needs") provides suggestions for how to proceed when a group member needs additional assistance in learning a skill or practicing it outside the sessions.

Every 3 to 6 months, the group progress notes can be used as part of the ongoing assessment of the social skills training intervention. This assessment will help the group leaders in planning how long to spend on specific skills, choosing skills to teach in the future, and determining what efforts need to be made to increase participation in role plays and homework assignments.

MONITORING HOMEWORK

Homework assignments are designed to encourage group members to practice the skills they are currently learning in the social skills training group. The clinician regularly gives a specific assignment (each session or each week) to use the skill outside the group and follows up by asking whether group members have completed the homework and how it went. In Chapter 4, suggestions are given for assigning homework and for helping group members complete their homework. On the Social Skills Group Progress Note in Appendix B, spaces are provided for recording homework assignments and whether they were completed.

Clinicians can also ask group members to keep track of their homework on the Social Skills Homework Record in Appendix B. It contains blanks for the following information:

- A brief description of the homework assignment
- Due date for the homework
- Name of the staff member or family member who is assisting with homework (optional)
- Date, time, and location that the skill was practiced
- Brief description of what took place
- Self-rating of effectiveness

For clinical and assessment purposes, the Social Skills Homework Record provides the following: a written reminder of the assignment for the group member, a written record of whether the homework was completed and how well the person felt the process went, a document that a staff member or family member can use to help the person with his or her homework. Collecting the completed Social Skills Homework Record helps the clinician to evaluate how often the social skills are being used outside the group and how effective the person feels when using the skills.

EVALUATING EFFECTIVENESS AT USING SPECIFIC SOCIAL SKILLS

One of the major goals of social skills training is to help people to be more effective in actual situations that require the use of social skills. To gather information about social skills effectiveness, the clinician can use some of the methods for assessing social skills described in the beginning of this chapter: interviewing the person about situations when he or she used the social skills that were taught in the group, informal observation of the person in situations that may require use of social skills, obtaining the perspective of significant others, and observation of role-play tests. The clinician can also ask the person to regularly complete the Social Skills Homework Record described earlier.

The Social Skills Effectiveness Self-Rating Scale, contained in Appendix B, can provide additional information. When administered at baseline, 3 months, 6 months, and 12 months, it can be used to assess changes in how effective the person feels at dealing with situations that require the use of specific skills. Before giving the scale to the person at baseline, the clinician needs to fill in the names of the skills that will be taught in the group and give an example of a situation when this skill may be necessary. Similarly, at follow-up assessments, the clinician will need to fill in the names of the skills that have been taught so far in the group and give examples of situations that require the use of those skills. The individuals are then asked to rate how effective they feel they are at dealing with these kinds of situations. Although self-ratings are imperfect, it is essential to elicit people's perspectives regarding their own effectiveness at using social skills. If they feel ineffective, they are less likely to have the confidence to use the skills and the training will have little if any impact in their lives.

SUMMARY

Social skills training is a structured learning model that the clinician tailors to the individual, based on careful assessment. This chapter has provided suggestions for how clinicians can evaluate people's social skills, both at baseline to determine their specific needs for social skills training and at regular intervals to assess their progress during treatment. Several forms are provided in Appendix B to aid clinicians in the assessment process: Social Functioning Interview, Social Adaptive Functioning Evaluation (SAFE), Social Skills Checklist, Social Skills Goals Rating Scale (clinician version and self-rating version), Social Skills Training Group Progress Note, Social Skills Homework Record, and Social Skills Effectiveness Self-Rating Scale. The chapter also described how to use role-play tests such as the Maryland Assessment of Social Competence to provide a more systematic and objective assessment of specific social skills.

4

Teaching Social Skills

Deficits in social skills are important components of social dysfunction in schizophrenia. Poor skills, such as the inability to initiate conversations, express feelings, and resolve conflicts, may be determined by a variety of factors in schizophrenia. These include biological factors, lack of access to good role models, loss of skills because of low morale, and persistent psychotic symptoms. Despite the multiple origins of skills deficits, clinical techniques based on social learning theory can be effective for teaching new social skills to clients.

In this chapter we describe the steps of social skills training. The specific methods used to train skills are based on several learning concepts, which are described first. We then describe the techniques for teaching social skills and helping people put the skills into practice in their everyday lives.

SOCIAL LEARNING THEORY

Social learning theory (Bandura, 1969) refers to a set of observations and principles concerning the natural development and learning of social behavior. According to this theory, social behaviors are acquired through a combination of observing actions of others and the naturally occurring consequences (both positive and negative) of one's own actions. Social learning theory builds on the earlier work of Skinner (1938, 1953) on the effects of positive and negative consequences (*operant conditioning*) on behavior. Five principles derived from social learning theory are incorporated into social skills training: modeling, reinforcement, shaping, overlearning, and generalization.

Modeling

Modeling refers to the process of observational learning, in which a person learns a new social skill by watching someone else use that skill. Although good social skills are modeled in many individual and group therapy treatments for schizophrenia, social skills training is unique in its emphasis on explicit and frequent modeling of social skills for clients. In social skills training, therapists frequently model specific social skills in role plays, directly drawing the attention of the participants to the process and discussing the specific steps of skills that are demonstrated.

Group leaders liberally use modeling in role plays to demonstrate targeted social skills, which are then practiced by clients in role plays. Thus, the learning that occurs through observing the behavior of the leaders is crucial to the success of social skills training. The power of modeling is that many clients have difficulty changing their behavior based on the verbal feedback of others, but they are capable of behavior change after observing skills modeled by group leaders.

Reinforcement

Reinforcement refers to the positive consequences following a behavior that increase the likelihood of that behavior occurring again. Two types of reinforcement can be identified: positive reinforcement and negative reinforcement.

Positive reinforcement involves providing a valued or desired outcome (e.g., verbal praise, money) following a behavior. Negative reinforcement refers to the removal or reduction of some unpleasant stimulus (e.g., criticism, anxiety) following a behavior. Positive reinforcement in the form of verbal praise from the leaders and other group participants is used in social skills training to reinforce both effort in the group and the performance of specific components of social skills. Throughout each social skills session, leaders provide and elicit from other group members abundant amounts of positive feedback about specific social skills performance to help each member improve his or her skill level. The high level of positive reinforcement in social skills groups and strict avoidance of put-downs or criticism make participation in the group an enjoyable, nonthreatening learning experience.

Positive reinforcement can also be used to encourage attendance at social skills training groups. For example, providing refreshments or linking privileges to attendance at the group may foster participation. As clients practice and become more skillful in their social interactions, their anxiety around others decreases, which provides negative reinforcement for using their new social skills.

Shaping

Shaping is the reinforcement of successive steps toward a desired goal. Most skills that are taught in social skills training are too complex and difficult for clients to learn in a single trial. If complex skills are broken down into component steps and taught one at a time over multiple trials, effective social skills can gradually be shaped over time.

Progress in social skills for clients with schizophrenia often occurs in small increments. The ability to shape gradual changes in clients' social skills requires that leaders be attentive to even very small, seemingly insignificant changes in behavior. If specific reinforcement for these small changes is provided, additional improvements can be made, and work can begin on other component behaviors. By adopting a shaping attitude, social skills trainers recognize that changes in social behavior occur gradually over time, with ample encouragement provided at each step along the way.

Overlearning

Overlearning refers to the process of repeatedly practicing a skill to the point at which it becomes automatic. In social skills training, clients repeatedly practice targeted social skills in role plays in the group, as well as for homework assignments outside the group. Familiarity with specific social skills is not sufficient for learning, however. The leaders' goal is to provide group members with so many opportunities to practice a skill that it becomes second nature to use the skill in the appropriate situations. For this reason, behavior rehearsals and role plays are frequently used in social skills training to facilitate overlearning.

Generalization

Generalization is the transfer of skills acquired in one setting to another, novel setting. Clearly, in order for social skills training to be effective, clients must both learn specific social skills and be able to use these skills in their naturally occurring encounters. The generalization of social skills is the ultimate test of skills training. Therefore, skills training methods are designed to maximize the ability of group members to transfer skills learned in the session to situations outside the session.

Generalization of skills is programmed using two methods. First, after being taught a skill in the session, members are given homework assignments to practice the skill outside the session in their natural environment. Homework assignments are then reviewed in the subsequent skills training session.

Second, clients may be prompted to use targeted skills in the natural setting by the skills trainer or another involved person. This *in vivo* prompting of specific social skills can take place in the context of planned trips (e.g., community outings) or spontaneously, as occasions arise. Programming the generalization of social skills is a critical ingredient in skills training that necessarily takes place outside the traditional group or individual therapy session. Furthermore, as discussed later, attending to issues of generalization often requires the involvement of other people in the client's immediate environment to ensure that targeted skills will be reinforced when they occur.

STEPS OF SOCIAL SKILLS TRAINING

Social skills training is a structured format for teaching interpersonal skills that follows a specific sequence of steps. These specific steps, followed on a routine basis within and across sessions, are what distinguishes social skills training from other rehabilitation approaches. Multiple sessions are usually necessary to thoroughly teach a skill. The steps of social skills training are listed in Table 4.1.

Each of these steps is described in the following paragraphs and is included in "Social Skills Group Format" in Appendix A. For ease of communication, we describe the use of skills training in a group format with two leaders. Later in this chapter we also address how to use social skills training with individuals, couples, and families.

TABLE 4.1. Steps of Social Skills Training

1. Establish a rationale for the skill.
2. Discuss the steps of the skill.
3. Model the skill in a role play and review the role play with the group members.
4. Engage a group member in a role play using the same situation.
5. Provide positive feedback.
6. Provide corrective feedback.
7. Engage the group member in another role play using the same situation.
8. Provide additional feedback.
9. Engage other group members in role plays and provide feedback, as in Steps 4 through 8.
10. Assign homework that will be reviewed at the beginning of the next session.

Step 1: Establishing a Rationale

To motivate group members to learn a new skill, a rationale for its importance must first be established. Broadly speaking, there are two strategies for establishing the rationale for learning a new skill: The leader can elicit the rationale from group members, or the leader can provide reasons for the importance of the skill. With most groups, a combination of both strategies is most effective.

The reasons for learning a new skill can be elicited from group members by asking leading questions about the importance of the skill. For example, when teaching the skill Starting a Conversation with a New or Unfamiliar Person, the leader can pose questions such as "Why might it be helpful to be able to start a conversation with somebody?" or "What's so important about being able to start a conversation?"

Typical responses to these questions include "That's how you get to know other people" and "If you want to make new friends, you have to know how to start a conversation." For another example, when introducing the skill Expressing Positive Feelings, the leader can raise questions such as "Why is it helpful to be able to express positive feelings to another person?" and "What happens when you express a positive feeling to someone about a specific behavior of that person?" These questions tend to elicit answers such as "It makes other people feel good" and "If you let people know what they did that you liked, maybe they will do it again."

When eliciting the rationale from group members, it may be helpful to ask questions regarding the disadvantages of *not* using a specific skill. For example, when developing the rationale for giving other people compliments, the leader might pose the question "What happens if you like someone a lot, but you never compliment that person about anything? How does it make him or her feel?" Asking group members about the disadvantages of not using a skill is another way of helping them see the advantages of learning that skill.

In most groups, the importance of learning a specific social skill can be addressed by asking the group members suggestive questions. The leader may also choose to amplify reasons given by group members or provide additional reasons. In some groups of clients, however, cognitive impairments may limit their ability to generate reasons for learning a particular skill. In groups such as these, the leader may elect to provide the rationale for the skill directly, rather than to elicit it from the group members.

When explaining the importance of a social skill, the leader should make his or her explanation as brief as possible. Then, to check on the understanding of group members, the leader should prompt members to paraphrase the rationale. Correct understanding can be reinforced, misperceptions can be corrected, and the leader can then move on to the next step of skills training.

Part II includes a wide variety of skills that can be taught using social skills training. For each skill, a specific rationale is provided and the component steps are listed.

An example of providing a rationale for the skill Expressing Unpleasant Feelings is provided here.

Example of Providing a Rationale

LEADER: Today we are going to work on the skill of Expressing Unpleasant Feelings. By "unpleasant" I mean feelings that are difficult or that don't feel good to have. Can anyone give me an example of an unpleasant feeling?

BOB: Mad.

LEADER: Yes, Bob. Feeling mad or angry is a good example of an unpleasant feeling. (*Writes down "anger" on the posterboard, and adds to the list as group members add other feelings.*) What are some other examples?

JUANITA: Feeling scared?

LEADER: Yes, feeling scared, or frightened, or anxious are examples of unpleasant feelings. Can you think of any other examples?

LIONEL: Boredom.

LEADER: You're right, Lionel, feeling bored is another example of an unpleasant feeling. Any other examples?

YOKO: Like when I want to hit someone.

LEADER: How do you feel when you want to hit someone, Yoko?

YOKO: Pissed off.

LEADER: Right, feeling pissed off or angry is another good example of an unpleasant feeling. You all came up with some good examples of unpleasant feelings: anger, anxiety, boredom. What happens when you have an unpleasant feeling, such as anger, and you hold it inside yourself for as long as you can?

YOKO: You feel even worse.

LIONEL: You explode.

LEADER: Yes. Holding unpleasant feelings inside you for a long time often feels really bad. And sometimes when you hold it in too long, one tiny little thing will just set you off. It's like the straw that breaks the camel's back.

What happens if you're feeling really upset about something and you just fly off the handle, like you yell or shout or scream, or even hit someone?

BOB: Trouble.

LEADER: Right, Bob. Yoko, what happens when you lose control over your anger?

YOKO: I lose privileges or get the other person mad at me.

LEADER: Good point, Yoko. Negative consequences often happen if you express your anger in a destructive or hostile way. What happens if you have an unpleasant feeling about something and you express it in a *constructive* way to someone else?

BOB: It's better.

LEADER: That's right. What about the situation? What if somebody's done something that annoys you, and you try to express an unpleasant feeling constructively to that person, telling the person what he or she did that annoyed you?

JUANITA: Maybe he'll change.

LEADER: Yes, Juanita, letting someone know what he or she has done that's upset you can help that person change his or her behavior, and maybe that situation will be prevented from happening in the future. So we can see that never expressing unpleasant feelings or expressing them in a hostile way has lots of disadvantages, but there are a number of advantages to expressing unpleasant feelings in a constructive way.

Step 2: Discussing the Steps of the Skill

When the rationale for learning the skill has been established, the leader introduces and discusses each step of the skill. The purpose of breaking down a skill into its component steps is to facilitate the teaching process by helping members focus on improving one step at a time. The steps of the skill should be written down and posted in a prominent location in the room so that all participants can see them. It is also helpful for group members to have large-print handouts of the steps of the skills.

The leader briefly discusses each step of the skill, eliciting from group members the importance of each step or directly explaining it. When discussing a step, the leader points to that step on the poster or flipchart. The discussion of the different steps of the skill requires only a few minutes.

Here we provide an example of discussing the steps of the skill, following the same group working on Expressing Unpleasant Feelings.

Example of Discussing the Steps of the Skill

LEADER: When learning how to express unpleasant feelings constructively, it can be helpful to break the skill down into a number of steps. The first step in expressing an unpleasant feeling is to look at the person and to speak in a firm voice tone. Why do you think it can be important to look at a person?

JUANITA: So you know they're listening.

LEADER: Right, you want to look at the person to make sure you have his or her attention. What's so important about speaking in a firm voice tone?

LIONEL: Then that person really knows you mean business.

LEADER: That's right, Lionel. If you have an unpleasant feeling about something and you express it with a meek, quiet voice tone, then the other person might not think you really mean what you're saying. The next step is to tell the other person what you're upset about. What's important here is to make sure that you're as specific as possible. Why do you think that might be important, Bob?

BOB: So the other person knows what you're mad about?

LEADER: Yes. If you tell the other person exactly what you're upset about, it will help him or her to understand better. The next step is to tell the other person how it made you feel. What we are talking about here is making a specific feeling statement, such as "I felt mad," or "I felt angry," or "I was upset." Why do you think making a feeling statement might be important, Yoko?

YOKO: So the person knows how you felt.

LEADER: Yes, making a clear feeling statement helps the other person know exactly how his or her behavior affected you. Being as specific as possible helps the other person understand better. The last step of Expressing Unpleasant Feelings is to suggest a way of preventing the situation from happening again in the future. Why is this an important step?

JUANITA: That way you could change the situation.

LEADER: Right.

YOKO: But what if the person doesn't want to change?

LEADER: Telling the other person how he or she could change the situation in a constructive way often works very well. However, you're right, Yoko, it doesn't work *every* time. I have found that if you use these steps, though, the chances are good that you can change the situation. There are some other strategies that we can talk about later that you can use when dealing with somebody who doesn't want to change a problem situation.

YOKO: OK.

Step 3: Modeling the Skill in a Role Play and Reviewing the Role Play with Group Members

Discussion of the steps of the skill is immediately followed by the leaders modeling the skill in a role play. This demonstration is intended to help participants see how the different components of the skill fit together into an overall performance that is socially effective. Demonstrating the skill helps translate the abstract steps of the skill into a concrete reality.

It is best if the leaders plan in advance of the session the role-play scenario they will model in the group. Role-play situations should be selected that have high relevance to the participants, may occur frequently, and are realistic. The role play should be brief and to the point. Many role plays for basic skills, such as Expressing Unpleasant Feelings, Making Requests, and Starting a Conversation with a New or Unfamiliar Person, may last as little as 15–45 seconds. More complicated skills, such as Compromise and Negotiation, Maintaining Conversations, or Listening to Others, may require longer role plays. If the group is conducted by two leaders, then both of them should participate in the role play, with one of them demonstrating the skill and the other taking the role of the partner. When the group is conducted by a single leader, he or she should enlist a group member to play the role of the partner in the role play. In the latter case, a participant should be selected who is cooperative and likely to respond appropriately to the leader during the role play.

Prior to beginning the role play, the leader tells the group members that he or she will demonstrate the skill and that their task is to observe which steps of the skill they see the leader use. The role play is then conducted. Immediately after the role play the leader reviews the different steps of the skill with group members, eliciting a response, for each step, as to whether it was performed. After reviewing the different steps, group members are asked to provide an overall evaluation of whether the leader was an effective communicator during the interaction.

Clients with schizophrenia sometimes get confused when observing or participating in role plays. This confusion can be due to a lack of clarity regarding when a role play begins and ends. To help clients differentiate between pretend and real interactions in the group, it is helpful if the leader explicitly points out the beginning and the end of each role play.

There are several strategies the leader can use to signify the beginning and end of a role play; usually some combination of strategies works best. First, the leader can make a clear verbal statement to initiate and terminate the role play, such as "Let's begin the role play now" and "Stop, let's end the role play here." Second, the leader can use hand signals to signify the beginning and end of a role play. For example, forming a "T" with one's hands, the signal used to stop a game for "time" in many professional sports games, can be used to indicate the end of a role play. Third, having the role-play participants change positions in the group for the role play can help to make it clear when a role play begins and ends. For example, the two role-play participants can stand or sit in the middle or in front of the group during the role play and then return to their seats after the role play is completed. Thus, a specific physical space in the group is reserved for active role playing. The strategy of repositioning role-play participants has the added advantage of introducing an element of theater or drama. By increasing the theatrical quality of role plays, the leader can attract the attention of less interested or cognitively impaired clients. Finally, encouraging participants in role plays to get up and move around the room can be energizing for all group members.

We provide an example of modeling and reviewing the skill, as follows.

Example of Modeling the Steps of the Skill and Reviewing the Role Play with Group Members

LEADER A: Now that we've talked about the different steps of Expressing Unpleasant Feelings, we'd like to demonstrate this skill for you in a role play. In this role play, we are going to pretend that I'm watching a TV program that I enjoy. In the middle of watching this TV program, someone comes in and changes the channel to watch a different program. Sandra [Leader B] will be playing the role of the person who comes in and changes the TV channel. I'm going to express an unpleasant feeling to Sandra about her changing the TV program. What I'd like you to do is to see which steps of the skill you see me do. (*Points to poster with steps of skill.*) Any questions?

JUANITA: No.

LEADER A: OK. (*Moves two seats to the center of the group and positions a third seat opposite from him for the imaginary TV.*) Let's pretend that I'm sitting here watching TV. (*Points to the empty seat to designate the TV.*)

Let's pretend I'm watching a baseball game. Sandra, I'd like you to come in and change the channel. This can be your seat (*pointing to the adjacent seat*). Let's start the role play *now*. (*Sits back in his chair and pretends to enjoy watching TV.*)

LEADER B: (*Walks up to TV.*) Oh, a boring sports program. I think I'd like to see what's on the news. (*Changes the channel.*)

LEADER A: Hey, Sandra! You just changed the TV channel that I was watching. It annoys me when you change the TV station like that without checking it out with me ahead of time. I'd appreciate your talking to me first if you want to change the station. Then maybe we can work something out.

LEADER B: I'm sorry. I didn't realize you were really watching it.

LEADER A: Well, I was. I would like you to turn it back to the game.

LEADER B: OK. (*Turns back channel.*)

LEADER A: Let's stop the role play *now*. (*turning to group members*) Let's talk about what you saw in that role play. (*Points to poster with steps of skill.*)

How about my eye contact? Was I looking at Sandra just then?

LIONEL: Yes, you were looking at her.

LEADER A: Right, and how about my voice tone? Did I speak with a firm voice tone?

JUANITA: Yes, you sounded pretty firm to me.

LEADER A: Good. How about telling her what I was upset about? Was it clear what I was upset about?

LIONEL: Yes.

LEADER A: What did I actually say I was upset about, Bob?

BOB: Changing the channel.

LEADER A: Right. And how about telling her how I felt? Did I make a feeling statement?

JUANITA: Yes, you did.

LEADER A: What was the specific feeling statement I made, Yoko?

YOKO: You were annoyed.

LEADER A: Right. And did I suggest a way of preventing this from happening in the future?

YOKO: You told her to check with you before changing the channel.

LEADER A: That's right. Overall, was I effective in getting my point across?

BOB: Yes.

LEADER A: Did I sound hostile, Yoko?

YOKO: No, you did a pretty good job.

LEADER A: Good. That was an example of how to constructively express an unpleasant feeling.

Step 4: Engaging a Group Member in a Role Play

The modeling of a specific skill is always followed immediately by a role-play rehearsal of the same skill by a group member. The leader explains that he or she would like each group participant to have a chance to practice the skill. A role play is then set up with a group member and a leader. Instructions are given to the group member, and the role play is conducted.

When a skill is introduced for the first time, it is preferable for participants to practice the skill using the same role-play situation that was modeled by the leaders. The purpose of these initial role plays is to familiarize participants with the specific steps of the skill, while minimizing the adaptations necessary to use the skill in different situations. Thus, it is best at this point not to modify the role-play situation significantly. Minor alterations can be made, however, such as having the participant identify a specific TV program that he or she could pretend to be watching during the role play.

When engaging clients in role plays, the leaders begin with an individual who is likely to be cooperative and more skilled. This will enable more skilled group members to serve as role models for less skilled group members who practice the skill in role plays later in the group. We recommend making a direct request to the client to do a role play rather than offering the open-ended question "Who wants to do a role play?" Making a direct request, such as "I would like you to try a role play," is usually more effective at engaging clients than leaving the decision up to the group members themselves.

An example of the step of engaging a group member in a role play is provided next.

Example of Engaging a Group Member in a Role Play

LEADER A: I would like each of you to have a chance to practice this skill in a role play. Juanita, let's start with you. I'd like you to do a role play of this same situation with the TV.

JUANITA: OK.

LEADER A: Good. Let's set up this role play situation the same way we did before. (*Helps Juanita position her chair in the middle of the group with an empty chair for the TV.*) Let's pretend you're watching a TV program. Juanita, what's a TV program that you like to watch?

JUANITA: *Who Wants to Be a Millionaire.*

LEADER A: OK, let's pretend that you're watching *Who Wants to Be a Millionaire*, and Sandra is going to come into the room and change the channel. When Sandra changes the channel, I'd like you to express an unpleasant feeling to her, using the steps of the skill the way I just did. Any questions?

JUANITA: I guess not.

LEADER A: Good. Let's start the role play *now.*

LEADER B: (*Walks into the room and looks at the TV.*) I think I'd like to watch the news. (*Changes channel.*)

JUANITA: What did you do that for?!

LEADER B: I just wanted to watch a different program.

JUANITA: Well, I was watching that program, and you changed the channel. Change it back!

LEADER B: But I wanted to see something different.

JUANITA: Well you just can't do that.

LEADER A: Let's stop the role play now. You did a good job on that role play, Juanita. Let's get you some feedback.

Note. It is important to end the role play with a brief, positive statement about the participant's performance. The imperfections in Jaunita's role play will be addressed in the step of providing corrective feedback.

Step 5: Providing Positive Feedback

Role-play rehearsals by group participants are always immediately followed by positive feedback about what specifically the person did well. Something genuinely positive must be found in even the poorest role-play performance.

Although it is important to encourage effort in participating in role plays, specific feedback about the participant's performance is necessary if behavior change is to take place.

Positive feedback can be provided both by the leaders eliciting it from other group participants and by providing it directly to the participants. To elicit positive feedback from other group members, it can be helpful after the role play is completed to inquire, "What did you like about the way _____ did that skill just now?" and "Which steps of the skill did you see _____ doing?" Specific feedback about aspects of the skill that were performed well are then given directly to the participant by other group members. The positive feedback provided by group members can then be supplemented by additional positive feedback from the leader.

Leaders must be vigilant to ensure that all feedback given at this stage is positive. Negative or corrective feedback is immediately cut off. The goal at this stage of feedback is to reinforce the group member's effort in the role play and to provide some specific feedback about what was done well.

Group members soon learn that positive feedback always precedes corrective or negative feedback, and this rapidly becomes accepted as a group norm.

Positive feedback should be as behaviorally specific as possible. The feedback may pertain to the specific steps of the skill identified on the poster or other specific nonverbal and paralinguistic skills. If the group member's role-play performance was rather poor, and leaders are concerned that group members will have difficulty in identifying aspects of the role play to praise, a leader can steer the group toward providing feedback about a specific aspect of the performance that was done well. For example, a leader could ask, "What did you like about _____'s *eye contact* in that role play?"

The process of providing positive feedback after a role play is usually relatively brief, lasting between 30 seconds and a couple of minutes. An example of this step of social skills training follows.

Example of Providing Positive Feedback

LEADER A: (*speaking to group*) What did you like about the way Juanita did that role play just then?

LIONEL: She spoke her mind!

LEADER A: Yes, she did seem to speak her mind. Lionel, what did you think of Juanita's voice tone? Was she firm?

LIONEL: Yes, she was pretty firm.

LEADER A: And what about her eye contact? Yoko, was Juanita looking at Sandra [Leader B] during that role play?

YOKO: Yes, she was looking right at her.

LEADER A: That's right. Juanita, you spoke firmly, and you had good eye contact in that role play. Bob, did Juanita make it clear what she was upset about?

BOB: I thought so.

LEADER A: What was she upset about?

BOB: She didn't like it when Sandra changed the channel on her.

LEADER A: That's right. (*speaking to Juanita*) You did a good job in that role play. Your eye contact and voice tone were good, and you made it clear that you were concerned when Sandra changed the TV channel while you were watching the TV.

Note. Just as the feedback must strive to be both specific and genuine, leaders should be careful to avoid hedging their compliments by using phrases such as "pretty good" and "not bad."

Step 6: Providing Corrective Feedback

Providing positive feedback immediately after the role play sets the stage for giving corrective feedback aimed at improving the participant's performance in the next role play. Corrective feedback should be brief, noncritical, to the point, and as behaviorally specific as possible. The aim is to identify the most critical aspects of the role-play interaction that need to be changed in order to enhance overall performance.

As with positive feedback, corrective feedback can be elicited from other group members and provided by the leader as well. At times it may be preferable for the leader alone to provide corrective feedback in order to maximize the member's ability to focus on those critical elements. Corrective feedback should not include an exhaustive list of all the problems in the group member's performance. Rather, it should focus on one or two of the most critical components of the skill.

Using phrases such as "Your role play would be even better . . . " can be helpful in suggesting modifications in a role play. Similarly, constructive feedback can be obtained from other group members by asking questions such as "Are there ways that _____ could improve his or her skill in this role play?"

The following is an example of providing corrective feedback.

Example of Providing Corrective Feedback

LEADER: How do you think Juanita could have done a better job of expressing an unpleasant feeling in this situation?

YOKO: She sounded a little bit hostile.

LEADER: What do other group members think? Did Juanita sound really mad?

BOB: Yes, I think so.

LEADER: Did Juanita make a specific verbal feeling statement about how she felt when the TV channel got changed?

YOKO: I can't remember.

LIONEL: No, she didn't.

LEADER: Juanita, I didn't notice that you made a feeling statement in that role play. Making a specific feeling statement can be helpful when expressing unpleasant feelings, because it lets the other person know exactly how you felt when they did something.

Note. The leader may also have addressed Jaunita's hostility in the role play. However, it is common for people to sound more hostile when they are not *verbally* expressing their feelings. The use of verbal feeling statements, such as "annoyed," "angry," and "upset" often make people actually sound less hostile. Therefore, the leader decided to focus on teaching Juanita to make a verbal feeling statement, with the expectation that it would make her sound less hostile and would be less likely to lead to an argument. In addition, it is desirable to limit the amount of corrective feedback to just a few points.

Step 7: Engaging the Group Member in Another Role Play of the Same Situation

Identifying the specific components of a social skill that were deficient in a role play leads naturally to making suggestions for improving performance in a subsequent role play. In this step of social skills training, the participant is engaged in another role play of the same situation and is requested to make one or two small changes based on the corrective feedback that has just been given. Although corrective feedback may be given about a number of different components of social skills, the specific instructions given to the participant before the next role play are limited to one or two components that are most salient and that the client is most likely to be able to change.

In offering feedback to group members about their role-play performances, contributions are elicited from group members and provided by the leaders. However, only the leader provides specific instructions to a participant about which social skill components to change in the next role play.

This ensures that the instructions given to the participant about how to improve his or her performance in the next role play are clear and within the realm of the person's capability. As when engaging group members in role plays, it is best if the instructions for the second role play are made in the form of a request (e.g., "I would like you to . . . "), instead of a question (e.g., "Would you mind . . . ?").

An example of how to engage a group member in a second role play of the same situation is provided here.

Example of Engaging a Group Member in a Second Role Play of the Same Situation

LEADER A: Juanita, I would like you to try another role play of this same situation. As before, I would like you to practice expressing an unpleasant feeling when Sandra [Leader B] changes the TV channel while you're watching your program. What I'd like you to do a little bit differently this time, however, is to include a specific verbal feeling statement about how you felt when the channel was changed.

JUANITA: I thought I made my feelings pretty clear just then.

LEADER A: Your voice tone and facial expression did communicate some unpleasant feelings. However, I'd like you to be even more clear in explaining how you felt by also using words to describe your feelings.

JUANITA: OK.

LEADER A: How would you feel if somebody changed the channel while you were in the middle of watching a program? (*Points to posterboard with different feeling statements.*)

JUANITA: I'd feel mad.

LEADER A: Good. Then what I'd like you to do in the next role play is to include the statement that you feel mad when someone changes the channel like that. Any questions?

JUANITA: No.

LEADER A: OK, let's set up this role play as before. (*Juanita and Leader B get up from their seats and position themselves in the center of the room.*) All right, let's start the role play now.

LEADER B: (*Walks into the room and looks at TV.*) I think I'd like to watch the news. (*Changes channel.*)

JUANITA: Hey, you changed the channel.

LEADER B: I thought I'd watch a different program.

JUANITA: I was watching that channel. It really makes me mad when you just go up and change the channel like that. Change it back!

LEADER B: Sorry about that.

LEADER A: Good. Let's stop the role play now.

Step 8: Providing Additional Feedback

As with the group member's first role play, the second role play is immediately followed by the provision of positive and corrective feedback. When providing positive feedback, it is best to first praise the group member for any improvements he or she made in response to the specific suggestions offered by the leader immediately prior to the role play. For example, if the leader requested the individual to speak more loudly in the next role play, and she succeeded in improving her voice volume, the leader would first provide positive feedback to the participant about her improved loudness.

After providing positive feedback for specifically targeted social skill components, the leader provides or elicits other positive feedback for steps of the skill that were performed well. As always, feedback should be behaviorally specific, to the point, and sincere. If the participant did not show improvement in the specific component of the skill targeted by the leader, then positive feedback is provided for other components of the skill that were performed well. Corrective feedback for the second role play should also be stated in constructive terms and be as behaviorally specific as possible. Corrective feedback is most helpful when it is provided sparingly, with an eye toward improving social skill performance still further in another role play. Too much corrective feedback can be discouraging to the participant, who may have difficulty remembering it all.

At this juncture in social skills training, the leader must make a decision about whether to engage the individual in a third (or even fourth) role play of the same situation, or whether to move on to the next group member. Several factors must be weighed in making this decision. The first and most critical factor is whether any improvement has taken place from the first to the second role play. If absolutely no improvement has occurred across the two role plays, then no demonstrated learning has taken place and it is essential to engage the group member in another role play. Additional teaching strategies, such as prompting and coaching, are described later in this chapter and can be used in subsequent role plays to maximize the chances of improving the group member's performance.

The second factor in determining the need for an additional role play is cooperation. If the participant was easily engaged in the role play and has made clear progress but still needs to improve further, he or she can readily be engaged in additional role plays to make further gains. The third factor is whether there is enough time to permit more than two role plays while still allowing for engagement with the other group members in two role plays as well. If time permits, the group member is willing, and minimal improvement was made after the second role play, the leader should try to engage the member in a third role play, and even possibly a fourth role play.

When engaging an individual in a series of role plays, it is best to work on changing one component first, then to move on to changing a second and even third component of the skill. When group members are able to experience gradual improvement in their performance of the social skill and positive feedback is used to reinforce these gains, participants often feel rewarded for their hard work and experience a greater sense of self-efficacy in being able to learn the skill. Even when several role plays are required to improve a single component of a social skill, participants usually do not feel discouraged, because positive change is duly noted and abundant reinforcement is provided. Through the process of repeated role plays and feedback, more effective social behavior is shaped.

When a group member has engaged in a final role play and the leader has decided not to do another role play of the same situation, a little more corrective feedback may be given, but is not necessary. The primary purpose of giving corrective feedback is to make specific suggestions for how to improve social skill performance. These suggestions are most likely to be useful when they are immediately followed by an opportunity to practice the skill again in a role play. Therefore, corrective feedback may serve a lesser purpose for the final role play. After the final role play, it may be helpful to the participant for the leader to praise his or her effort in the role plays and to point out improvements that were made over the succession of behavior rehearsals.

An example of the step of giving additional feedback follows.

Example of Providing Additional Feedback

LEADER A: Juanita, I really like the way you included the specific feeling statement in that role play. Bob, do you remember what feeling statement Juanita made?

BOB: I think she said she felt mad.

LEADER A: That's right. I thought you made it very clear how you felt when Sandra [Leader B] changed the TV channel. (*turning to other group members*) What else did you like about the way Juanita expressed an unpleasant feeling in that role play?

YOKO: She was clear about what she was upset about.

LEADER A: And what was that?

YOKO: She didn't like it when the TV channel got changed in the middle of her program.

LEADER A: Yes. What else did you like about Juanita's role play? Was her voice tone firm?

LIONEL: You bet! I wouldn't mess with her.

LEADER A: Yes, Juanita, you did have a firm voice tone. How about Juanita's facial expression? Bob?

BOB: She looked pretty serious.

LEADER A: Yes, I thought so too, Bob. (*turning to Juanita*) Juanita, I think that you did a really good job in that role play just then. You had a serious facial expression and spoke in a firm voice tone. You were clear about what you were upset about, and you made a specific feeling statement.

JUANITA: I guess I did.

LEADER A: (*turning to other group members*) Does anyone have a suggestion for how Juanita could do an even better job in that situation?

LIONEL: She let it be known: "Don't mess with me!"

LEADER A: I agree, Lionel, Juanita was pretty clear about her feelings. How about the way she ended the role play? Does anyone remember what she said?

YOKO: She said, "Change it back!"

JUANITA: Yes, I told Sandra to turn the channel back.

LEADER A: Yes, that's what I remember, too. What do other group members think about that? Do you think that would be an effective way to get Sandra to change the channel back?

YOKO: I don't know; it might turn off the other person.

LEADER A: How come?

YOKO: Well, I thought she sounded a little hostile, like she was saying, "Turn it off *or else!*"

LEADER A: That's a good point, Yoko. If you want someone to change his or her behavior, sometimes it's more effective to make a request than to demand something. What do other people think? Would it be better to make a request?

BOB: Yes.

LIONEL: Maybe, but that might not work either.

LEADER A: That's true, Lionel, but I've found that people tend to be more responsive to requests than demands. (*turning to Juanita*) Juanita, I'd like you to try one more role play of this situation. I'd like you to do it just the way you did it last time, with one exception. At the end I'd like you to make a request for Sandra to change the channel back rather than a demand. OK?

JUANITA: OK.

LEADER A: So what are you going to try to do in this role play?

JUANITA: Express an unpleasant feeling and not be so demanding.

LEADER A: That's right. I'd like you to make a request that Sandra change the channel, not a demand.

JUANITA: Right.

LEADER A: Let's set up the role play again. (*Juanita and Leader B move into their positions.*) Let's start the role play now.

LEADER B: (*Walks up to imaginary TV.*) I think I'd like to watch the news now. (*Changes channel.*)

JUANITA: Hey, you changed the TV channel, and I was in the middle of watching something.

LEADER B: So?

JUANITA: It really makes me mad when you change the channel when I'm watching a program.

LEADER B: Sorry about that.

JUANITA: I'd like you to change the TV channel back to the program I was watching.

LEADER B: OK.

LEADER A: Let's stop the role play now. (*turning to group members*) What did you notice that Juanita did differently in that role play compared to the previous one?

LIONEL: She made a request.

LEADER A: Yes, you did make a request, Juanita. I thought you stated it in a positive, effective manner. (*turning to group members*) What else did you like about Juanita's role play just then?

YOKO: I thought she was pretty clear, and she didn't sound as hostile this time.

LEADER A: I agree, Yoko. (*turning to Juanita*) I thought you made it clear that you were upset, but you did not sound hostile.

JUANITA: It seemed a little more polite.

LEADER A: Yes. Bob, did you think that Juanita was clear about what she was upset about?

BOB: Yes, changing the TV.

LEADER A: That's good feedback, Bob. (*turning to Leader B*) Sandra, you were on the receiving end of those different role plays. Which one did you like most?

LEADER B: Juanita, I liked your last role play most. You were clear about what you were upset about, you made a specific feeling statement, and you made a suggestion about what I could do to correct the situation.

JUANITA: OK.

LEADER A: You did a nice job with those role plays, Juanita. I thought you really got your point across in that last role play very effectively without sounding hostile.

JUANITA: I didn't really feel hostile—maybe a little bit mad.

LEADER A: You did a good job, Juanita. Let's move on, and give someone else a chance to practice this skill.

Step 9: Engaging Other Group Members in Role Plays and Providing Feedback

The social skills training format is established with the first group member and continues with each of the other members of the group. The same principles of role plays, behaviorally specific feedback and abundant praise for even small improvements, apply to each group member. For the initial role play, we recommend beginning with a member who is either more socially skilled or more cooperative than the others. However, we caution against engaging subsequent group members based on these criteria. Overall, in the life of a group, it is best if no particular order is followed for engaging members in role plays.

Step 10: Assigning Homework That Will Be Reviewed at the Beginning of the Next Session

At the end of the session, the leader gives the group members a homework assignment to practice the skill before the next skills training session. The importance of homework can not be overemphasized. Although role plays in the group give members an opportunity to practice new social skills, generalizing these skills to real-world settings is crucial to the success of social skills training. Therefore, homework assignments to practice targeted social skills are given at the end of every social skills training session, and difficulties in completing homework assignments are addressed immediately as they arise.

When homework is assigned, it is important that participants understand the rationale behind an assignment and even be involved in determining the nature of the assignment for themselves. This can be explained in a straightforward manner, such as by saying, "Now that you have had an opportunity to practice this skill in some role plays here in the group, it's important for you to try the skill on your own in situations you naturally encounter in your everyday life. It's very helpful for me to know which steps you're having success with and which ones are a problem for you. For this reason, I will be very interested in learning what happens when you try to use the skill outside the group." Once the rationale for homework has been established, it need not be repeated in every group. However, when a group member does not complete a homework assignment, the leader should first ask questions to assess the group member's understanding of the rationale for giving homework.

To maximize the chances that a homework assignment will be completed, it is important that the assignment be clear, as specific as possible, and within the realm of the person's capability. When possible, individualizing homework assignments can facilitate follow-through. For example, asking group members to identify specific situations in which they could practice the skill is more effective than instructing them in a general way to practice the skill on their own. A final consideration is the use of written materials or other documentation regarding the completion of homework assignments. Some social skills trainers find it helpful to provide homework sheets for participants to record completion of their homework assignments. These sheets are distributed at the end of each group, and group members bring the completed sheets back to the next group. The use of homework sheets, such as the one provided in Appendix B, is often appropriate in working with participants who have fewer impairments. Cognitively impaired or highly symptomatic individuals are able to complete their homework sheets more consistently when they have the assistance of a staff member or a family member.

An example of providing a homework assignment follows.

Example of Assigning Homework That Will Be Reviewed at the Beginning of the Next Session

LEADER: I'm very pleased that all of you did such a good job working on this skill today. Before we meet next time, I would like you to do a homework assignment. The assignment is to find at least one situation where you could try out the skill of Expressing Unpleasant Feelings. Remember that skills training can be effective only if you try the skills we practice here in the group in real situations you encounter on your own. Do you have any questions about this assignment?

YOKO: Sandra [Leader B] was always nice and friendly in the role plays we did in group. But people aren't always like that. What do we do if the other person gets on our case?

LEADER: That's a good question, Yoko. I have found that if you try to express an unpleasant feeling in a constructive manner and avoid getting hostile, most people will respond positively and will hear you out. That doesn't mean that they'll always do what you ask them to, but it usually doesn't worsen the situation.

LIONEL: But what if it does?

LEADER: In general, it is best to avoid getting into an argument with someone who is hostile to you when you express your feelings. If this happens, we'll see if anybody can come up with some good ideas on how to handle that type of difficult situation.

LIONEL: OK.

LEADER: Let's talk a little bit about some situations where you might be able to use the skill of Expressing Unpleasant Feelings. Bob, what is a situation that might happen in the next couple of days where you might be able to use this skill?

BOB: I'm not sure.

LEADER: Are there any people you sometimes have conflicts with, or issues that come up again and again? Such as with your roommate?

BOB: My roommate sometimes bothers me when he plays the radio too loud.

LEADER: That's a good example, Bob. For your homework assignment, I'd like you to express an unpleasant feeling to your roommate about his playing the radio too loud. When might be a good time to talk to him about this, Bob?

BOB: Over dinner?

LEADER: That sounds like a good time to me. At our next group meeting, Bob, I'll be interested in hearing how your conversation with your roommate went.

BOB: OK.

LEADER: Juanita, how about you? What is a situation you might encounter in the next few days where you could express an unpleasant feeling? . . .

Reviewing Homework

Except for the very first social skills training session, all sessions begin with a review of the homework assignment given at the end of the previous session. The review of homework serves several purposes. It provides information about whether group members were able to identify appropriate situations in which the targeted skill could be used and whether they were successful in using that skill. In addition, the homework assignment helps to identify real-life situations that can be used in role plays in the group to continue working on the skill. The overall strategy for the group is to first acquaint members with the steps of the skill by using standardized role-play situations. Then, in subsequent sessions, real-life situations that group members have encountered or expect to encounter are practiced in the group.

The review of homework begins with the leader asking group members about specific situations when they tried to use the particular skill. During the homework review, leaders assess both whether group members are able to identify appropriate situations in which they can use the skill, as well as the members' ability to use the skill effectively. An individual group member is then instructed either to show what happened in the situation (if he or she tried to use the skill) or to try practicing how he or she might have used the skill (if the person forgot to use the skill). The leader encourages the participant to describe the situation in sufficient detail in order to determine if it is suitable for using the skill. It is preferable to avoid a full recitation of what happened in the situation and to focus instead on getting the participant to show what happened in a role play. After the role play is completed, positive and corrective feedback are given, and if further improvements can be made, additional role plays of that situation are conducted.

When the participant reports that he or she has successfully used the skill and demonstrates good performance of the skill in the role play, the leader inquires as to whether the participant's goals in the situation were achieved. Positive consequences of using the skill are pointed out, and the group member's effort at using the skill is recognized. If the group member used the skill but did not meet with success, the leader can lead a brief discussion focused on identifying other strategies that might have been used to achieve the goal in the situation.

When reviewing homework, the leader is sometimes confronted with the problem of individuals who did not follow through on the assignment. With these group members, the goal is to help them identify appropriate situations that they have encountered, or may encounter in the near future, in which they could use the skill. These situations are then used to set up role plays in which the member practices the skill in the group. At the end of the session, when providing the next homework assignment, the leader explores obstacles to completing homework with those individuals who did not do their homework and arrives at a plan for circumventing those obstacles.

The following example illustrates how homework is reviewed and how role plays in the group can be structured, based on the homework. This vignette includes the same group as the previous vignettes, but it takes place in the session after the skill Expressing Unpleasant Feelings was first introduced.

Example of Reviewing Homework

LEADER: I'd like to start by finding out how your homework assignment went. I asked each of you to try to find at least one situation where you could use the skill of Expressing Unpleasant Feelings. What kinds of situations did you come up with?

YOKO: I got into a fight with my mother.

LEADER: That sounds like that might be a good situation in which to use the skill, Yoko. Could you tell us a little bit more about what happened?

YOKO: Well, my mother keeps saying we'll go out for lunch, but then every time it comes around to the date, she calls up and cancels. She always says, "Something else came up."

LEADER: That's certainly an appropriate situation in which to express an unpleasant feeling. Did you try to express a unpleasant feeling to your mother about this?

YOKO: I tried, but it didn't work out very well.

LEADER: Let's set up a role play of this situation and see what happened. Yoko, who would be a good person to play your mother in this role play?

YOKO: Juanita.

LEADER: OK. Juanita, I'd like you to play the role of Yoko's mother. Yoko, where did this situation take place?

YOKO: Over the telephone. She called me at 11:30 yesterday and said she couldn't make our lunch appointment.

LEADER: All right, so in this role play, your mother, played by Juanita, will call you to tell you she can't make lunch. Yoko, I'd like you to respond just the way you responded to your mother yesterday when she called. Any questions?

YOKO: No.

JUANITA: No.

LEADER: I'd like both of you to pretend to be talking on the telephone. Juanita, you start the role play by calling Yoko and telling her you can't make your lunch appointment. (*Sets up role play.*) Let's start the role play now.

JUANITA: (*Pretends to talk on the telephone.*) Hello, Yoko. I'm sorry, but I can't make lunch today. Something's come up.

YOKO: You have to cancel lunch again?! Something always seems to come up! Why can't I ever count on you? Why can't you think of somebody other than yourself?

JUANITA: I'm sorry, Yoko, but you're not the only person in the world.

YOKO: But I should count!

LEADER: OK, let's stop the role play now. Let's give Yoko some feedback. What do you like about the way Yoko handled that situation?

LIONEL: (to Yoko) I thought you came right out and told your mother what you were unhappy about.

LEADER: That's true, Yoko, you got to the point. Bob, what did you think about Yoko's voice tone? Did she sound firm?

BOB: Yes, she did.

LEADER: Yes, I thought you sounded quite firm, Yoko. Was this role play similar to the situation that occurred?

YOKO: It was a little bit similar, but I got madder when it really happened.

LEADER: And how did your mother react?

YOKO: She got madder, too, and then I hung up on her.

LEADER: I see. I noticed that in this last role play you didn't make a specific feeling statement about how you felt when your mother canceled your lunch appointment.

YOKO: I guess I never said how I really felt. But she knew I was mad.

LEADER: I'd like you to do a second role play of the situation, Yoko, and this time include a very clear feeling statement to your mom about her canceling your lunch appointment.

YOKO: OK.

LEADER: Are you ready to do another role play, Juanita?

JUANITA: Yes.

LEADER: OK. Let's start the role play now.

JUANITA: (Pretends to talk on the telephone.) Yoko, I'm calling to tell you I can't make our lunch appointment. I'll have to reschedule.

YOKO: Mom, it really makes me mad when you cancel our lunch appointments like this.

JUANITA: I'm sorry, Yoko. Something just came up.

YOKO: Well, it makes me feel mad.

JUANITA: Sorry.

LEADER: Let's stop the role play now. What did you notice that Yoko did differently in the second role play compared to the first one?

BOB: She said she felt mad.

LEADER: That's right, Bob. (turning to Yoko) You made a very clear feeling statement to your mother about how you felt when she canceled your lunch appointment. I thought you did a good job making your feelings known just then. I'd like you to try this role play just one more time, Yoko, and this time make one more small change. When you have an unpleasant feeling about a situation, sometimes it's helpful to suggest a way for the other person to prevent the situation from happening again, like in the last step of this skill. In this next role play, I'd like you to make a suggestion to your mother about how to prevent the situation from happening again.

YOKO: All right.

LEADER: Good. When you express an unpleasant feeling to your mother in this role play, make a clear feeling statement like you did before, and also suggest how to prevent the situation from happening again. Are you ready, Juanita?

JUANITA: Yes.

LEADER: OK, let's start the role play now.

JUANITA: (*Pretends to talk on the telephone.*) Yoko, honey, I'm sorry I can't make our lunch appointment today.

YOKO: Mom, I really feel mad when you keep canceling our lunch appointments like this.

JUANITA: I'm sorry, Yoko, something just came up.

YOKO: Well, I still feel mad, Mom. Next time I'd like to set up a time to get together where nothing can interfere with our plans.

JUANITA: That sounds like a good idea, Yoko. Lunchtime is often busy. Maybe we should get together for dinner.

YOKO: I'd like that.

LEADER: Let's stop the role play now. You did a great job, Yoko. What did you like about Yoko's last role play?

LIONEL: She tried to solve the problem.

LEADER: That's right. I thought that talking to your mother about how to prevent the situation from happening again was very constructive. How about the other steps of this skill? Did Yoko speak in a firm voice tone?

BOB: Yes.

LEADER: And did she make a clear feeling statement?

BOB: Yes.

LEADER: And was she clear about what upset her?

LIONEL: She didn't like her mother canceling her lunch appointment.

LEADER: That's right. Juanita, what did you think about Yoko's last role play?

JUANITA: I thought she sounded real serious and that she got her message across. But at the same time, she didn't put me off. She seemed to want to try to change the situation, and I liked that.

LEADER: Yes. Yoko, I agree with Juanita. You came across that you were upset about the situation, but you tried to take steps to prevent it from happening again. Nice job, Yoko. Bob, in our last session we gave you a homework assignment to express an unpleasant feeling to your roommate about playing his radio too loud. I'd like to know how that went. . . .

Note. When engaging group members in role plays based on actual situations they have encountered, the leader may allow them to participate in role plays with each other, rather than with one of the leaders. An advantage of this approach is that it allows members a little more leeway in structuring role plays that are similar to the actual situations they experienced, because they can select any person in the group who reminds them of the other person in the situation. A disadvantage is that the leader retains less control over the role play when it involves two clients rather than just one. Clinical judgment must be exercised when the leader is determining whether to allow members to participate in role plays together. When the role play involves two group members, the leader can give instructions to the second one about how to respond in the situation.

PACING OF SOCIAL SKILLS TRAINING

There is no golden rule for determining how long to spend teaching each skill over the course of social skills training. Several factors must be weighed in determining when it is best to introduce a new skill. First, it is important that all or most group members demonstrate some improvement in the social skill that has been the focus of training. Second, the amount of interest generated by continued work on a skill needs to be considered. If group members are beginning to feel restless when working on a particular skill, and definite gains have been made, it may be time to move on, even if there is still room for some improvements. Third, the overall ability level of clients has some bearing on how long to spend on each skill. More severely impaired clients typically require more time and practice to acquire targeted social skills.

Most groups of clients benefit from spending at least two or three sessions working on a particular social skill, and some may require more sessions. After the group has moved on to new skills, old skills should be reviewed periodically to ensure that the gains made do not dissipate. In addition, skills should be reviewed whenever problematic issues arise for group members. For example, if there have been several incidents of heated arguments, it may be more beneficial for the group leaders to teach Expressing Angry Feelings rather than Starting a Conversation with a New or Unfamiliar Person, which may have been next on the schedule.

SYSTEMATICALLY FOLLOWING THE MODEL OF SOCIAL SKILLS TRAINING

To obtain optimum results from social skills training, it is critical to systematically follow the model described in this chapter. Clinicians who are new to conducting social skills training groups may find it challenging at first to coordinate the materials, follow the steps of conducting a group, and maintain a positive communication style. Even experienced leaders may find themselves inadvertently taking short cuts or drifting away from the systematic methods of conducting the group. Two checklists are provided in Appendix A to help group leaders obtain feedback about the extent to which they are following the steps of conducting social skills training sessions. Both checklists contain a list of general structuring and positive engagement skills (e.g., "created a welcoming atmosphere" and "provided ample positive feedback for participation") and a list of the specific steps of social skills training (e.g., "established a rationale for using the skill" and "discussed the steps of the skill with group members"), which are rated as being performed by the group leader "not at all," "partially" or "fully." One checklist is designed to be completed by an objective observer ("Social Skills Group Observation Checklist") and the other is designed to be completed by the group leader him- or herself ("Social Skills Group Leader Self-Rating Checklist"). Both checklists foster valuable discussions about the steps of social skills training and how to stick to the basic model, which can be very useful to group leaders, team leaders, and supervisors to help put strengths and problem areas into focus. The completion of one or both of these checklists every 3 months will help group leaders as they develop or maintain their skills for conducting social skills training groups. It should be noted, however, that the checklists were not designed to be research instruments or to be used in comparing the performances of different group leaders.

ADDITIONAL TEACHING STRATEGIES

Up to this point we have described how social skills are taught using a combination of modeling, role-play rehearsal, positive and corrective feedback, and homework. These methods are the core of social skills training. However, additional teaching strategies can be useful in helping group members learn skills when verbal instructions alone are ineffective at producing behavior change. These strategies should be used as frequently as necessary to facilitate skill development.

The primary goal is to ensure that some improvement in social skill takes place within each social skills training session. Four different teaching strategies are described in the following discussion: supplementary modeling, discrimination modeling, coaching, and prompting.

Supplementary Modeling

Modeling is one of the most powerful teaching tools available to clinicians. In addition to leaders modeling to demonstrate a newly introduced skill, they can provide *supplementary modeling* at any time throughout the group. The primary distinction between initial and supplementary modeling is that the latter is provided for an individual member, and the leader plays the role of that person in a role play.

Supplementary modeling is usually employed when verbal instructions alone to change a particular social skill component do not result in the desired change. Rather than relying on additional verbal instructions, the leader explains to the participant that he or she would like to demonstrate what he or she means in a role play. The participant is instructed to pay close attention to the specific component of the skill that is demonstrated in the role play.

The leader explains that he or she will play the role of the client in the role play. When the role play has been completed, the leader gets feedback from the participant about the specific skill component that was demonstrated. This is immediately followed by the participant practicing the skill in a role play, with special attention paid to the targeted skill component. When the group member has completed the role play, positive and corrective feedback are provided as usual.

An example of supplemental modeling is provided in the following vignette, with group member Bob participating. He has just completed his second role play of the skill Expressing Unpleasant Feelings. Before this role play, the leader instructed him to make a clear verbal feeling statement in the role play. However, Bob forgot to include this specific feeling statement in the second role play. The leader has elicited positive feedback for aspects of the skill that Bob performed well. The example begins with the leader providing corrective feedback to Bob, followed by the use of supplemental modeling to demonstrate the skill for him.

Example of Supplementary Modeling

LEADER A: I noticed in your role play, Bob, that you did not include a feeling statement about how you felt when Sandra [Leader B] changed the TV channel.

BOB: I guess I forgot.

LEADER A: Yes, that sometimes happens. I would like to show you what I mean by making a feeling statement. In this role play, I'm going to play the part of you, and Sandra is going to play the same role she played before; that is, she's going to change the channel while I'm watching it. I would like you to watch me during this role play and pay particular attention to the feeling statement that I make. Do you have any questions?

BOB: No.

LEADER A: What are you going to look for really closely in this role play?

BOB: To see if you make a feeling statement.

LEADER A: Right! OK, let's set up this role play. (*Exchanges places with Bob in order to take his part in the role play. Chairs are rearranged accordingly, and the role play commences.*)

LEADER B: I think I'd like to watch the news now. (*Changes TV channel.*)

LEADER A: Excuse me, I was watching my TV program. It really annoys me when you change the TV station in the middle of a program that I'm watching. I would appreciate it if you would check with me first before changing the station while I'm watching TV.

LEADER B: All right, sorry about that.

LEADER A: All right, let's stop this role play now. (*Leaders move out of their positions.*)

LEADER A: Bob, did you notice what feeling statement I made in that role play?

BOB: You said you felt annoyed.

LEADER A: Good! That's right. How about the other steps of the skill? Were my voice tone and eye contact good?

BOB: Yes.

LEADER A: Did I make it clear what I was upset about?

BOB: Yes, changing the channel.

LEADER A: And did I suggest how the situation could be changed?

BOB: Yes, you told her to check with you first.

LEADER A: Right. Now, Bob, I'd like you to do this role play one more time and to make a clear feeling statement, just as you saw me do in this role play just now. (*Bob and Leader B move back into the center of the group, and the role play begins.*)

Discrimination Modeling

Discrimination modeling refers to a method of highlighting a specific component of a social skill by modeling the skill in two role plays, one immediately following the other. The role plays are identical except for the one component to be highlighted. This component is performed poorly in the first role play and competently in the second role play. Group members are asked to observe both role plays and to attend to which skill component is different.

Discrimination modeling can be a useful strategy when one is discussing with group members the specific components of the social skill. It can also be used when a group member has difficulty modifying a particular skill component based on verbal feedback from the leader or other group members. In addition to asking group members to identify the component skill that is different across the two role plays, group members can be asked to judge which of the two role plays was more effective.

Discrimination modeling can also be a very effective method for highlighting the importance of specific nonverbal and paralinguistic behaviors, such as eye contact and voice volume. By exaggerating poor performance of these component skills, in contrast to good performance, the value of the skill can be easily appreciated by all the group members. Discrimination modeling can also be used to highlight verbal steps of the skill, but it is most effective for the nonverbal and paralinguistic elements.

Example of Introducing Discrimination Modeling

LEADER: We've talked about how voice tone and loudness can be an important part of social skill. We would like to demonstrate this importance in a couple of role plays. We're going to do two role plays of the same situation.

We would like you to pay attention to how my behavior in the two role plays is different. When we have completed with the two role plays, we will ask you to explain how they were different and whether I was a more effective communicator in one role play than in the other.

After this introduction, the leader first demonstrates poor voice tone in a role play by speaking very quietly and meekly. Then, in the second role play, he or she strives to speak in a strong, clear, assertive voice tone.

After the two role plays are completed, the leader can stimulate a brief discussion among group members by asking questions such as "What did I do differently in the second role play compared to the first one?" "Was I more effective in one role play than another? Why?" "What did you think about how I came across in the first role play?" "How was this different in the second role play?" "Which role play did you like better? Why?" The discussion of the two role plays need not be an extended one. Usually several minutes are sufficient to underscore the importance of the skill component in question.

Coaching

Coaching refers to the use of verbal prompts to a participant during a role play to perform specific components of a social skill. Coaching is most often used when verbal instructions before the role play are unsuccessful in producing the desired change in social skill. Rather than simply providing additional verbal instructions and hoping that the participant will be able to do better in the next role play, the leader helps the participant through the role play by providing verbal prompts as necessary.

Coaching can be done spontaneously when it is apparent that the group member has forgotten a step of the social skill in the role play. The member can be prompted to use a specific skill by whispering the reminder in his or her ear during the role play. After the participant has completed the role play, feedback is provided as usual. Then the participant is engaged in another role play of the same situation, this time without the coaching (or a lessened amount of coaching). The basic goals of coaching are to enable the participant to perform the skill with help and then to decrease the amount of help provided in subsequent role plays.

The first time coaching is used, the group member may express some surprise, and it may evoke mild laughter from other group members. However, members quickly become accustomed to coaching and appreciate the help they receive in performing the skill. It is preferable if coaching is used *after* verbal instructions alone have not resulted in behavior change. Otherwise, overreliance on coaching can interfere with the assessment of the member's ability to perform the skill. In addition, a highly symptomatic individual may not be a good candidate for coaching because of his or her paranoid reaction to someone speaking into his or her ear.

An example of how to coach is provided here. In this example, Lionel is practicing the skill Expressing Unpleasant Feelings. In a first role play, Lionel forgot to make a feeling statement. The leader instructed Lionel to make a feeling statement before the second role play, but Lionel forgot to include this statement. The example begins right before the third role play.

Example of Coaching

LEADER A: Lionel, I would like you to try another role play of this situation. In this role play, I'd like you to pay special attention to expressing your feelings about the TV channel being changed. How do you feel when someone changes the channel while you're in the middle of watching a program?

LIONEL: I don't know. It bothers me, I guess.

LEADER A: Good. In this role play I'd like you to tell Sandra [Leader B] that it bothers you when she changes the channel. OK?

LIONEL: OK.

LEADER A: (*Lionel and Leader B move to the center of the room, and chairs are rearranged accordingly.*) Let's begin the role play now.

LEADER B: I think I'd like to watch the news now. (*Pretends to change TV channel.*)

LIONEL: Hey, what did you do that for?

LEADER B: I wanted to watch the news.

LIONEL: You can't do that, I was in the middle of watching my program.

LEADER B: I wanted to see something else.

LIONEL: You can't do that.

LEADER B: Why not?

LIONEL: Because I was watching something. (*Leader A kneels down next to Lionel and whispers into his ear, "It bothers me. . . . "*) It bothers me when you change the channel.

LEADER B: I'm sorry.

LIONEL: Would you change it back?

LEADER B: OK.

LEADER A: Let's stop the role play now. Lionel, I really liked the fact that you made a clear verbal statement in that last role play. You told Sandra that it bothered you when she changed the channel like that. I'd like you to try this role play one more time, and this time I'm not going to coach you. I'd like you to remember to include a feeling statement, just the way you did in this last role play. Any questions? . . .

Prompting

Prompting is the use of nonverbal signals during a role play to improve a component of a social skill. Prompting is most useful for changing nonverbal and paralinguistic features of a social skill, such as eye contact and voice volume.

Prompting is unlike coaching, in that the meaning of specific signals may not be clear to the participant unless they are discussed prior to the role play. Therefore, immediately before the role play, the leader discusses the specific prompt he or she will use in the role play and how the participant should respond.

A common hand signal used in prompting is for the leader to point to his or her eye to indicate that the participant should increase eye contact during the role play. Another common hand signal is to motion one's thumb upward to indicate that the participant should speak more loudly during the role play. Both of these hand signals are provided as needed throughout the role play, with the leader standing directly behind the person with whom the group member is interacting in the role play. As with coaching, prompting is used to facilitate performance during the role play and is then faded in subsequent role plays. An example of how to set up a role play with prompting is provided in the following exchange.

Example of Prompting

LEADER: Bob, I noticed that it is sometimes hard for you to speak loudly enough in your role play.

BOB: Yes.

LEADER: For the next role play, I would like to arrange a signal to help you to remember to speak up. During this role play I'm going to stand behind Sandra [Leader B] where you can see me. Whenever I want you to speak up, I'll point my thumb up, and I'll keep doing that until you are speaking loudly enough. (*Demonstrates signal.*) If your voice trails off again, then I'll just use the same signal again. Is that clear?

BOB: I understand.

DIFFERENT TRAINING MODALITIES

Thus far in this chapter we have described how to conduct social skills training in a group format. Although there are obvious advantages to the group format, other formats for skills training can be suitable as well. Social skills training conducted with individuals, families, or couples can be an excellent way of supplementing or improving the generalization of group-based social skills training. Some considerations for addressing these other formats for social skills training are addressed in the following discussion.

Individual Format

Individual social skills training can be used either to supplement group-based training or alone. It can also be used in combination with other therapeutic techniques, such as psychoeducation and stress management training. Sometimes clients are reluctant to attend social skills training groups, and a limited number of individual skills training sessions can help prepare them for participating in a group. In such cases, it can be beneficial for the clinician, if he or she is not the group leader, to attend some of the early group sessions with the client. This strategy can gradually ease the person into the group with a minimum of stress.

When individual skills training is conducted on a long-term basis, several modifications in skills training procedures may be necessary. To avoid the repetition of the therapist always engaging in role plays with the individual, it can be useful to elicit the occasional help of another person to participate in the role plays. Trips with the therapist into the community to practice social skills may also provide necessary variations in the training procedures.

Another consideration when using an individual format is the content of the session. In group skills training, sessions are devoted exclusively to training specific social skills. In individual skills training, sessions may focus on skill development, but they may address other topics as well. For example, skills training sessions can address topics such as education about the psychiatric illness, strategies to manage stress (e.g., relaxation techniques), methods for coping with persistent symptoms, or leisure and recreational activities. Thus, social skills training can either be the dominant form of therapy provided or one of a variety of strategies in a clinician's armamentarium of techniques.

Couple and Family Format

Social skills training for couples or families can be an effective strategy for improving communication and decreasing stress. It has been well established that people with schizophrenia are highly susceptible to the negative effects of critical and emotionally laden communications from family members ("expressed emotion"; Butzlaff & Hooley, 1998). More effective communication skills can be taught using skills training techniques, thereby decreasing the stress on everyone in the family.

Treatment manuals are available that describe the rudiments of social skills training with families and couples (Falloon, Boyd, & McGill, 1984; Mueser & Glynn, 1999). Typically, skills training approaches with families emphasize work on conflict resolution and skills for expressing positive feelings and making requests. The emphasis is on developing more effective communication skills using the same procedures as when one is conducting social skills training groups. Skills training with families is usually combined with other therapeutic techniques, such as psychoeducation.

When one is working with families, the focus is on *all* family members, not just the client. Because family sessions usually occur on a weekly basis or less frequently, participants tend to acquire skills at a slow rate. Therefore, family-based social skills training is usually not a satisfactory alternative to more intensive group-based social skills training. However, family and couple sessions can provide a useful complement to group skills training. Furthermore, when relatives review the skills that are taught in group sessions, they can then prompt and reinforce clients' use of these skills in their day-to-day interactions. Meeting regularly with relatives and other significant persons to review the skills taught in groups is an effective strategy for programming the generalization of social skills to the natural environment.

SUMMARY

Social skills training is a set of teaching strategies designed to systematically help individuals develop more effective skills for interacting with others. Skills training techniques are based on a number of learning principles, including *modeling* (observational learning), *reinforcement* (verbal praise for effective components of a social skill), *shaping* (reinforcing successive approximations toward a desired goal), *overlearning* (repeatedly practicing the skill until it becomes automatic), and *generalization* (the transfer of skills from the training setting to another setting via homework).

Social skills can be taught in a variety of formats, ranging from group treatment, individual psychotherapy, or family or couple therapy. Social skills training is taught following a sequence of steps: (1) Establish a rationale for learning the skill, (2) discuss the component steps of the skill, (3) model (demonstrate) the skill, (4) engage a group member in a role play, (5) provide positive feedback, (6) provide corrective feedback, (7) engage the group member in another role play, (8) provide additional feedback, (9) engage other group members in role plays and provide feedback, (10) assign homework, which will be reviewed in the next session.

Skills trainers may utilize a number of additional methods for helping clients acquire better social skills, including *supplementary modeling* (modeling the skill in additional role plays for the client), *discrimination modeling* (modeling good versus poor performance of the skill in subsequent role plays to highlight differences), *coaching* (providing verbal prompts to the client during the role play), and *prompting* (providing nonverbal prompts to the client during the role play).

Social skills training incorporates a diverse set of clinically based strategies into a structured teaching format. The methods can be adapted to teach skills to a wide variety of people who have schizophrenia, while ensuring that the learning process is enjoyable and rewarding for both clients and clinicians.

5

Starting a Skills Group

As described in Chapter 4, social skills training utilizes a structured format that can be adapted for use with individuals, couples, families, and groups. Providing social skills training to people with schizophrenia in a group format has several advantages. For example, groups can provide clients with a variety of models as they see both group leaders and peers practicing the skills being taught. Clients also receive support and feedback from both of these sources. Another advantage of the group setting is that it can encourage clients to socialize with their peers. This is particularly important for individuals with schizophrenia because their symptoms often make it difficult for them to interact with others. Participating in a group can help foster a sense of community among the clients that may, in turn, reduce the sense of social isolation that many feel and provide an opportunity for friendships to develop that may be pursued outside the group setting. In addition, social skills training in groups is both an efficient and cost-effective approach to rehabilitation, as several clients can participate in a group led by two leaders. This chapter provides practical advice necessary for beginning a social skills group.

PRACTICAL CONSIDERATIONS WHEN PLANNING A GROUP

The importance of preparation for a group cannot be overemphasized. In the planning phase of any project, one must begin by clarifying a rationale for its creation. Planning for a social skills group is no different; it is important to be clear as to why there is a need for such a group and what its objectives will be. Paying careful attention to pregroup tasks and concerns will greatly increase the likelihood of having a successful group. The following questions are important to consider when one is planning a social skills group.

1. Who will participate in the group? Clients with the same skill deficits or those with different deficits? Clients in the hospital or those living in the community? Higher- or lower-functioning clients? Clients with or without a substance use disorder?

2. What are the goals of the group? What will clients gain by participating in it?

3. How long will the group be conducted? Will it be time-limited or open-ended?

4. How many clients will be in the group? Where will the group meet? How often will it meet? How long will each meeting last?

5. What characteristics and background are you looking for in a group leader? Who will lead the group, and how will the responsibilities of leading be divided?

6. What client screening and selection procedures will be used? What is the rationale for using these procedures?

7. How will clients be prepared for participation in the group? How will leaders articulate the group goals to clients? How will clients set individual goals? What ground rules will be established by the group leaders at the outset?

8. What evaluation procedures will be used? What follow-up procedures?

9. How will other staff be involved in reinforcing the skills taught in group? How can they encourage generalization of skills to outside the group?

The answers to these questions will depend on a number of factors, including the group composition, size, setting, frequency, duration, and logistics. Guidelines for addressing these and other issues related to starting a group are provided in the rest of this chapter.

GROUP COMPOSITION

It is usually easier to conduct social skills training when group members function at a similar level. Group leaders should make every effort to identify clients with similar deficits during the assessment process, as a group will run more smoothly when its members are focusing on related goals.

However, often it is not feasible to match all clients on skill level and/or need. Most clients can still benefit from being in groups with members with differing abilities. Therefore, it is important for the leaders to learn ways to balance the needs of all the members of the group regardless of skill level. For example, clients who are making progress slowly in group can learn from, and be encouraged by, the improvement being made by more advanced clients. The more advanced clients often experience the satisfaction of helping others having difficulty, which can boost their self-esteem and provide valuable practice in using the skills with others. Further strategies for tailoring the group to meet the specific needs of all of its members and troubleshooting for specific populations are discussed in Chapters 7 and 8. Clients who are actively using drugs and alcohol present unique challenges and tend to do better in groups that are specifically focused on substance abuse. Chapter 9 provides detailed instructions about conducting such groups.

Group Size

The ideal size for a group is between 4 and 10 clients, with size determined mainly by the functional level of impairment (e.g., severity of positive or negative symptoms, level of independent living). A small group size allows leaders to provide more focused teaching, including more explanation about role plays, modeling, and role-play rehearsal for clients who may have difficulty concentrating because of symptoms or cognitive deficits. However, if the group consists of primarily less-impaired clients, then as many as 10 clients can be accommodated. The limiting factor in group size is that group leaders must ensure that all clients have ample opportunity to practice targeted skills, as well as to reap the benefits of having a variety of models to observe.

Duration of Groups

Deciding how long a group should run and whether it will be time-limited or ongoing requires that the group leaders take several factors into account. External constraints must be considered, such as the type of facility they are working in, whether the group members are in a hospital setting or living in the community, and the length of time clients are available, as well as their level of functioning. In addition, group leaders need to determine the breadth of the group's focus. Will it be a group that is designed to improve clients' general social skills functioning, or will it be focused on a specific goal, such as improving friendship skills?

For example, leaders conducting groups in long-term inpatient facilities may have greater flexibility to work on improving a broad range of social skills. However, a short-term group that takes place in a day hospital and is designed to improve client assertiveness cannot work on a range of skills. In addition, the level of client functioning will impact the leaders' ability to work on a range of skills. Leaders working with highly impaired clients will need to focus on basic skills such as Listening to Others, Making Requests, Expressing Positive Feelings, and Expressing Unpleasant Feelings, whereas those working with less-impaired clients will have freedom to work on a greater number of skills.

Frequency and Length of Meetings

When determining how many times a week to hold group meetings, it is important for group leaders once again to ask themselves the following questions: What is the focus of the group? Will it be time-limited or ongoing? How impaired are the group members? As a rule, it is best if time-limited groups meet two or more times a week. This provides clients with ample opportunities to practice the skills being taught. The more time clients spend in groups practicing the skills, the greater the likelihood that they will be able to incorporate the skills and use them outside the group. Ongoing groups may also provide multiple weekly training sessions, or in some cases, they may employ weekly sessions as a maintenance or booster strategy.

Determining how long each group meeting should last depends primarily on the level of impairment of the group members. Meetings should be shorter for highly symptomatic or cognitively impaired persons than for less symptomatic clients. For example, a group composed of highly symptomatic clients who can be expected to have difficulties in concentrating may last only 20 minutes, whereas a less symptomatic group may last up to 1 hour or longer. In a group with clients of varying levels of symptomatology, group leaders must be sensitive to the individuals' needs at any given meeting. Such a group could be scheduled for 1 hour, but it could be shortened if necessary.

LOGISTICS

The major logistics that need to be considered when one is planning a social skills group include the setting and timing of the group.

Setting

As a rule, it is wise to hold meetings within a naturally occurring group setting such as an inpatient unit, a day treatment program, or a structured living residence. In this way, the group members will already be at the location of the meeting and will not require that any additional support services be coordinated, such as transportation and the supervision for transport. In addition, clients are usually more relaxed and comfortable in these familiar surroundings.

When groups are held where clients spend much of their time, the leaders can also incorporate the setting into role-play scenarios. Practicing role plays in familiar surroundings may also increase the chances that clients will connect what was taught in group with events happening outside the group in the same environment. The closer the role plays mirror real life, the greater the likelihood that clients will be able to use the skills outside the group setting.

Choosing a room that is conducive to learning social skills is another task that requires some foresight on the part of the group leaders. The room should be far enough away from high-traffic areas, such as the dayroom of a hospital, so as to shield group participants from distractions. Ideally, the room should have a door that closes it off from the rest of the facility and should be large enough that group members can participate in role plays without feeling closed in or cramped.

Timing

When deciding on a time to hold the group meetings, it is important that the group leaders choose a time that does not conflict with other scheduled activities which the clients are involved, especially recreational activities. Social skills training should be used to enhance clients' skills when they participate in other activities. Clients need to be encouraged to take part in activities outside the group so that they can practice what they have learned. Moreover, early mornings are usually not good times for many clients.

Once a location and time are chosen, it is best not to change them. Frequent changes in the time and location can be disorienting and quite stressful for some clients. The group needs to enhance these clients' level of comfort by providing a sense of structure and continuity, which may enable them to participate more fully in the group.

INCENTIVES FOR PARTICIPATION

All of the time and energy focused on planning for the group will have been of little value if leaders cannot get clients to attend the groups. Therefore, building in incentives for client participation is an important consideration when planning for a group. Some incentives that have been successfully used include providing special privileges for those who regularly attend the group, holding a monthly pizza party, or scheduling special recreational activities for those who actively participate in the groups. Coffee, soft drinks, and cookies can be served at the conclusion of each session as an ongoing incentive. Leaders can tailor the incentives to meet the needs and desires of the group members.

SELECTING GROUP LEADERS

Group leaders can come from a variety of clinical backgrounds. Counselors, activity therapists, occupational therapists, case managers, social workers, nurses, psychologists, and psychiatrists have been successfully trained to lead social skills groups. The formal degrees and job titles of the group leaders appear to be less important than other characteristics, such as warmth, clinical experience, and an interest in the clients served.

Highly structured teaching techniques are employed by group leaders. Leaders take an active role throughout the group by modeling the skill being taught, role playing with group members, and providing feedback to group members. The leaders do not focus their attention on group process or encourage the general sharing of feelings, unless they are directly related to the skills being taught. The emphasis is on helping clients develop new skills through experiential learning and group feedback.

The qualities that are needed to successfully lead a group fall into two categories. The first category comprises qualities that are not specific to social skills training but are required of any person who works with psychiatric clients, such as warmth, empathy, enthusiasm, flexibility, good social skills, willingness to listen, and the ability to provide structure and reinforcement.

The second category includes skills that are more specific to social skills training with clients who have schizophrenia. Leaders function more like teachers or coaches than psychotherapists. They must be comfortable with imposing and sticking to a structure. Most important of all is the ability to persistently focus on small units of behavior without losing patience. Other specific skills include the following:

1. Knowledge of basic behavior principles
2. Knowledge of schizophrenia, including characteristic symptoms and related impairments
3. Ability to present material in an easy-to-understand format
4. Ability to plan and present role-play scenarios
5. Ability to engage group members in behavioral rehearsals
6. Ability to elicit and provide specific feedback about verbal content, and about nonverbal and paralinguistic elements of the role plays
7. Ability to be active and directive in coaching and prompting clients to make desired changes in role plays
8. Ability to assign homework that is tailored to the individual needs of the clients
9. Ability to manage problematic behaviors that may occur during group.

CO-LEADING GROUPS

It is preferable that social skills groups be conducted by two leaders, because it is challenging for one person to teach the skills, set the pace, and maintain control of the group on a continuing basis. In addition, the use of co-leaders can greatly facilitate the demonstration and modeling of new skills, as well as aid in the coaching of clients during role plays.

Conducting social skills training is demanding and requires that the group leaders complete a number of tasks. Table 5.1 provides a list of tasks that need to be accomplished during groups. These tasks can be grouped under two specific headings: group facilitator tasks and role-play confederate tasks. Usually the co-leader who takes on the role of facilitator is responsible for structuring and pacing the session, introducing the skill being taught, and assigning homework. The leader who takes on the job of the role-play confederate is responsible for participating in role plays with group members as well as providing an overview of the group, reviewing group rules and expectations, and introducing new group members. Leaders should meet before each session to agree on tasks and go over strategies for conducting the particular group. Leaders often find it helpful to alternate between the two roles (within or across sessions) to prevent boredom and burnout.

LEADER TRAINING

Written materials and didactic presentations are helpful in training prospective group leaders. Another important component of their training, however, is the direct experience of both observing and co-leading groups with an experienced therapist. Although it is advisable that prospective group leaders participate in supervision during their training period, it may not be feasible.

Therefore, prospective group leaders should become familiar with the information provided in this book so that they can incorporate its many suggestions into their repertoires, and then use the book as a reference guide.

TABLE 5.1. Tasks for Group Leaders

1. Review group rules and expectations.
2. Provide group rationale and format.
3. Introduce new group members.
4. Introduce the skill to be taught.
5. Structure and pace the session (i.e., set up role-play scenarios, elicit feedback about role-play performance, monitor group participation and disruptive behaviors, etc.).
6. Model the skill for the group and participate in role plays as the confederate.
7. Assign homework.

SELECTING CLIENTS FOR GROUP

Almost any client who exhibits difficulties in interpersonal situations is a potential candidate for social skills training. Determining which clients will be able to successfully participate in group requires that the leaders consider several issues. First, it is important that the clients symptoms be as stable as possible. Group members who are actively experiencing hallucinations or delusions may be distracted and have more difficulty in following what is being taught in groups, especially if those symptoms are temporarily exacerbated. If the symptoms are particularly distressing, these clients may even become disoriented or disruptive. Second, it is desirable if clients are able to interact in a small group setting without talking to themselves, pacing, being disruptive, or exhibiting other problem behaviors. Finally, it is best if clients are able to communicate using simple sentences, focus their attention for at least a few minutes without interrupting, and follow simple instructions.

Some clients, however, will not be able to meet the demands that participation in the group requires. Because schizophrenia is an illness characterized by periodic symptom exacerbations, it is not uncommon for previously stabilized clients to have episodes of increased symptomatology. During these periods, it is the group leaders' responsibility to weigh the needs of the individual client with those of the group as a whole. If a symptomatic client becomes so disruptive that one or both of the leaders are primarily focused on managing that client's behavior and cannot accomplish the group goals for the day, then the client should be asked to take a break from group until the symptoms are better under control. In many cases, both individual and group needs can be accommodated. For instance, a client who has become agitated and is unable to remain seated, but who is quiet, may be able to remain in group. The group leader can arrange the seating so that the agitated client can come and go as he or she needs without interrupting the group. However, a client who is delusional and is prone to loud outbursts about his or her delusions will require more intensive supervision and frequent redirection and is, therefore, less likely to be able to remain in group.

PREPARING CLIENTS FOR PARTICIPATION IN GROUP

It is important that the group leaders meet with prospective members prior to their beginning group. The leaders' goals for this meeting are to orient the clients to social skills training and to assist them in setting individual goals for the group. In addition, therapists can use this meeting as an opportunity to build rapport with the individual clients and to screen out clients who may not be ready to attend group. Because building rapport is important for both co-leaders, it is preferable for both to be present at the initial meeting with the client.

Group leaders should plan to spend between 15 and 30 minutes meeting with each client. If a client has difficulty in concentrating for that length of time, two shorter meetings can be arranged. The first few minutes of the meeting can be spent making small talk in order to put the client at ease and begin to build rapport. The leaders can then describe the rationale for skills training. Appendix A provides an example of some of the information that the leader will want to convey. Leaders should bear in mind that not all clients will be able to absorb the same amount of information when the group is described; the leaders must be able to gauge for each client how much information to provide and at what level the language should be.

After the leaders have described the rationale and feel confident that the client has understood, they should begin the process of helping the client to set goals for the group. Prior to the meeting, therapists should familiarize themselves with previous assessments of each client's functioning, particularly regarding interpersonal and expressive deficits. Armed with this information, a leader is in a good position to guide the client in choosing appropriate and realistic goals. Questions such as those in Table 5.2 can be used to guide the leaders in the goal-setting process.

Not all clients will be able to identify specific goals to work on. Therefore, before meeting with the clients, the group leaders should consult staff or family members about goals they would set, based on their observations of the clients's behavior, and review client charts for any goals already set by the treatment team. It is helpful for the leaders to come to the meeting with a mental list of common goals that are relevant to most clients, such as living independently and having more money.

Other clients, however, may identify very ambitious goals, such as finding a girlfriend, getting a skilled job, getting married, and buying a house, all within the upcoming year. In these cases, the leaders' job will be to assist the client with breaking the goal down into manageable steps, such as assessing conversational and friendship skills and targeting areas that the client needs to improve before being able to achieve these goals. It is important that leaders not discourage clients from pursuing their goals, even those that are very ambitious. However, leaders need to be alert for goals that appear to be delusional, such as be-

TABLE 5.2. Individual Goal Assessment

Name: _____

Date: _____ Age: _____ Sex: _____

Education (highest level completed): _____

Current occupation: _____

Work history: _____

_____

What activities are you involved in on a daily or weekly basis? _____

_____

Are there any activities that you are currently not participating in but would like to? _____

_____

Who are the people you spend most of your time with? _____

_____

Are there people whom you do not currently spend time with but would like to? _____

_____

Identify two goals that you would like to achieve within the next 6 months (short-term goals).

_____

_____

Identify two goals that you would like to achieve within the next year (long-term goals).

_____

_____

coming the CEO of a large corporation or a rock star. Leaders must become adept at compassionately steering clients away from those goals that they deem to be delusional while assisting them in breaking down the more ambitious goals into manageable steps.

Occasionally leaders will meet with a client who is not yet ready to attend group. When this occurs, the leaders should stay in contact with the client until he or she is stabilized enough to benefit from treatment. Regular contact can take the form of a brief informal conversation with the client at around the time of the group session. Group leaders should also maintain frequent contact with staff members, mental health providers, or family members who have regular contact with the client so they can receive their input as to the client's progress toward attending group.

WORKING WITH OTHER MENTAL HEALTH PROFESSIONALS TO GENERALIZE SKILLS

One of the primary goals of social skills training is to get clients to generalize the skills learned in group to situations outside the group. This is a particularly difficult task for clients with schizophrenia who have significant cognitive and attentional deficits. For these clients, participation in groups alone is rarely sufficient for the skills to be generalized outside the group setting. For maximal skill acquisition to take place, clients need help in practicing the targeted skills in their everyday environments. To accomplish this, others who are involved in a client's care must be included as part of the greater social skills training team, such as mental health professionals, family members, and other support staff.

Clients with schizophrenia often have difficulty in independently identifying situations outside the group where they can use the new social skills. Other mental health professionals who have frequent contact with the clients, such as case managers, inpatient staff members, employment counselors, and other staff at community residences, can help clients identify situations where it is appropriate to use the specific skills and can help them implement what they have learned. Therefore, staff working with clients need to be kept abreast of the skills taught in group. To accomplish this, it is essential to establish a collaborative relationship with professionals and agencies involved in the day-to-day treatment of the clients participating in a social skills group.

Establishing relationships with other professionals is a rewarding, but not always easy, task. It requires patience, flexibility, and commitment on the part of the leaders. In many cases, the integration of social skills training into a hospital setting, day treatment program, or supervised living situation requires a formal orientation of the staff to the program. As with the introduction of any new therapeutic intervention, it is not unusual for there to be some resistance or suspicion on the part of the staff. The leaders must address directly any discomforts or concerns that may arise among the staff members and work toward building enthusiasm among them for the skills training approach.

The leaders should explain how social skills training and the techniques involved can be useful not only in addressing clients' skill deficits, but also in helping staff member respond to clients' problematic behaviors. It is also helpful for group leaders to have an idea of what problems the staff members are currently experiencing in working with the clients and then be able to explain how skills training can be used to specifically address those problems. Some common problems facing staff at community residences include frequent arguments among the clients and refusal to do chores or to take prescribed medication. These problems, although common, make the staff's job more stressful, and any assistance in managing them is usually very well received.

There are many ways that group leaders can orient staff members to the philosophy and principles of social skills training. Appendix A provides an example of what might be covered in a written overview of social skills training. In addition, supplementary readings on behavioral principles and social skills training are helpful; however, these should not be the only means used to orient the staff. Workshops outlining the principles of behavioral training and social skills techniques offer an interactive and efficient way to provide information to the staff. It is usually most effective to combine instructive workshops with written materials. A list of supplemental readings can be found in Appendix A.

Group leaders should remain in contact with the staff through regularly scheduled meetings. The group leaders can use these meetings as a way to monitor how well staff members are integrating what is being taught in group with what is happening outside the group. It is important that the leaders set the expectation from the start that the staff members will be practicing the skills with the clients. These meetings can also be used to tell staff members about the topics being covered in group and other behaviors that occurred in group that might be of some interest to them. In addition, these meetings can be used as times when staff members can bring up any issues or problems that they may be experiencing relating to the skills training or ask questions about how to handle problems that arise in their setting. Table 5.3 provides the format around which the staff meetings can be structured.

Leaders will find that the type of relationship they establish with other professionals working with the clients in their group can often determine whether a group ends up a success or a failure. Developing and maintaining a collaborative relationship with other professionals is a critical component of the social skills training approach and should therefore be awarded as much time and energy as planning and conducting the group itself.

TABLE 5.3. Staff Meetings

1. Discuss the skill that the clients were taught during last week's group. Identify positive aspects of each client's performance and suggest areas for improvement.

2. Review the need for *in vivo* practice to help clients generalize the skill they are learning in group. Discuss situations for prompting and how to set up role plays if the relevant situations do not spontaneously arise.

3. Discuss any new skill that will be taught before the next staff meeting. Hand out copies of the steps of the skill, and role play an example of using the skill. Describe how the skill can be modeled by the staff members themselves.

4. Discuss opportunities for practicing the new skill. Elicit ideas from staff members about when the skill can be used in the clients' environment. If indicated, role play how staff members can prompt clients to use the specific skill and provide positive feedback when the clients use the skill.

5. Hand out homework for staff members to complete with clients during the next week.

6. Discuss general problems that staff members have experienced during the past week with clients. With the assistance of the staff members, identify ways that the problems can be addressed using the social skills model.

7. Elicit suggestions for further social skills needed by the clients to be used in future groups.

SUMMARY

In this chapter we discussed issues related to starting a social skills group. We addressed practical considerations that are necessary when planning a group, detailed important characteristics to seek out when selecting group leaders, and presented guidelines for selecting clients and preparing them for group participation. We concluded the chapter with a discussion centering on the importance of developing collaborative relationships with other mental health professionals.

6

Using Curricula for Social Skills Training Groups

In this chapter we address curriculum planning for social skills groups. In contrast to other group psychotherapy approaches, social skills training groups employ preplanned curricula and teaching aids (such as posters and blackboards). Therefore, the selection of a curriculum and development of new curricula are central to the success of skills training groups. In this chapter we first focus on the content of skills training curricula by identifying the basic skills that serve as building blocks for other skills. Guidelines for developing short- and long-term lesson plans based on these skills are provided, as well as examples of curriculum menus. Although a wide range of curricula for skills training are provided in Part II, leaders often need to develop additional skills to address specific problems and achieve goals. To facilitate this process, we describe procedures for the development of new curricula for skills training groups. In addition, we discuss the importance of problem-solving training and how to implement it in a group setting. Finally, we address a variety of issues related to teaching curricula, including sensitivity to sociocultural differences, balancing training in verbal and nonverbal/paralinguistic skills, and training in social perception skills.

USING AN EXISTING CURRICULUM

The curricula provided in Part II are grouped in nine broad skill areas: Four Basic Social Skills, Conversation Skills, Assertiveness Skills, Conflict Management Skills, Communal Living Skills, Friendship and Dating Skills, Health Maintenance Skills, Vocational/Work Skills, and Coping Skills for Drug and Alcohol Use. These skill areas do not need to be taught in a particular order. Leaders are encouraged to teach the skills that are most relevant to the goals and skill levels of the clients with whom they are working. There are a few skills, however, that we consider to be basic social skills that all clients can benefit from, regardless of their personal goals. These basic skills are Expressing Positive Feelings, Making

Requests, Listening to Others, and Expressing Unpleasant Feelings. The skills are usually taught in this order, with the most difficult skill, Expressing Unpleasant Feelings, being taught after the clients have learned other skills and have more experience with the group process. These four skills serve as the building blocks for the other skills because they provide clients with the practice and tools necessary to master some of the more complicated skills. For example, the skill of Listening to Others is essential for the successful mastery of more complex skills such as Compromise and Negotiation, and Disagreeing with Another's Opinion without Arguing. Similarly, mastery of the skill Making Requests helps clients to learn skills such as Asking for Information and Asking Someone for a Date. In addition, leaders can use these basic skills to help clients become familiar with the process of social skills training. Table 6.1 contains the four basic skills and their steps.

GUIDELINES FOR USING SKILL SHEETS

Each social skill that is included in Part II has its own individual skill sheet that serves as a guide for teaching that skill. As no two groups are the same, the skill sheets are intended to provide a framework for teaching those skills, which leaders can tailor to meet the specific needs of the participants. Table 6.2 provides an example of one of the skill sheets located in Part II.

As illustrated by Table 6.2, the skill sheets are divided into five sections. The first section identifies the specific social skill being addressed (Compromise and Negotiation). The second section contains a rationale for teaching the skill. Based on this rationale, the lead-

---

TABLE 6.1. The Four Basic Social Skills

Listening to Others

Steps of the skill
1. Look at the person.
2. Let him or her know that you are listening by nodding your head or saying something like "Uh-huh" or "OK" or "I see."
3. Repeat back what you heard the other person saying.

Making Requests

Steps of the skill
1. Look at the person.
2. Say exactly what you would like the person to do.
3. Tell the person how it would make you feel.

Expressing Positive Feelings

Steps of the skill
1. Look at the person.
2. Tell the person exactly what it was that pleased you.
3. Tell him or her how it made you feel.

Expressing Unpleasant Feelings

Steps of the skill
1. Look at the person. Speak calmly and firmly.
2. Say exactly what the person did that upset you.
3. Tell the person how it made you feel.
4. Suggest how the person might prevent this from happening in the future.

TABLE 6.2. Sample Skill Sheet for Conflict Management Skills: Compromise and Negotiation

SKILL: Compromise and Negotiation

RATIONALE: Often, people find that they disagree with each other, even when they want to do something together. At these times it is helpful to work out a compromise. In a compromise, each person generally gets some of what he or she wants, but usually has to give up something. The goal is to reach a solution that is acceptable to all involved.

STEPS OF THE SKILL:
1. Explain your viewpoint briefly.
2. Listen to the other person's viewpoint.
3. Repeat the other person's viewpoint.
4. Suggest a compromise.

SCENES TO USE IN ROLE PLAYS:
1. You want to go to lunch with your friend at the pizza parlor. He or she does not want pizza that day.
2. Your case manager asks you to schedule an appointment for 2:00 P.M. on Wednesday. You have plans to go on a day program outing at that time.
3. You and your friend want to go see a movie. You want to see an action movie, and your friend wants to see a comedy.
4. In planning an outing for the community residence, the counselors suggest bowling. You would rather go out for ice cream.
5. You want to visit your family next weekend. They have other plans.

SPECIAL CONSIDERATIONS WHEN TEACHING THIS SKILL: Not all clients will understand what it means to negotiate and come to a compromise. Therefore, it is important that the group leaders spend time explaining these concepts *before* beginning a role play. For example, to negotiate something, both parties have to state what it is that they want to get out of the interaction. Once all the wishes have been listed, both parties must review the list and decide upon a compromise. A compromise usually occurs when both parties get *some* of what they wanted.

ers can generate discussion about the importance of the skill so that group members can appreciate why learning the skill will help them achieve their personal goals. Group leaders should use this section to help clients identify the relevance of the skills for dealing with situations and events that occur in their own lives. For example, questions that may be asked when discussing the rationale for the skill Compromise and Negotiation include "Why might it be helpful to be able to negotiate and compromise?" "Can you think of a recent situation where using this skill would have been useful?" and "Have you ever had a disagreement with someone that you weren't able to resolve? What happened?" Clients are motivated to work actively on learning new skills when they can understand how the skills are related to current issues or events affecting their lives. It should be noted, however, that the length of time spent on this section depends on the level of functioning of the group members. Less time should be devoted to the rationale for a skill in groups with clients who experience severe symptoms, as they often have difficulty in sustaining attention. Groups whose clients have less social impairment may benefit from a more involved discussion that emphasizes their personal goals.

The third section of the skill sheet provides the steps of the skill. Group leaders are encouraged to review each step with the members and elicit comments from the participants about the importance of each step. For example, the first step of the skill Compromise and Negotiation (Table 6.2) directs the person to explain his or her viewpoint briefly. Leaders can ask group members questions such as "Why is it important to explain your viewpoint?" and "Why it is helpful to be brief when doing so?" After having elicited reasonable answers for the first step of the skill, leaders then move on to each of the other steps and do the same thing. The fourth section includes examples of scenes that the leaders can use when modeling or setting up role plays. It is not necessary to use the particular scenes provided on the skill sheet when leading the group. These examples are offered to give leaders ideas for role plays and to provide a starting point for practicing the skill through the use of role plays. As group members become more proficient in using the skill, leaders can tailor the scenes so that they are directly relevant to situations experienced by the group members (see Chapters 4 and 7). The last section of the skill sheet includes special considerations for teaching the skill, including suggestions for how to deal with issues that may arise in the group when teaching the skill. It is important for leaders to familiarize themselves with the information provided on the skill sheets before beginning a new skill. This will allow them the opportunity to anticipate questions or issues that may arise during the group so that they can be better prepared when teaching the skill.

DEVELOPING CURRICULUM MENUS AND LESSON PLANS

Developing curriculum menus and lesson plans is an important component of skills training. Both menus and lesson plans aid leaders in the process of mapping out strategies to address long- and short-term group goals. A curriculum menu is a list of specific skills related to a general topic area that will be the focus of the skills training group. Curriculum menus are useful when planning long-term group goals such as Anger Management, Coping with Substance Use, Managing Positive Symptoms, and Vocational Maintenance.

Table 6.3 provides examples of these and other menus for social skills training groups. Leaders may choose to develop other social skills menus by combining different skills, putting menus together (e.g., Making Friends and Developing Romantic/Intimate Relationships), or developing additional skills for a particular menu (addressed later in this chapter).

Leaders are encouraged to develop lesson plans before beginning a social skills group in order to construct a tentative timetable for accomplishing the specific tasks of the group. These lesson plans may include suggestions for conducting the group, such as the order in which the skills will be taught, the approximate length of time that will be spent on each skill, and examples of possible role plays to conduct. Lesson plans assist leaders in modifying the skills identified in the curriculum menus according to the level of functioning of the group, providing a framework for monitoring the group's progress in achieving its goal. For example, a lesson plan designed for a group of higher-functioning clients with goals related to improving anger management skills will differ from the plan for a group of lower-functioning clients with similar goals. Lesson plans may differ in the number of sessions each group spends on a skill, as well as in the level of difficulty of the role-play situations.

Tables 6.4 and 6.5 provide sample lesson plans for a group with goals related to Anger Management. As can be seen, more sessions are allocated for each individual skill in groups whose clients experience severe symptoms (Table 6.4) than in the groups with clients with less social impairment (Table 6.5). In addition, leaders working with the lower-functioning group may decide that before working on the skills in the lesson plan, it is necessary to re-

TABLE 6.3. Examples of Curriculum Menus

Anger Management

   Expressing Unpleasant Feelings
   Leaving Stressful Situations
   Responding to Untrue Accusations
   Expressing Angry Feelings
   Disagreeing with Another's Opinion without Arguing
   Responding to Unwanted Advice

Coping with Substance Use

   Offering an Alternative to Using Drugs and Alcohol
   Requesting That a Family Member or Friend Stop Asking You to Use Drugs and Alcohol
   Leaving Stressful Situations
   Compromise and Negotiation
   Solving Problems

Using Leisure and Recreation Time

   Finding Common Interests
   Making Requests
   Refusing Requests
   Asking for Privacy
   Compromise and Negotiation
   Asking for Information
   Listening to Others
   Starting a Conversation with a New or Unfamiliar Person
   Getting Your Point Across

Managing Positive Symptoms

   Listening to Others
   Checking Out Your Beliefs
   Leaving Stressful Situations
   Letting Someone Know That You Fell Unsafe
   Making a Doctor's Appointment on the Phone
   Asking Questions about Medications
   Complaining about Medication Side Effects
   Responding to Untrue Accusations

Vocational Maintenance

   Listening to Others
   Following Verbal Instructions
   Responding to Criticism from a Supervisor
   Asking for Feedback about Job Performance
   Joining Ongoing Conversations at Work
   Disagreeing with Another s Opinion without Arguing
   Asking for Information
   Asking for Help
   Solving Problems

Developing Romantic/Intimate Relationships

   Giving Compliments
   Accepting Compliments
   Expressing Positive Feelings
   Asking Someone for a Date
   Expressing Affection
   Refusing Unwanted Sexual Advances
   Compromise and Negotiation
   Requesting That Your Partner Use a Condom

TABLE 6.4. Partial Lesson Plans for Anger Management in a Group with Clients Who Experience Severe Symptoms

Session   1: Generate a list of early warning signs of anger that people commonly experience (e.g., heart racing, muscles tense, jaw clenched, desire to punch something, etc.). Have the group members discuss the items listed.

Session   2: Generate a list of situations that commonly induce angry feelings in most people. Have the group members discuss the items listed.

Session   3: Generate a list of coping strategies for dealing with angry feelings. Have group members discuss the items listed.

Session   4: Introduce the skill Leaving Stressful Situations. Leaders model an example of using the skill and then practice the skill with each group member, using the same role-play scene.

Session   5: Continue with the skill Leaving Stressful Situations. Leaders practice the skill with each group member and begin to tailor the role-play scenes to specific situations that the group members have experienced.

Session   6: Continue with the skill Leaving Stressful Situations. Group members can begin to practice the skill with each other, using role-play scenes.

Session   7: Finish with the skill Leaving Stressful Situations. Group members can practice the skill with each other, using role-play scenes that are relevant to their experiences.

Session   8: Introduce the skill Expressing Angry Feelings. Leaders model an example of using the skill and then practice with each group member, using the same role-play scenes.

Session   9: Continue with the skill Expressing Angry Feelings. Leaders should practice the skill with each group member and begin to tailor the role-play scenes to specific situations that the group members have experienced.

Session 10: Continue with the skill Expressing Angry Feelings. Group members can begin to practice the skill with each other, using the same role-play scenes.

Session 11: Finish with the skill Expressing Angry Feelings. Group members can practice the skill with each other, using role-play scenes that are relevant to their experiences.

Note. Leaders continue to proceed at similar pace with the remaining skills listed on the curriculum menu for Anger Management.

view some of the more basic skills, such as Listening to Others and Getting Your Point Across.

Although it is important to be flexible, leaders are advised to plan the group's curriculum 1–3 months in advance, depending on how well the leaders know the participants and how well they function in the group. If clients are highly symptomatic or vary widely in their functioning, it is more difficult to predict how long it will take to teach a specific skill, as well as which skill will be needed next. Planning the specific curriculum 1 month in advance is usually sufficient in these cases. If the group is composed of clients with less social impairment or if the leaders are well acquainted with the clients' abilities to master new skills, a 3-month lesson plan is feasible. Of course, all curriculum plans must be flexible; it is preferable to shift to a skill that is more relevant to the clients than to stick with one just because it is on the schedule.

ADDING SKILLS TO EXISTING LESSON PLANS

Leaders need to be ever vigilant in monitoring how well the clients are responding to the specific lesson plan designed for the group and must be ready to modify it whenever necessary. By observing clients' behavior in and out of group meetings, and getting feedback regularly from significant others (e.g., staff members, relatives) who know about the clients' social behavior outside the group, leaders can add skills that will meet the ongoing needs of the group members. Often an interaction that occurs in group will indicate that the members need to learn a specific skill in order to deal with a problem. For example, if clients repeatedly argue with each other in group, teaching Disagreeing with Another's Opinion without Arguing, or Compromise and Negotiation, may be beneficial. If the leaders note that clients have difficulty in conversing with each other beyond a simple greeting, they can teach skills related to maintaining conversations. If clients are observed making demands of each other, the leaders may consider reviewing Making Requests.

Self-reports by clients are also useful in choosing relevant skills to teach. A client may report that he or she is upset by a roommate who is very messy, which may be addressed by reviewing Expressing Unpleasant Feelings in the group. If relevant information does not come spontaneously, the leaders can elicit feedback from the group members, asking them about what problems they are currently experiencing. For example, if several clients report that a new resident at their community residence is demanding that they lend him their personal belongings, the leaders may decide to include Refusing Requests as a skill to be taught in the near future.

TABLE 6.5. Partial Lesson Plans for Anger Management in a Group with Clients with Less Social Impairment

---

Session 1: Generate a list of early warning signs of anger that group members have experienced, as well as a list of situations that commonly induce angry feelings. Have the group members discuss the items on both lists.

Session 2: Generate a list of coping strategies for dealing with angry feelings (encourage group members to list strategies that they have personally used). Have group members discuss the items listed.

Session 3: Introduce the skill Leaving Stressful Situations. Leaders model an example of using the skill and then practice with each group member, tailoring the scenes to specific experiences.

Session 4: Continue with the skill Leaving Stressful Situations. Group members practice the skill with each other, using role-play scenes that are relevant to their experiences.

Session 5: Finish with the skill Leaving Stressful Situations. Leaders practice the skill with each member while increasing the difficulty of the role-play scene.

Session 6: Introduce the skill Expressing Angry Feelings. Leaders model an example of using the skill and then practice with each group member, tailoring the role-play scenes to specific experiences.

Session 7: Continue with the skill Expressing Angry Feelings. Group members can begin to practice the skill with each other, using role-play scenes that are relevant to their experiences.

Session 8: Finish with the skill Expressing Angry Feelings. Leaders practice the skill with each member while they increase the difficulty of the role-play scene.

Session 9: Introduce the skill Responding to Criticism from a Supervisor. Leaders model an example of using the skill and then practice with each group member, tailoring the scenes to specific experiences.

Session 10: Continue with the skill Responding to Criticism from a Supervisor. Group members can begin to practice the skill with each other, using role-play scenes that are relevant to their experiences.

Session 11: Finish with the skill Responding to Criticism from a Supervisor. Leaders should practice the skill with each member while they increase the difficulty of the role-play scene.

Session 12: Introduce the skill Responding to Untrue Accusations. Leaders should model an example of using the skill and then practice with each group member, tailoring the scenes to each member's specific experiences.

Note. Leaders continue to proceed at the same pace with the remaining skills listed on the curriculum menu for Anger Management.

Staff members who are involved in the clients' treatment or living situation are also a good source of information. They may describe problem behaviors such as smoking cigarettes in a nondesignated area or refusing to keep medical appointments. If staff members do not spontaneously provide information, however, the leaders can probe by asking about specific problem areas. For example, staff members may report situations such as clients accusing each other of stealing things, in which case the leaders can teach the skills Locating Missing Belongings and What to Do If You Think Somebody Has Something of Yours.

PROBLEM-SOLVING TRAINING

There are some situations in which clients cannot adequately deal with a problem by using a social skill or a combination of social skills. For example, many clients need to make decisions about complicated issues such as where they will live, how they will resolve legal problems, or how they can reestablish relationships with family members. At such times, it is helpful to use a step-by-step method of solving problems. Teaching the skill of Solving Problems is more complicated than teaching most of the other skills in the curriculum.

The skill has six steps: (1) define the problem, (2) use brainstorming to generate possible solutions for the problem, (3) identify the advantages and disadvantages of each possible solution, (4) select the best solution or combination of solutions, (5) plan how to carry out the solution(s), and (6) follow up on the plan at a later time. Learning to complete these steps requires significant concentration, sequential thinking, and the ability to speak objectively about problem situations. However, it is worth the extra effort of the group leaders to teach this skill, because clients who improve their problem-solving ability may experience significant benefits with far-reaching effects on their ability to manage daily life challenges and achieve personal goals.

Even clients who have difficulty with generalizing this skill outside the group may benefit from using problem solving in the group to address specific conflicts or goals.

Because of the complexity of the skill, problem solving is best taught after group members have covered the basic social skills and have experience with some of the more complicated skills, such as Compromise and Negotiation.

Although formal teaching of the skill usually takes place later in the course of the social skill training group, leaders can use this method from the beginning of training, both with clients and with other staff members. For example, group leaders can use problem solving to help clients overcome obstacles to attending the group (e.g., figuring out the mode of transportation, how to fit the group into their schedule, etc.) and to deal with crises that occur in the group (e.g., how to restore confidence in group safety after two members have had a heated argument).

Leaders model problem-solving skills during groups, engaging clients as much as possible in the process and pointing out that they will be learning this skill at a later date. By demonstrating that a step-by-step approach can successfully resolve a problem or deal with a crisis, group leaders serve as powerful models and help motivate clients to learn the steps of the skill. Using the same rationale, the group leaders can begin early on to model the use of the skill with other staff members. For example, the leaders can use the problem-solving skill to help staff members develop strategies to increase a particular client's attendance at group.

When teaching problem solving, leaders follow the same format as in teaching other skills, beginning with a discussion of how this skill may be relevant in the lives of the clients. Throughout the teaching of problem solving, the leaders choose to work on problems that are important to the group members, beginning with those that are relatively easy to solve. The leaders begin by modeling the steps of problem solving in one session so that clients can see how the overall skill works. Subsequently, several sessions are spent teaching the clients the six steps of the skill. For clients who experience severe symptoms, the leaders may want to spend some entire sessions focusing on some of the more difficult steps of the skill. As the clients become more familiar with problem solving, they can work together to solve a problem in a single session.

In groups composed of clients with less social impairment, it is helpful to have a chairperson who assumes the task of systematically guiding the clients through the completion of the steps. The chairperson accomplishes this by reading aloud to the group the instructions for each step, eliciting input from group members and keeping the discussion focused on the task. It is also helpful to have a secretary or recorder, who writes down the results of each step and keeps a record to which other group members can refer. When conducting training in problem solving, group leaders will find it helpful to use a preprinted problem solving worksheet such as the one provided in Appendix A. A sample skill sheet for solving job-related problems is presented in Part II (pp. 261–268) in the section titled "Vocational/Work Skills."

It is very helpful to simultaneously teach problem solving to staff members while teaching it to the clients. Staff members can be valuable role models for clients by responding to their problems using this step-by-step, solution-oriented approach. Problem solving is an especially useful skill for staff members because its emphasis is on helping clients develop their own solutions to problems, giving clients more responsibility for solving their problems and achieving personal goals. This relieves the pressure on staff members to always come up with the answers, at the same time providing clients with some much-needed experience in determining how to handle problems.

DEVELOPING A NEW CURRICULUM

In some instances, the leaders may identify a problem that is not addressed by the existing curriculum. When this occurs, leaders can design new skills to address the particular problem. We have found that the following steps are useful for developing a curriculum for new social skills. The first step involves talking about and defining the problem that is not being addressed. Once the problem has been identified and defined to everyone's satisfaction, the leaders move to the second step, which involves deciding what general skill might be able to resolve the problem situation. The third step requires leaders to develop a rationale for learning the skill. The fourth step involves brainstorming possible steps for the skill. When selecting the steps, it is important to remember that it is best if the skill has three to four steps, each of which is relatively brief. The fifth step involves developing role-play scenes for practicing the skill. Once these steps are completed, leaders move on to the sixth step, which involves trying out the new skill in their group. After piloting the skill(s), leaders can make any revisions needed (the seventh step). Leaders then devise a skill sheet that can be added to the curriculum that is taught (the eighth step).

We illustrate the process of developing new skills with an example from a community residence. Staff members had reported that the residents were getting into arguments and fights because they were falsely accusing one another of stealing their belongings. Staff members at the residence explained to the leaders that in most of the cases the accusing resident had simply misplaced the item in question. After reviewing their social skills curriculum, the leaders decided that this problem was not adequately addressed in the current curriculum and that new skills were needed to help residents deal with the problem of missing belongings. To address this need, the leaders developed two new skills: Locating Your Missing Belongings and What to Do If You Think Somebody Has Something of Yours. Steps for each of the skills were developed, as well as the corresponding role-play scenes. Once the leaders felt comfortable with what they had developed, they tried out the skills in their groups and then asked staff members for feedback regarding whether the skills were addressing the identified problems. Feedback from the staff members indicated that both of the skills were successful at addressing the issues. If the staff members had informed the leaders that the new skills were not addressing the problem effectively, the group leaders would have needed to analyze the problems further and make modifications to the skills or develop alternative skills that might be more successful. Table 6.6 provides a summary of the steps involved in developing new curriculum.

SPECIAL CONSIDERATIONS

Sociocultural Issues

Social skills are the interpersonal behaviors that are socially sanctioned in a given community, and are therefore influenced by the specific sociocultural features of that community. For the purpose of this discussion, *sociocultural factors* refer to the social norms, roles, values, and beliefs that identify membership in a specific racial or ethnic group, subculture, or socioeconomic class. These factors may affect such skills as how a person uses or does not use eye contact, the distance a person stands from another, how assertive a person is, and how much affect is contained in one's voice.

TABLE 6.6. Summary of Steps Involved in Developing a New Curriculum

Step 1: Define the need that is not being addressed.
Step 2: Identify a skill that would address the need.
Step 3: Develop a rationale for the skill.
Step 4: Decide how best to break down the skill into clear and concise steps.
Step 5: Devise role-play scenes to practice the skill.
Step 6: Pilot the skill in the group.
Step 7: Revise the skill as necessary.
Step 8: Make a record of the new skill, using the same format used for the other skills, and add it to the existing curriculum.

As we have emphasized earlier, the ability to perceive and conform to specific social norms in a given community is a crucial component of social competence. A major error that leaders can make when conducting social skills groups is to operate under the assumption that different cultural groups employ the same verbal and nonverbal patterns of communication. Problems often arise when the communication styles of the leaders do not match the styles of the clients with whom they are working. What is appropriate or adaptive for one group or in one setting may be inappropriate, or even maladaptive, for another group or setting. Clients who learn from models that are out of touch with the nuances of their particular sociocultural group or who are reinforced for behaviors that are maladaptive are unlikely to develop the social skills that are necessary for effective living within their community. Leaders need to be sensitive to the sociocultural factors relevant to the clients with whom they are working and must be able to modify the skills taught so that they accommodate the differences in lifestyles, values, norms, and preferences. Being sensitive to sociocultural factors will increase the likelihood that clients will use the skills being taught and that they will have successful experiences with these skills.

There are several ways that leaders can enhance their understanding of the sociocultural factors that affect the groups with whom they work. They can elicit information about social values and norms from group members through discussions centering on what life was like growing up in their neighborhoods and communities. Leaders can also seek out resources that will aid them in their ability to identify the specific sociocultural needs of their clients. Seeking out individuals who have frequent contact with clients, such as staff members and family, can be helpful, as can having frank discussions with co-workers who share the same background as the clients. In addition, attending training sessions or workshops on multicultural issues, or seeking consultation with knowledgeable individuals, can be helpful.

Social Perception Training

Difficulties with social perception are common among individuals with schizophrenia (Bellack et al., 1996; Mueser et al., 1996). These individuals often misread the verbal and nonverbal cues in their social environment. Leaders need to be aware of their clients' ability to accurately perceive another person's feelings through reading his or her facial expression, body language, or voice tone. Because accurate social perception is such an important component of being socially skilled, leaders should weave training in social perception throughout each group session.

Social perception training involves teaching individuals how to identify the behavioral components that accompany different emotions. Behaviors such as eye contact, voice quality, facial expressions, and body language provide important clues to how a person is feeling. By pointing out nonverbal and paralinguistic behaviors that occur during role plays in the group, and by discussing the role of these behaviors in interactions, leaders use real-life models that illustrate the wide range of behavioral cues that people provide. For example, when teaching the skill of Expressing Angry Feelings, leaders can elicit from the group the many behaviors that can indicate that a person is feeling angry or upset. Leaders can ask questions such as "What might a person's face look like if he or she were angry?" "What sorts of things would you notice about his or her body language?" "How would his or her voice sound?" and "What different types of behavior might he or she show?" Depending on the level of functioning of the clients, leaders may then want to ask every member what behavior changes they notice in themselves when they are feeling angry (e.g., speaking in a louder or more angry voice tone). It is helpful if group leaders write the clients' responses to these questions on a board or flipchart so that they can be displayed and referred to throughout the lesson. Leaders and group members can then use the list to provide helpful feedback to individuals who are practicing the skill through the use of role plays.

Group members who have very poor social perception skills can benefit from training in the group that helps them focus on one nonverbal or paralinguistic component at a time. For example, before conducting a role play, the leader may instruct one member to listen closely to another member's voice tone during the role play to determine whether it conveys a negative feeling. Then, immediately after the role play, the leader can ask the group member whether the voice tone of the person in the role play conveyed a negative feeling. If the client's observation is consistent with that of other group members, then praise is given for accurate social perception. If the group member's observation is significantly different from that of other group members, corrective feedback is given, and the client is instructed to watch for the same behavior in another role play. By giving individual clients specific assignments to attend to particular social perception behaviors, leaders are able to provide more focused training in social perception skills for those clients who most need it, while continuing to teach other skills to the group at large.

SUMMARY

In this chapter we discussed how to plan the curriculum for a social skills training group. We reviewed the organization of skill sheets provided in Part II and described how different skills can be combined into menus to address general topic areas such as managing conflict, dealing with substance abuse, and friendship and dating skills. We addressed how to develop specific lesson plans tailored to the functional level of the group participants. Steps for developing new social skills not covered in Part II were provided. We also provided strategies for conducting training in problem solving. We concluded the chapter with a discussion of how to integrate training and social perception skills into social skills training groups.

7

Tailoring Skills for Individual Needs

Individuals with schizophrenia differ greatly in the specific problems they experience and in their personal goals for treatment. Likewise, they exhibit a wide range of social skill assets and deficits. Some clients have limited social skills deficits and may need to improve their skills in only a few areas, whereas others are more severely affected and require extensive training in many skills over long periods of time. Although social skills training is provided following a standardized structure of modeling, role play, feedback, and homework, the content and format of groups are flexible and can be tailored to respond to the specific needs of the individual.

Using the assessment techniques described in Chapter 3, the leaders can identify the specific abilities and deficits of each client in the social skills training group. Once the primary deficits are identified, the most effective way to tailor an individual's program is to work directly with him or her to set specific goals that have personal relevance. If clients feel that skills training is irrelevant or uninteresting, they will not be motivated to participate actively and may even stop attending groups altogether. Bearing in mind the individual assets, deficits, and goals of each client, however, the leaders can adapt skills training procedures to meet the needs of each person. In this chapter, we describe how to tailor social skills training to address a variety of problems common in clients with schizophrenia.

THE ROLE OF ASSESSMENT
IN SETTING INDIVIDUAL CLIENT GOALS

In Chapter 3 we described the assessment of social skills, beginning with general questions about the client's activities and moving to more specific probes concerning his or her social functioning. Appendix B contains several useful forms for assessment, including the Social Functioning Interview, the Social Adaptive Functioning Evaluation, and the Social Skills Checklist. If it is determined that the client has an interpersonal problem that is due to a social dysfunction, specific deficits in social skills must be identified. Understanding the nature of the skills deficit, including such factors as the circumstances under which the deficit is evident, will help the leaders target specific behaviors to modify.

Table 7.1 contains some examples of social skills deficits that are frequently identified by leaders during the assessment process and some possible goals related to addressing the deficits. In some examples, these goals may be broken down into smaller, more specific steps based on the individual client and his or her circumstances.

Setting goals for social skills training is a collaborative process; clients should be encouraged to take the lead in setting all goals, although many will need group leaders to assist them. It is important for clients to identify goals that they would like to achieve and that have meaning for them. Clients' goals vary considerably, from staying out of the hospital to taking college-level courses. If group leaders can help clients understand that social skills training can assist them in achieving their own goals, they will participate more actively in the group and be more likely to practice the skills they are learning outside the group. The process of skills training must feel relevant to clients in order for them to put forth the effort required to participate in the group. When clients are assisted in articulating their goals and when leaders keep those goals in mind in designing and conducting the group, the clients are far more likely to be engaged, to participate actively, and to benefit from the social skills training intervention. The clients' progress in achieving their goals should be regularly assessed throughout the treatment process, as described at the end of this chapter.

Table 7.2 provides examples of how goals can be broken down into specific, attainable steps. Of course, the specific steps and time frame for goal attainment will vary, depending on the individual client's capabilities and levels of functioning. In addition, it is very important to define goals that can be achieved. Clients with schizophrenia often have had multiple experiences in failing to achieve personal goals and may give up altogether in pursuing their ambitions; it is crucial that skills training reverses this pattern of failure, helping clients to realize that progress toward goals and an improved quality of life are possible.

TABLE 7.1. Goals Related to Specific Social Skills Deficits

Problems in social functioning	Possible goals for social skills training
No friends, socially isolated	To start conversations on a regular basis (e.g., daily)
Lack of interest in leisure activities	To participate in at least one form of recreation
Gives in to unreasonable demands	To refuse inappropriate requests
Becomes physically aggressive when angry	To express anger appropriately (i.e., verbally)
Speaks in a monotone	To vary voice tone and expression
Speech is delusional and tangential	To stay on the conversational topic
Makes frequent demands	To make positive requests of others

TABLE 7.2. Breaking Down Goals into Smaller Steps

Goal	Possible steps to achieve goal
Make friends	Start a conversation with one person at work Attend the next social event at the drop-in center. Introduce self to one person.
Shop for clothes independently	Choose one item of clothing to purchase. Shop with the assistance of a relative. Establish size needed, approximate price. Select item for purchase.
Respond effectively to criticism from employer	Use reflective listening when receiving supervisory feedback. Ask clarifying questions to obtain more information. Request suggestion for improvement.
Use public transportation to all locations	Obtain schedule for buses stopping nearby. Choose a relatively close destination that does not require transferring buses. Ask friend to accompany on first trip.

USING CLIENT GOALS TO DESIGN SOCIAL SKILLS TRAINING GROUPS

At every stage of a social skills training group, the leaders need to keep in mind the abilities and goals of the clients. The specific goals of each client are especially important when designing a group, which involves decisions about specific skills to teach, role plays to assign, and expectations about homework.

Choosing Appropriate Skills to Teach

As much as possible, it is important for the leader to choose the curriculum for a social skills group based on the needs and goals of its members. However, almost all clients who are entering social skills training can benefit from first learning certain very basic skills that can serve as a core curriculum to which other skills can be added. As described in Chapter 6, the four basic skills are Expressing Positive Feelings, Making Requests, Listening to Others, and Expressing Unpleasant Feelings.

Teaching this core curriculum in the beginning phase of the group serves at least three purposes. First, it is easier to orient the clients to the group format by teaching skills that are basic and not too complex. Many group members have participated in groups in the past in which the format was quite different and need time to adjust to the expectations of a skills group. The process of learning basic skills is also more likely to give clients an opportunity to have a successful experience in the group. Second, the core skills are excellent building blocks for later, more complex skills. For example, Expressing Positive Feelings is very useful in skills related to conducting conversations, making friends, and living in the community. The skill of Expressing Unpleasant Feelings is helpful as a basis for teaching conflict resolution and assertiveness. Third, teaching these basic skills provides the leaders and the group members with a common vocabulary, a way of referring to fundamental aspects of social skills.

In some instances, such as in conducting a group with clients with severe impairments, it may be most effective to focus primarily on the four basic skills without adding many others. For a severely impaired group, the leaders might spend a month on each of these skills and then teach them again in rotation. Even though the skills are being repeated, the leaders can vary the subject matter and complexity of role plays and homework to keep the group members engaged. Overlearning skills by repeatedly practicing them beyond the first few successes is advantageous because it promotes durability of the skills and their transfer to real-life situations, which is especially critical for lower-functioning clients who experience persistent symptoms or cognitive difficulties.

In most groups, the leaders can build upon the skills of the core curriculum by adding skills that relate to the goals of the individuals in the group. The key to the process of selecting relevant skills is being able to link individual goals to specific social skills. With experience, the leaders learn to translate problems into goals and to relate goals to specific skills. For example, if a client is having difficulty in getting along with his or her roommate, the leaders might help him or her to establish a goal of decreasing arguments. Achieving this goal could be facilitated by learning the four basic skills (Expressing Positive Feelings, Expressing Unpleasant Feelings, Making Requests, and Listening to Others) plus the following: Giving Compliments, Compromise and Negotiation, Disagreeing with Another's Opinion without Arguing, and Finding Common Interests.

Table 7.3 provides several examples of skills that might be chosen to help clients

TABLE 7.3. Matching Individual Goals with Social Skills

Goal	Skills
Make a friend	Expressing Positive Feelings Giving Compliments Accepting Compliments Starting a Conversation with a New or Unfamiliar Person Finding Common Interests Maintaining Conversations by Asking Questions Maintaining Conversations by Giving Factual Information Listening to Others Ending Conversations
Talk to physician about reducing medication	Asking Questions about Health-Related Concerns Listening to Others Making Complaints Making Requests Disagreeing with Another's Opinion without Arguing
Apply for a volunteer position	Interviewing for a Job Listening to Others Staying on the Topic Set by Another Person Asking for Information
Improve assertiveness	Making Requests Making Complaints Asking for Information Refusing Requests Expressing Unpleasant Feelings Expressing Angry Feelings Making Apologies Leaving Stressful Situations

achieve specific goals. As can be seen in this table, many types of goals can be matched with learning the four basic skills. In addition, different goals can be matched with the same social skills. Thus, the leaders can include clients with different goals in the same group because their goals are all furthered by learning the same skills. The actual steps of the skills would be taught in the same way, but the role plays and homework assignments would be tailored differently.

Structuring Role Plays

One of the major considerations in planning role plays is the level of functioning of the group members. If the clients are high-functioning and have good concentration and ability to attend to details, they can benefit from complex role plays that may involve a relatively detailed description of a specific scene and may require the client to modify some aspect of the skill he or she has been learning. For example, to practice the skill of Refusing Requests, the leaders might ask a high-functioning client to role play by saying, "I'd like you to show me how you would refuse a request from your friend Humberto who is asking to borrow your new blue sweater to wear to a mixer at the drop-in center. Keep in mind that although you like Humberto and would like to help him out, you don't really want to lend your sweater."

If the group members are relatively low-functioning, it is best to keep role plays more basic, with simple descriptions of the scene and uncomplicated instructions about using the steps of the skill. For example, the leaders might ask a low-functioning client to role play Refusing Requests by instructing him or her as follows, "I'd like you practice saying 'No' to me when I ask you if I can borrow a whole pack of cigarettes; remember to look at me and to use a firm, clear voice."

In general, the leaders plan role plays to introduce and model a new skill, to demonstrate how to do a homework assignment, and to model how the skill can be varied in different situations. The subject matter selected for role plays must be relevant to the real-life situations of the clients in the group. For example, if the group is composed of clients who are all working at least part-time, the subject of the role plays might be related to an on-the-job situation, such as how to start conversations with new coworkers or how to ask for feedback about job performance. If the group members are inpatients in a psychiatric hospital, the role plays would be more relevant if they involved a situation that might occur on the ward, such as how to respond to another client who demands cigarettes or how to make a request of a busy nurse.

In addition to planning variety in role plays, the leaders must always be alert for opportunities to use role plays that are specific to the goals of an individual client. For example, suppose the leaders are aware that a client has had difficulties in planning an activity with a friend; when teaching Compromise and Negotiation, they can suggest a role play such as the following: "Let's say that you are talking to Sally about where you want to go on Saturday night. She wants to go to a movie and you want to go for pizza. I'd like you to use the steps of this skill to work out a compromise." The client would be more motivated to participate in this role play than in one that seems unrelated to his or her goal.

The leaders can also get ideas for role plays from the group members themselves. Asking members questions such as "What kinds of situations have come up in the last few days when you needed to ask someone for help?" can yield a wealth of relevant subject matter for role plays for Making Requests. Family members and staff members can also provide examples of situations that clients have encountered that would lend themselves to role plays. Leaders' observations of problems in the group meetings can also lead to relevant role plays. For example, if a group is learning Expressing Unpleasant Feelings and the leaders observe two members arguing about one sitting too close to the other, that situation can be suggested for a role play. The leader can give instructions, such as "Humberto, I just noticed that you seemed upset with Joe for moving his chair closer to you. I'd like you to use the skill of Expressing Unpleasant Feelings to let him know how you feel about what he did."

Table 7.4 contains examples of role plays that a leader might suggest to make skills more relevant to the individuals in the group.

Assigning Homework

The ultimate goal of social skills training is to enable clients to communicate more effectively in their naturally occurring interactions. For a skill to help clients achieve their goals, they must be able to practice that skill outside the group. Homework assignments to practice targeted skills are most effective when they are designed to help clients progress toward their goals. Although all clients in a group may be working on the same skill, each of them can receive a different homework assignment, tailored to his or her individual abilities and goals.

The leaders can vary the setting and complexity of the homework assigned. For lower-functioning clients who are just beginning to learn a skill, it is preferable to start with assignments in familiar environments with people they already know. As clients show an abil-

TABLE 7.4. Choosing Role Plays Relevant to Individual Goals

Skills being taught	Individual goals	Role plays
Making Complaints	Shop independently	The woman at the clothing store gives you the wrong size.
	Increase self-assertion	The person at the fast-food restaurant gives you the wrong order.
Listening to Others	Improve relationship with roommate	Ask roommate to tell you about his or her day.
	Increase ward privileges	Ask counselor about requirements for next level of privileges.
Expressing Positive Feelings	Develop an intimate relationship	Give your date a compliment about something he or she does well.
	Increase leisure opportunities at community residence	Tell staff member how much you enjoyed the last bingo game.
Eating and Drinking Politely	Achieve a promotion at work	You get catsup on your face while eating with supervisor.
	Feel comfortable going out for coffee with friends	When out with a new friend, you find your coffee is very hot, but you want to drink it.

ity to perform the simpler assignments, the leaders can make these assignments more complicated, including directing clients to less familiar environments and asking them to interact with people they do not know as well. For example, in teaching the skill of Giving Compliments, the assignments might start by asking clients to give compliments to staff members, then progress to giving compliments to other clients, then to a sales clerk in a store where the client shops often.

For higher-functioning clients who have demonstrated proficiency in a certain skill in the group, the leaders can assign homework that involves an unfamiliar setting or engaging with strangers. Gradually increasing the complexity of homework assignments will keep higher-functioning clients feeling challenged and will maintain their engagement in the social skills training process. For example, with high-functioning clients learning the skill of Making Requests, the homework assignments might progress from requesting a staff member to make a change in an appointment time, to requesting a roommate to turn down the stereo, to requesting an employee of a fast-food restaurant to supply more napkins and catsup packets for customers.

Examples of homework assignments are included in Table 7.5.

MANAGING THE RANGE OF SKILL LEVELS

It is usually advantageous to have groups composed of clients with similar levels of concentration, symptomatology, and ability to follow role-play instructions. In most circumstances, however, a range of skill levels, goals, and motivations exists among the clients in the group. By keeping in mind the individual differences, the leaders can nevertheless overcome major obstacles by planning curricula, role plays, and homework assignments that

TABLE 7.5. Homework Assignments Related to Client Goals

Skills	Goals	Homework assignments
Making Requests	Improve relationship with staff	Ask staff member to help with budget.
	Make friends	Ask person at drop-in center if you can sit with him or her at lunch table.
	Get a promotion at work	Ask boss for a more difficult assignment.
	Shop at local store	Ask clerk for cost of item.
Expressing Angry Feelings	Improve marital relationship	Tell spouse that you are angry that he or she forgot to pick you up.
	Avoid explosive anger	Tell roommate about anger due to unequal housekeeping chores.
Compromise and Negotiation	Improve enjoyment of living at home	Suggest compromise regarding how late you can play the radio.
	Increase self-assertion	Suggest compromise about where to go on group outing.
	Avoid unpleasant tasks on job	Suggest compromise about task assignments.

will be appropriate to each group member's level of functioning, as described earlier in this chapter. In addition, it is helpful for leaders to devise strategies for dividing tasks of running the group and for responding to the needs of both the lower-functioning clients and higher-functioning clients in a social skills group.

Dividing Tasks between Co-Leaders

A common problem exists when some group members function at a fairly high level and others are having difficulty with poor concentration or intrusive symptoms. Leaders can take this into consideration when dividing responsibilities for running the group, which is described in Chapter 5. One leader can focus on teaching the skill and setting up role plays, while the other leader can focus on redirecting the client(s)who may be distractible. The redirecting leader can use coaching (see Chapter 4) to help focus a client's attention on what is happening in the group. Coaching involves the use of verbal prompts to perform specific components of a social skill. For example, sitting next to the client and speaking quietly, the leader can say something like "Alice is doing a role play of Expressing Positive Feelings; let's watch how she does it."

Responding to the Needs of Lower-Functioning Clients in the Group

Lower-functioning clients usually have more difficulty in concentrating, focusing on the group, and carrying out instructions regarding role plays. These individuals can nonetheless benefit from learning the same skills as the higher-functioning clients, if the instructions and role plays are simplified. The leader can review all steps of the skill when addressing the group as a whole, but direct the lower-functioning clients to focus on only one or two steps at a time. The leader can also choose simple role plays that will allow the lower-functioning clients to practice the skill without being overwhelmed by detail.

Coaching is also helpful in assisting lower-functioning clients in performing specific steps of a skill. For example, the leader can sit next to a group member and quietly remind him or her to "look at the person" while role playing Expressing Positive Feelings. This enables the lower-functioning clients to practice successfully along with the rest of the group. More strategies for working with low-functioning clients are provided in Chapter 8.

Responding to Needs of Higher-Functioning Clients in the Group

Clients with a higher level of functioning may complain that the group is not challenging enough or not relevant to their needs. In spite of their protests, they can often benefit from mastering the social skills being taught. The leaders can remind the higher-functioning clients of the rationale for learning the skill and how it relates directly to their goals. The leaders can also design more challenging role plays that call for more complex responses and that relate more directly to their specific goals. Homework can be made more challenging, so that the higher-functioning clients are expected to use the skill in more difficult real-life situations. As mentioned in Chapter 5, many higher-functioning clients enjoy participating in a group with mixed abilities by serving as models and as confederates in the role plays with other clients because it provides an opportunity to feel pride in their abilities.

KEEPING ALL MEMBERS INVOLVED IN THE GROUP PROCESS

Although the focus of the group is usually on the person performing the role play, it is important to keep the non-role-playing group members engaged in some aspect of the group throughout the session. Because of attentional deficits and distraction by symptoms, many clients tend to tune out when they are not directly involved in a role play. When this happens, they are no longer benefiting from the group process and may, in fact, become increasingly distracted and out of touch with what is going on around them. To prevent this tuning out process, the leaders must be aware of the level of involvement of each group member. When a member is uninvolved for a significant period of time, the leaders can try one of the following strategies.

Assigning Specific Tasks

The leaders can directly assign tasks to individuals in the group. For example, the leaders can ask a client to read the steps of the skill or to act as the confederate in a role play. They can also give specific assignments to individual clients regarding what to watch for or listen for during the role play. For example, a leader may say, "Juan, I would like you to watch during this role play to see if Jennifer looks at Paul while she's talking to him." After the role play is completed, the leader can ask, "Juan, did you see whether Jennifer was looking at Paul?"

Checking for Understanding

For a variety of reasons, such as attentional impairment, there are times when clients may not understand what is happening in the group. To increase the comprehension of such clients, it is helpful for the leaders to periodically check on the clients' understanding by asking questions. This is especially important when clients are participating in role plays or are observing others' role plays.

Leaders can check on whether clients understand their own role plays by first asking them to repeat the instructions (e.g., "Please tell me what I am asking you to do in this role play.") Leaders can also ask questions about the role play, such as "What is the skill we are working on in this role play?" "Whom will you be doing the role play with?" "What happens first in the role play?" "What happens next?" Good questions to check for comprehension are "What is your goal in this role play?" and "What do you want to accomplish?" The answers to these questions will reveal a great deal about what the client understands.

Leaders should also check on whether clients understand what they are expected to do when observing others' role plays. They can ask clients to repeat the instructions and can ask questions such as "Who is doing the role play?" "What is the role play about?" "What will you be watching for while Samuel and Tamika are participating in the role play?" "What is Samuel's goal in this role play?"

Making Role Plays Lively

Sometimes the leaders may observe members of the group who are uninvolved, looking off into space, not watching the role plays, maybe even dozing.

When assigning specific tasks and checking for understanding does not improve the situation, the leaders can try making the role plays more engaging.

Some additional techniques to make the role plays more fun include introducing humor, adding movement, using theatrical techniques, and using current events or elements of the popular culture.

To introduce humor in a role play of Disagreeing with Another's Opinion without Arguing, the leaders can set up role plays in which the confederate is instructed to mix up important facts, such as praising a famous football player for his skills in batting or insisting that Bill Cosby was the best president America has ever had. In groups in which the members are aware of current events, the leaders can use topical examples in their role plays, such as asking the members to tell each other something they read in the newspaper recently as a way of practicing Listening to Others or thinking of compliments they might give the star of a currently popular television show to practice Expressing Positive Feelings.

To add movement to a role play of Starting a Conversation, the leader might suggest that the client stand up, walk out of the room, and pretend to be entering a party where he or she will strike up a conversation with someone standing near the food table. To loosen things up when introducing the skill of Eating and Drinking Politely, the leaders can use discrimination modeling (see Chapter 4) by first presenting a humorous example of not following the steps of the skill, perhaps gobbling their food or talking with their mouths full. When practicing the skill of Finding Common Interests, the leaders can suggest that clients ask each other about television shows they enjoyed when they were children or teenagers, perhaps even asking if they remember the theme songs from their favorite shows. When leaders make the role plays fun and engaging, even the members distracted by symptoms are more likely to pay attention and become involved.

To make social skills groups more lively and enjoyable, group leaders may occasionally want to use games and activities that encourage social interaction. For example, *Shake Loose More Memories* (Shelley & Wheeler, 2000) is a card game that can be used to encourage conversations about common experiences, and *Guesstures* (Milton Bradley Company, 1990) is a type of simplified charades game that can be used (without the timer or the game board) to call attention to nonverbal communication. There are several examples of commercially available games for older clients in Chapter 8 that can also be adapted to use with any social skills group.

ONGOING ASSESSMENT OF PROGRESS MADE IN GROUP

Chapter 3 contains information about assessing social functioning and social skills in clients with schizophrenia. It is also helpful for group leaders to regularly assess the progress made by individuals in social skills groups. Even when the leaders do not have the resources available for doing extensive assessments, a broad measure of progress every 3 to 6 months helps the leaders to evaluate whether the skills are being learned, whether the clients are using them outside the group, and whether the skills are helping clients to achieve their goals. The answers to such questions aid leaders in planning how long to spend on specific skills, choosing skills to teach, and determining what efforts need to be made to increase participation in role plays and homework assignments. Information gleaned from regular assessments can also help the leaders give feedback to other treatment staff members. For example, if the clients in a community residence are not using the skills outside the group, the leaders might use this information to encourage staff members to spend more time actively assisting the residents to practice the skills.

As noted in Chapter 3, Appendix B contains several forms that leaders can use to help assess the progress being made in group: the Social Skills Goals Clinician Rating Scale, the Social Skills Goals Self-Rating Scale, the Social Skills Training Group Progress Note, and the Social Skills Homework Record.

Are the Clients Learning the Skills?

As skills are being taught, it is important to assess whether the clients are actually learning them. When group members cannot perform the steps of a skill in the group session without being prompted, it indicates that they have not adequately learned the skill and require further assistance. The leaders must first determine whether there have been sufficient opportunities for clients to practice; perhaps the group needs more sessions focusing on the skill in order to learn it. If the leaders spend more time on the skill but find that learning is not taking place in spite of sufficient opportunity to practice, they can try other strategies, such as actively coaching individual group members, modifying the role plays to make them more relevant, giving some group members extra opportunities to do role plays in the group, or adding more homework assignments.

In some instances clients have difficulty learning a skill because it is too complex. The skill may need to be broken down into more manageable segments. For example, if low-functioning clients have difficulty in learning Compromise and Negotiation, the leaders can try separating the steps and practicing them in three different group sessions as follows: Step 1 (explain your viewpoint briefly); Steps 2 and 3 together (listen to the other person's viewpoint and repeat the other person's viewpoint); Step 4 (suggest a compromise).

After the group members have shown the ability to perform the steps separately, the leaders can ask them to practice the whole skill. If the clients are still unable to perform the skill without prompting, the leaders can return to a more basic skill, such as Listening to Others.

Are the Clients Using the Skills Outside the Group?

The success of social skills training hinges on the transfer of skills from the group setting to the outside world. Leaders can determine whether clients are using the skill outside the group in several ways: by asking the clients directly for examples of instances when they used the skill, by reviewing their homework assignments, and by asking others who have opportunities to observe the clients, such as family members, day treatment staff members, or community residence staff members. If the clients have learned to perform the steps of the skills while in the group but are not able to use them elsewhere, the leaders can try modifying both the role plays and the homework assignments to more accurately reflect the kinds of situations that occur in the clients' environment.

It is especially important to role play situations that occur frequently and that matter to the clients. Real-life examples are more likely to result in practice outside the sessions. For example, while teaching the skill of Making Requests, group leaders in a community residence discovered that residents were not using the skill outside the group; in fact, they were getting into frequent arguments with staff members because of the unpleasant manner in which they demanded their daily spending money. The residents were becoming discouraged by these arguments and reported feeling under increased stress. The leaders decided to implement a role play of clients politely requesting their spending money, which they practiced repeatedly in the group. The assignment was then given to practice this skill in an actual situation in the community residence. Subsequently, staff members reported that the clients improved greatly in their ability to make requests outside the group.

Are the Skills Helping the Clients to Achieve Goals?

If the clients are learning specific skills and using them outside the group, the question remains as to whether these skills are helping them to achieve their personal goals. Because the achievement of goals is one of the strongest motivations for clients to participate in the group, if the skills are not helping clients to progress, they will often lose interest. To determine whether the skills are furthering the clients' goals, it is important to review the goals that were established during the initial assessment (see Chapter 3 and Chapter 5) and to determine whether any steps have been accomplished that would lead to the eventual achievement of those goals.

Sometimes it is necessary to ask whether the skill is helpful on its own or whether additional skills are needed to make it effective. For example, Richard, a client with the goal of being able to ask his physician to change his medication regimen, found it very difficult to use the skill of Making Requests when it came time to actually talk to his doctor. When the leaders taught the skill of Asking Questions about Health-Related Concerns, however, Richard was able to use it as a way of effectively introducing his request about medication.

In situations in which using a skill is leading to little or no progress in achieving goals, the leaders may also need to determine whether the client may be engaging in other behaviors that are interfering with his or her ability to achieve the desired goal. For example, if a client with the goal of making friends is correctly using the skill of Starting a Conversation with a New or Unfamiliar Person but is very poorly groomed, he or she will have little success in getting people to talk. Working on improving the client's grooming may lead to more success in using the conversation skills to achieve his or her friendship goals.

In other situations, it may be that the skill itself needs to be modified to be even more specific to the client's goal. This may mean the addition of a step or a key phrase. For example, a client living in an inner-city environment who had established the goal of refusing money to panhandlers found that simply using the skill of Refusing Requests was not working. However, adding a phrase such as "I don't have any money to spare" or "I can't give anyone money" improved her effectiveness.

SUMMARY

Although social skills training is a very structured approach, the procedures can be adapted to meet the needs of individual clients. Once the clients' goals have been established, the group leaders can help them break down the goals into smaller steps and identify the social skills that would be helpful in accomplishing those steps. In designing a group, the leaders can choose a curriculum based on the skills the clients need to learn, and they can structure role plays and assign homework using situations that are relevant to the clients' individual circumstances. The leaders can also make the role plays and homework more or less challenging, based on the clients' levels of functioning.

In some situations, the leaders can design a group for clients with similar needs and levels of functioning (for example, a group for high-functioning clients who are working and want to improve their communication skills with coworkers). However, there is often a range of skill levels, goals, and motivation among the clients in a group. Individualizing the role plays and homework assignments helps to overcome some difficulties related to different levels of functioning in clients. In addition, the leaders can assign specific tasks to different members of the group, such as reading the steps of the skill out loud or watching for a particular step in a role play, in order to keep them engaged.

Tailoring social skills training to individual needs is an ongoing process. Leaders need to set aside time regularly to review clients' progress and ask questions such as "Are the clients learning the skills?" "Are they using the skills outside the group?" "Are the skills helping them achieve their goals?" The answers to these questions will help the leaders know how to help each client meet his or her own personal goals.

8

Troubleshooting
Common Problems and Challenging Clients

As in any clinical intervention, social skills training requires the trainers to be familiar with strategies to prevent or deal with problems that may occur in this intervention. Many difficulties in social skills training can be anticipated and prevented by carefully planning the group and tailoring the treatment to individual needs. Efforts made at the planning stage serve to build a firm foundation for the training process and pay off countless times throughout the intervention.

Even with optimal planning, however, problems may arise in social skills groups. This chapter describes strategies for resolving some of the more common problems in conducting social skills training groups and the special problems related to working with clients who present special challenges, including the following:

- Clients who experience severe symptoms
- Clients with less pronounced social impairment
- Older adult clients
- Clients who have mild mental retardation
- Clients who have involvement in the criminal justice system
- Young adult clients

By applying the strategies described in this chapter, leaders will be able to keep their groups running smoothly and effectively.

GENERAL ISSUES

This chapter contains specific strategies for subgroups of clients who may present challenging situations for social skills group leaders. It is crucial, however, for group leaders to tailor the content and approach of *all* their groups according to the varying needs and abilities of the group members. Depending on the group members, the same basic social skills content areas can be presented with different levels of complexity and different expectations for the group members' performance. For example, in teaching the skill Starting a Conversation with a New or Unfamiliar Person with a group whose members have intellectual impairment, the leaders may concentrate on the basic steps of how to say "Hello," give one's name, and say "Good-bye." Role-play rehearsals can be brief and uncomplicated, and the leaders can limit feedback to the basics, such as "Did the person say 'Hello'?" and "Did the person give his name?" In contrast, in teaching the same skill to a group of young adults with no intellectual impairments, the leaders might teach more sophisticated conversation skills, including making small talk about musical groups or sporting events, using "I" statements, looking for ways to continue the conversation, and so forth. Role-play rehearsals may be longer, and the group leader may make the situation more challenging by introducing difficulties, such as having the confederate express a lack of interest in the initial topic chosen for small talk. Feedback might include additional factors such as voice inflection, use of gestures, and social reinforcers. The range of content can also be adjusted, depending on group members' cognitive abilities and what they will be expected to do in their community. For example, young adults living independently might be taught dating skills and job interview skills, whereas older adults living in a skilled nursing facility might focus on skills for strengthening their relationships with children and grandchildren, fellow residents, and care providers.

COMMON PROBLEMS IN CONDUCTING SOCIAL SKILLS TRAINING GROUPS

Following the Group Format

Prior to participating in social skills training, most people with schizophrenia will have experienced other group therapy approaches that were less structured, more insight oriented, and in which members were encouraged to "just let their feelings out." When first attending a social skills training group, people might be surprised at its structure and at its teaching approach. Because of their previous experiences, some people may think that the goals of a social skills training group are to express feelings as they arise and to discuss whatever is on their minds. Consequently, they may have difficulties in following the group format at first.

To counteract the tendency to see the social skills group as an insight-oriented therapy group, the leaders should provide a clear description and explanation of the format of social skills training groups in their initial interviews with people (see Chapter 5). The leaders can be specific about how social skills groups are different from other types of group therapy. For example, the leaders can explain how people who practice Expressing Unpleasant Feelings (such as anger) in the skills group often find it easier to express these feelings effectively when they experience them in real-life situations. Many leaders find it useful to give a brief description of the skills training format in a handout provided during the initial orientation. Appendix A contains an example of such a handout.

Even with good preparation, however, some people find it difficult to follow the group format. In such instances, it is helpful for the leaders to remind group members of the format at the beginning of each session. They may say something such as "Today we will be focusing on the skill of Giving Compliments. First we'll talk about why it's important to be able to give compliments, and then we'll discuss the steps of the skill. After that we will show you an example of how to give a compliment, and then everyone in the group will have a chance to practice giving compliments themselves." Throughout the session, the leaders can directly point out each phase of the format as the group progresses. For example, the leaders may say, "Now it's time for each person to have a chance to practice Giving Compliments. Steve, I would appreciate it if you could practice first."

When people deviate from the format, the leaders can gently but firmly redirect them to the task at hand ("Right now I'd like you to hold your comments while you watch Steve do a role play"). Praising group members who make progress in following the format is also beneficial. For example, to a person who previously interrupted role plays and has now begun to observe them quietly, a leader could say, "Miguel, I liked the way you waited until Steve finished his role play before you gave feedback."

Usually people are able to follow the group format after several sessions. If difficulties persist, however, it may be helpful to make a brief handout, listing the steps of the format. Table 8.1 contains an example of a handout that can be used with group members. A brief discussion of the steps of a typical social skills group session and the rationale for each step can be quite helpful. A copy of the format can also be posted in the group room, and the group leaders can refer to it as necessary.

Reluctance to Role Play

Like many people in the general population, some group members feel uncomfortable or awkward speaking in front of others. This may make them reluctant to role play. First, it is important for the leaders to acknowledge the person's feelings and that his or her discomfort is understandable. It is helpful to let the person know that many people feel shy when they first try role playing, but that they gradually get used to it and may even start to enjoy it. The person can be reminded that role plays are very brief and that everyone in the group will be doing them. Some people are concerned that they will be criticized or teased. The leaders can point out that the emphasis of skills training is on providing positive feed-

---

TABLE 8.1. Steps of a Social Skills Training Group Session

1. Review the last homework assignment.
2. Identify the skill that will be worked on in the group and talk about the reasons for using the skill.
3. Discuss the steps of the skill.
4. Watch a role play of the group leader using the skill.
5. Give feedback to the leader about how he or she used the steps of the skill.
6. Each group member does a role play using the skill.
7. Each group member receives feedback about how he or she used the steps of the skill.
8. Each group member has a chance to improve his or her performance in another role play.
9. Homework is assigned.

back and suggestions for helping people to be even more effective at using the skills. Negative comments and criticism are avoided in the group.

Second, reviewing the rationale for role playing is important. The most common rationale is that "People need to practice the skills they are learning so that they can really know how to use them. It's like learning to play the piano or play basketball. You have to practice to become skillful." The leaders can add that, by role playing, people usually feel more comfortable when a situation comes up in real life where they need to use the skill. It may be helpful to encourage group members to identify examples of specific situations in their lives when the skill would be useful.

Third, it often helps shy people to observe other group members role playing, so that they can see that role plays are, in fact, brief and that criticism is avoided. If a person is adamant about refusing to do role plays, he or she can build up to it by first giving feedback to other group members. Or some people may feel more comfortable serving as confederates in role plays first. These stages of participation can continue until the person is comfortable in attempting a brief role play. After letting the person observe other group members role playing, the leaders encourage him or her to give it a try, usually in a shortened version of a role play, perhaps just the first step. Whatever effort the person makes should be followed by praise, such as "I really liked the way you looked at Bernice" or "You used a calm voice; that was good." The leaders can keep the interaction brief and move on to the next person, first saying something like "Thanks for giving it a try; you did a good job on that first step of looking at the person." In later role plays, the leaders can gradually increase the number of steps they ask the person to do.

Difficulty with Providing Appropriate Feedback

When people are first involved in a social skills training group, they sometimes give feedback to each other that is either critical or vague. This is not surprising, as this is the kind of feedback most people have received in the past. Moreover, many people find it easier to find fault than to praise, and learning how to give helpful feedback takes time. With practice, however, almost anyone can learn to give feedback that is both positive and specific. There are many ways that the leaders can facilitate this.

In explaining the group format in the initial sessions, the leaders can describe how feedback will be given in the social skills group, being sure to include that feedback is specific about the steps of the skill, starts with positive comments, and gives suggestions (one at a time) for improvement. The leaders can provide brief examples of appropriate feedback, as described in Chapter 4. After explaining the desired format for feedback, the leaders serve as important models. In giving feedback, therefore, the leaders must be conscious of the need to always start with positive feedback after a role play. The group members will learn to expect that kind of feedback and can imitate the leaders. The leaders can also remind people to give positive feedback by saying something such as "Rosalita, I'd like you to give some feedback to Robin about how she did in that role play about Accepting Compliments. Remember to start with what she did well."

If a person starts to severely criticize someone in the group, the leaders need to interrupt the criticism as soon as possible. Because people with schizophrenia may be very sensitive to criticism (Bellack et al., 1992), it is better to nip criticism in the bud. The leaders can say something such as "Let's stop here, Rosalita. First I'd like you to tell me what Robin did well. Later we can offer a suggestion for improvement." If a mild criticism occurs after some positive feedback, the leaders can try reframing the critical feedback into a constructive suggestion immediately, such as "In accepting compliments, would you suggest that Robin remember to thank the person first?" It is also important to praise people who begin to make positive comments after having been critical in their previous feedback. For example, the leaders might say, "Thanks, that was very helpful feedback. You really noticed what Robin did well."

The leaders also serve as role models in providing feedback that is specific. Starting with general comments such as "Good job," "Nice work," or "Fine" is a good beginning, but the leaders need to follow with more specific feedback. For example, the leaders might say, "Good job, Robin. I especially liked the way you did Step 2. You said thank you for the compliment in a very sincere way." The leaders can also directly guide or instruct the group members to be more specific. This can be done by asking questions. For example, when it is Rosalita's turn to give feedback, the leaders might ask her, "How did Robin do on Step 1, looking at the person?" If Rosalita is vaguely positive about Step 1, the leaders can prompt her by saying, "Yes, I think Robin did well, too, but can you be more specific? Did she look directly at the person she was talking to?" When a group member gives specific feedback, the leaders can praise his or her efforts by pointing it out, saying something such as "Telling Robin that she looked right at Joe is very specific. That's very helpful feedback."

After the group has met for several weeks, a sense of cohesion usually develops, and group members become more supportive of each other's efforts. They may begin to offer positive feedback spontaneously and may even applaud group members who accomplish something that was very difficult for them in the past. If appropriate feedback does not occur after several weeks, it may be helpful to review what is meant by *constructive feedback* and to provide a written handout to group members and post a copy in the group room. See "Guidelines for Giving Constructive Feedback" in Appendix A for an example of such a handout.

Difficulty in Completing Homework

For people to get the most benefit from social skills training, they must practice the skills outside the group. Because practice does not usually occur spontaneously, it is important to assign homework for using a skill in real-life situations. Chapter 4 includes descriptions of how homework is assigned and reviewed and how role plays in the group can be structured based on the homework. An example of a homework assignment sheet can be found in Appendix B as a Social Skills Homework Record.

Even when people understand the rationale for doing homework and the assignment is written down, they often have difficulty in following through. The leaders need to be persistent, however, in giving the clear message that homework is important and will be pursued. Each group starts with a review of the homework assigned in the previous session. The leaders praise any efforts at completing the homework, even if the group members were not totally successful. When people report that they encountered difficulties, the leaders can ask for more details, helping them to problem solve how specific obstacles can be overcome.

It is best to start by assigning relatively simple tasks for homework, so that group members have a good chance of being successful. As they demonstrate that they can accomplish homework at the basic level, the difficulty of the assignments can gradually be increased. People are also more likely to put effort into their homework assignments when they are interesting and related to their personal goals. The leaders can tailor assignments with this in mind, as described in Chapter 7. For example, if a person has a goal of earning more spending money, his assignment for the skill of Making a Request may be to ask the manager of his apartment complex if there are any jobs that he can do for a fee. Group members should also be actively involved in deciding the details of their own assignments. For the skill of Giving Compliments, for example, the leaders can ask the group members, "Is there someone in your family to whom you would like to give a compliment?"

People who have difficulty with their memory and/or who have low motivation can benefit from someone actively helping them to complete their assignments. For example, if a person lives at home, a family member might be asked to prompt him or her about homework by saying something such as "It's two o'clock, the time you said you wanted to do your homework. Let's look at the assignment sheet together."

The family member can also participate in completing the assignment by being the person with whom the skill is practiced. For example, for the skill of Making a Request, the person's homework could be to make a request of a specific sibling who has agreed to the assignment. In residential settings, it may be more effective for the leader to assign the homework task to a specific staff member to prompt the resident to practice the skill. The staff member then takes responsibility for initiating the assignment and for recording the results. This method of assigning homework to family members and staff members is most effective when they receive guidance about how to prompt and reinforce people for using social skills (see Chapter 10 for details on staff training). For example, when a staff member or family member is involved in completing the homework assignment, that person should praise the group member on the spot for his or her efforts because immediate, specific praise is very reinforcing. Staff members and family members also have the advantage of being able to use a variety of *in vivo* situations and community outings as opportunities to help people practice the skills of the homework assignments.

The word *homework* has a negative connotation for some people for a variety of reasons. For some, homework brings back memories of doing poorly at school; for others, doing homework is experienced as demeaning because it is something "just for kids." For people who do not feel comfortable with the term *homework*, the leaders can substitute another term, such as *practice* or *home assignment*. For example, the leaders might say, "I'd like you to practice giving compliments before our next group; I've written down the details of what you'll be practicing on this sheet to help you remember."

Table 8.2 provides a summary of strategies for the common problems encountered in conducting social skills training groups.

TABLE 8.2. Strategies for Common Problems in Social Skills Training Groups

General principles

1. Encourage participation by each person according to his or her ability.
2. Set clear expectations.
3. Praise small steps toward improvement.

Specific problems	Strategies
Difficulty in following group format	At the beginning of group, remind members of format.
	As group progresses, point out each phase.
	Consistently redirect people when they go off the topic or interrupt others.
	Provide written handout or poster of format if problems persist.
Reluctance to role play	Acknowledge shy feelings.
	Engage person in observing others role play.
	Engage person in providing feedback.
	Start with a shortened version of role play.
	Gradually increase the number of steps to perform in a role play.
Providing vague or critical feedback	Consistently model appropriate feedback.
	Guide people by asking questions about specific steps.
	Stop critical comments.
	Reframe criticisms into constructive suggestions.
	Provide handout or poster about feedback if problems persist.
Difficulty in completing homework	Write down assignments.
	Start with simple tasks.
	Help plan where, when, and with whom assignments will be completed.
	Review previous assignment at beginning of each session.
	Problem solve about obstacles encountered in completing assignments.
	Consistently assign and follow up homework.
	Request assistance in completion from family or staff members.
	Tailor assignment to the individual.

PROBLEMS RELATED TO CLIENTS WHO EXPERIENCE SEVERE SYMPTOMS

Poor Attendance

One of the most fundamental problems leaders encounter when they conduct social skills training groups with people who are experiencing severe symptoms of schizophrenia is getting them to attend and/or to stay the entire length of the session. This problem is not unique to social skills training; most professionals working with people who have severe symptoms of mental illnesses report that it is an ongoing struggle for them to attend programs of any kind. There are several reasons for this problem. Many of the positive symptoms, such as auditory hallucinations and delusions, are often persecutory in nature and lead people to be suspicious of any new person or activity. People with schizophrenia often feel overstimulated by their environment, and this can interfere with good participation. The negative symptoms of schizophrenia, such as apathy (lack of interest) and anhedonia (difficulty in experiencing pleasure), also interfere with attendance. Finally, people may be reluctant to attend social skills training groups because of past experiences with group approaches that were less structured and more emotionally charged and therefore not suitable for people with schizophrenia.

From the very first contact, it is helpful for the leaders to express warmth and a positive expectation about participation in social skills training. The leaders need to convey the expectation that the group will help people to achieve personal goals and that they will enjoy attending. For people who express extreme reluctance, have short attention spans, or have a poor attendance record with other programs, it is desirable to set small goals for initial attendance. For example, for the first group, the leaders might ask a person to give it a try for 10 minutes and make very few demands during those 10 minutes. People who observe the process of the group are usually reassured by what they see and become more receptive to attending the group. As the person becomes more comfortable during short periods in the group, the leaders can gradually increase their expectations for how long the person will attend.

It is important to provide positive reinforcement for all efforts at attending the group. Even when a person attends for only a few minutes, it helps for the leaders to praise him or her, saying something such as "Thanks for coming today; I hope you come back on Thursday." Most people respond well to sincere praise and encouragement, which can come from a variety of sources, including the leaders, other treatment staff members, family members, and friends. Other reinforcers, such as money, food, increased privileges (in the case of an inpatient facility), recreational opportunities, or time with a favorite staff member also help provide motivation for increasing attendance. Some community residences develop a reward system whereby goals for attendance and participation are set each month, and people who achieve their monthly goals are invited to a party. Progress toward these attendance goals is recorded on a chart in the room where the social skills group is held. The party may include pizza and interactive games.

At times the leaders may feel discouraged when a particular person does not attend the group. However, it is important not to give up. With encouragement, even people who do not attend any other treatment programs may attend social skills groups. We have seen several situations in which people who had vigorously resisted attending a social skills group for months finally tried attending. This kind of breakthrough can occur for different reasons. One reason is that, even for people with severe forms of the illness, the symptoms of schizophrenia fluctuate. People who have a brief reduction of symptoms may experience a window of opportunity when they are able to think more clearly or feel less suspicious; at that time, they may be more willing to try coming to a social skills training group. Once they try attending, the chances are good that they will return.

Another reason people may begin attending after a long period is that it takes time to develop a trusting relationship with the group leaders. Therefore, it is important for leaders, especially those who are not regular staff members or who come from another agency, to establish relationships with people whom they want to join the group. For example, the leaders can regularly greet people who are not attending group, saying that they are glad to see them, and develop topics of conversation, such as sports, music, current events, books, movies, or television shows. It is also important to conduct the group consistently on the same days and at the same time; keeping the same routine helps people to count on the fact that the group will continue to occur. Leaders should avoid scheduling social skills groups at times that conflict with other activities, especially leisure and recreational activities or smoking breaks.

In residential settings where social skills training groups are conducted by in-house staff members, they can use their existing relationships with people to encourage them to attend groups and can enlist the help of their coworkers. It is also beneficial to have an additional staff member assigned to assist with each social skills group. The assisting staff member can remind people in advance of the scheduled group time and can gather or direct people into the group room. The reminders and requests for attendance should be upbeat and friendly and convey an expectation of attendance. When reminding a person about group, it is preferable to make a direct request, saying something like "It's 5 minutes until social skills group; I'd appreciate it if you could join us in the living room now" or "I'd like it if you could join us in social skills group; it would be great to have you attend today." However, making the request in the form of a "yes" or "no" question such as "Are you coming to the social skills group?" more frequently leads to the easier answer of "No," which is difficult to counter. In addition to gathering people for a group, staff members can also help by attending the group, even if they are not acting as leaders, because some people feel more secure when there is a trusted staff member in the room. In the group, staff members are always welcome to serve as confederates in role plays and can assist the leaders in designing role plays that relate to the person's natural environment.

Cognitive Difficulties

The cognitive impairments common to schizophrenia, such as distractibility, poor attention, impaired executive functioning, and memory problems, can interfere with some people's ability to benefit from groups. The repetition, overlearning, and behavioral rehearsal that are built into the social skills model can help to compensate for some of these cognitive difficulties. Several other strategies may also be used to address cognitive impairments.

The treatment room should be minimally distracting and located in a quiet area of the treatment facility. The room should be arranged to facilitate eye contact with the leader, and visual cues such as posters, schedules, and signs may be used to assist individuals with memory impairments. Smaller groups and shorter training sessions are sometimes indicated for people who have significant cognitive impairments.

In group sessions, the clinician who is not serving as the primary leader should constantly be scanning the group and may unobtrusively signal individuals who appear distracted to gently remind them to focus on the leader. Questions may be directed to individuals who appear distracted to prevent them from drifting away from the work of the group. If people have trouble paying attention to role plays, the leader should assign them the task of watching for specific target behaviors. For example, the group leader may say, "I would like you to report on Tony's eye contact at the end of the role play."

Group leaders should periodically remind people of the goals of the session in terms of what task they are working on. They should frequently ask people to repeat instructions and should ask questions designed to confirm comprehension of group materials. For example, the leader might ask, "What is Dan's role in the role play? What is Yolanda's role?

What are the goals of this skill?" If comprehension appears poor, the skills or skill components should be further simplified. For example, in one social skills group session, a group member expressed interest in doing a role play for Giving Compliments. She said she had just one question, however. She asked, "What is a compliment?" Her face brightened when the group leader explained that giving a compliment is telling people something you like about them, and she proceeded to enthusiastically participate in a role play.

In general, it is evident that cognitive difficulties are interfering with participation when group members have a delayed response to questions or requests, even when the leaders are speaking in a clear, simple manner and are checking for understanding. When the leader asks some group members a question eliciting feedback, for example, they may take such a long time to answer that it appears they lack the knowledge necessary for responding. These individuals, however, often volunteer appropriate and accurate feedback several minutes after the group leader has moved on to another topic. A similar phenomenon occurs with following through on role plays. For example, when the leader first asks some group members to participate in a role play, they initially appear unable to follow even the first step, but, when called on later for another reason, start doing the role play instead. It is extremely important for group leaders to be aware that many individuals with schizophrenia need extra time to process information and formulate answers. Almost all group members will be able to respond, however, if given some additional time or allowed to take their turns later.

Responding to Psychotic Symptoms

Many people with schizophrenia experience psychotic symptoms such as delusions or auditory hallucinations on a continual basis. For some people, voices may be a low background noise; for others, they may be loud and commanding. Regardless of the level of voices, however, many people experience voices as being in competition with the speech of real people and find it difficult to fully attend to what others are saying and doing.

To help improve comprehension, the leaders can begin by keeping the group relatively short, from 30 to 40 minutes, to better match the clients' limited ability to concentrate. It is also helpful to make sure that communication is brief and to the point. Excessive detail or discussion makes it difficult for a person to pick out the main points. When a person looks puzzled and asks, "What am I supposed to do?" after listening to the instructions for a role play, it is usually a sign that the leaders need to be more concise and to speak in shorter sentences. They may also need to simplify what the person is being asked to do. The leaders need to check regularly on whether people are comprehending by asking questions such as "Could you please repeat back what I said?" or "Tell me what you're going to do in this role play."

Clearly delineating the different stages of the group also helps to keep the person focused on what is happening in the session. Announcing, "Now it's time to give feedback about the role play that Maria and Clinton just did" or "Now it's Alice's turn to practice making a request for a cigarette" can be helpful. Gradually, even people experiencing severe symptoms can understand the format of the group and what is expected of them. In addition to clearly identifying the stage of the group, leaders will benefit by judiciously shortening certain stages of social skills groups. For example, spending less time on eliciting the rationale allows leaders to move directly to the more active stages of modeling and role playing, which hold people's attention better.

There may also be times when people's symptoms lead to difficulty in making themselves understood. For example, when one group member, Lyle, became excited or agitated about certain subjects, he would hurry his words and not pronounce them clearly, making it difficult to understand him. Leaders found it helpful to ask Lyle to slow down and to speak in short sentences.

The leaders also need to check on whether they are understanding someone correctly by asking questions and repeating back what they heard. An example of checking for comprehension is for a leader to say, "Let me see if I'm understanding you correctly; you're saying that you are upset because you think someone took your seat?" It is important to show an interest in what people say, even if they do not make sense immediately. However, the leaders must guard against spending too much time on one-to-one interactions that exclude the rest of the group. Individual conversations can be pursued after the group.

Distractibility

It is difficult for some people to focus their attention and to concentrate for significant periods of time, especially when symptoms are competing for their attention. To help group members maintain their concentration, it is important to keep other distractions to a minimum, such as street noise, people walking in and out of the room, telephones ringing, and people being called out of group. It is also important to keep communication brief and clear in the group; the leaders themselves must avoid long explanations and must redirect other group members who speak for long periods or in vague terms. Because "a picture is worth a thousand words," especially to people who are already distracted by symptoms, it is often preferable for leaders to show a simple example by demonstrating what they mean rather than giving a lengthy explanation.

To help keep group members' attention during the group, the leaders can design role plays that are brief, lively, and contain scenes that reflect people's real-life situations. The leaders can also stand in front of the group, like teachers, to explain the steps of the skills, provide rationales, and model the skills. They can also ask group members to stand during their role plays. This helps people to recognize whom to watch and listen to during the group. To gain attention, the leaders also need to speak in a voice that is pleasant, animated, and sufficiently loud. Speaking too softly or without authority will lose group members' attention.

Some group members can remain focused while they are participating in a role play themselves but become distracted when others are speaking or role playing. It is therefore useful for the leaders to assign specific tasks to group members observing role plays. These tasks of observation can vary from requiring a small amount of concentration (listening for the tone of voice) to a large amount (listening for the specific suggestion made in Step 3 of Expressing Unpleasant Feelings). When people who are experiencing psychotic symptoms are not engaged in specific tasks, the pull of competing stimuli becomes more powerful and their distractibility increases.

Disruptions

When people are particularly troubled by symptoms, they may respond with behavior that is highly disruptive to the rest of the group. For example, if a person is hearing voices that say that an alien force is trying to harm him, he might call out, "I need help! Someone is trying to hurt me!" Or a person who has visual hallucinations may report seeing fire coming in the window. Someone with active delusions may accuse the leaders of being members of the Mafia. The leaders should be understanding and empathetic about these symptom-based interruptions, but should also recognize that they are disorienting and distracting to the rest of the group and must be addressed.

When people have symptom-related outbursts, they are often afraid or alarmed by what they are experiencing. In situations in which a person is obviously distraught, the leaders' first goal is to reassure him or her. Many people feel reassured when the leaders remind them that the group is a safe place. It is also reassuring when the leaders say something to show that the person is welcome in the group, such as "We're glad you're here with us today." The next goal is to redirect the person in a kind but firm manner, reminding him or her of the focus of the group and assigning the person a specific task to perform. For example, a leader might say, "What we're doing in the group right now is focusing on how to give compliments. I'd like you to listen to Dorothea practice giving a compliment to Tito. Notice whether she looks at Tito when she speaks."

In some situations, the leaders can suggest that the person take his or her mind off the disturbing symptom by paying close attention to the group. A leader might say something like "I'm sorry you feel that someone wants to steal your jewelry. I don't think that is going to happen here. It would be a good idea to take your mind off the subject by concentrating on what we're doing in the group. Today we're talking about making requests." In other situations the leaders can omit the reference to "taking your mind off the subject" and simply suggest focusing on the topic of the group. In still other situations the outburst can actually be linked to the group topic, and the person can practice expressing his or her concern by using the skill being practiced. For example, in a group where Barbara shouts at Joe to get away from her because he was hired to spy on her, the leaders can say something such as "It sounds like you're worried about Joe's intentions toward you, and you would like him to move his chair away from you. Since we're working on the skill of Making Requests today, I'd like you to practice using the steps of the skill to ask Joe to move his chair. Remember to use a calm voice."

If the person persists in talking about hallucinations or delusions, a leader can suggest that they could talk about it together after the group, giving a specific time for the conversation. The leader might say something like "That's a very interesting point you're making, but let's wait to talk about that until the end of class at 2:15. Right now we need to keep working on the skill of Making Requests." It is important, however, for leaders to follow up by initiating a conversation after the group, or the person will lose faith that the leaders are really interested in his or her concerns.

In rare circumstances, some people may have such severe symptoms that it is impossible to reassure or redirect them. For example, after the leaders make two or more unsuccessful attempts to get a person to concentrate on the topic of the group, they might consider asking the person to take a short break from the group or excuse him- or herself from the rest of the group for that day, making sure to invite the person to return to the next meeting. There are three questions the leader can ask him- or herself to guide the decision about whether to ask a disruptive group member to leave: (1) Can I continue to conduct the group if the person stays in the group? (2) Can other group members concentrate if the person stays? (3) From what I know of the person's previous behavior, does this level of disruption usually escalate?

If the decision is made to ask the person to leave, it is important to refer to the specific behavior that was disruptive and to "leave the door open" for the person to attend the next group. The leaders should not ask the person to leave the group as a punishment, but rather as an acknowledgment that he or she is currently having difficulties that prevent effective group participation. It is also important to express the expectation that the situation can improve. For example, the leaders might say, "Since it's very hard for you not to shout during the group today, I'd like you to take a break from the rest of this session. But I'll look forward to seeing you on Wednesday."

Finally, there are social skills that people can learn that are specifically designed to address symptomatic behavior. After several disruptions, the leaders might choose to introduce one of these skills, such as Checking Out Your Beliefs, Letting Someone Know That You Feel Unsafe, Staying on the Topic Set by Another Person, Responding to Untrue Accusations, and What to Do When You Do Not Understand What a Person Is Saying. In rare instances, for example, if an individual's symptoms substantially worsen, his or her participation in the group may need to be terminated completely or for several sessions until additional treatment can be obtained. Decisions involving removals from the group should be made only after the leaders have made several efforts to redirect the person, and when it becomes clear that the disruptive behavior makes it impossible for other group members to learn or for the leaders to teach. In our collective experience, including working with severely ill inpatients, this happens very rarely.

Social Withdrawal/Low Level of Participation

In contrast to group members who are disruptive, there are those who are withdrawn and uncommunicative during the group. Some are withdrawn because of negative symptoms such as poverty of speech, apathy, and anhedonia. For these individuals, it is very difficult to become involved in any activity, including a social skills group. Other people are withdrawn as a response to positive symptoms. For example, if someone is hallucinating, hearing several voices at once, he or she may withdraw in order to cut down on the amount of stimulation experienced. In addition, some people are slow to become involved in social skills groups because they are apprehensive that they will make a mistake or will be criticized. This last group of people usually increase their participation over time as they see that the group environment is supportive rather than critical.

Some people are so withdrawn that they may not respond to questions or may refuse to participate. This lack of participation can be misinterpreted as laziness, rudeness, or hostility. It is helpful for the leaders to remind themselves that the behavior is due to the negative symptoms of schizophrenia and is not willful. The leaders must avoid seeing the person's lack of involvement as a criticism of the group or of their leadership. The most effective way to improve rapport with severely withdrawn individuals is to reward them for even the smallest efforts at involvement. The leaders' goal is for all group members to develop a positive association with the group; this process may be very gradual and often requires a great deal of persistence on the part of leaders.

To maximize positive interactions with very withdrawn people, the leaders must keep their communication pleasant and brief. It is also helpful to communicate initially by making statements that do not require people to respond. For example, the leaders might give a person a compliment ("I like your shirt today, David; purple is one of my favorite colors") or praise the person for attending ("I'm really glad you are in group today"). Asking questions that require an answer, such as "What kinds of situations do you encounter in which you have to make requests?" are often too demanding at first for a withdrawn person. When some kind of rapport has been established, the leaders can begin asking very simple questions that can be answered with "Yes" or "No" (such as "Did you hear Jose asking Robin a question in the role play?") and should positively reinforce any responses given. Gradually the leaders can begin to ask questions that are more open-ended.

Although the leaders may be very curious about the reason for a group member's being withdrawn, it is often ineffective to spend too much time asking the person why he or she is not more involved with other people or the group. Although some people can tell why they feel a certain way, it is more common for withdrawn individuals not to know why and to feel embarrassed that they cannot respond. Leaders should avoid offering interpretations about the reason behind a person's withdrawal, because it is extremely difficult to know what is going on in someone's mind. For example, a leader once suggested to a group member that perhaps he was uncomfortable because the group was too large. The person heatedly denied this, saying, "The reason I'm not participating in group is because everyone is speaking pornography, and I don't want any part of that." It is important to note that quiet, withdrawn group members are sometimes listening and processing what is going on in the group, in spite of appearances to the contrary. One person, who regularly attended group but remained silent and appeared distracted during the sessions, once surprised group leaders by responding to a general question with a very detailed answer, which showed that he had indeed been attending closely.

Table 8.3 provides a summary of strategies for responding to problems related to conducting social skills groups with people who are experiencing severe symptoms. Appendix A also contains guidelines for group leaders on communicating effectively.

PROBLEMS RELATED TO CLIENTS WHO HAVE LESS SOCIAL IMPAIRMENT

Difficulty in Accepting the Need for Improved Social Skills

Some people with schizophrenia have less impairment in their social skills, social perception, and information-processing ability. In fact, a minority of people with schizophrenia need little or no social skills training (Mueser, Bellack, Douglas, & Morrison, 1991), so it is important to conduct a thorough assessment, as described in Chapter 3, to determine whether specific individuals actually need social skills training. In many instances, however, even clients with less social impairment experience difficulties in one or more areas of so-

TABLE 8.3. Strategies for Problems Related to Clients Who Experience Severe Symptoms

General principles
1. Keep communication brief and to the point.
2. Be consistent in maintaining structure and holding group at same time and in same place.
3. Praise efforts and small steps toward improvement.
4. Teach and review basic skills frequently.

Specific problems	Strategies
Poor attendance	Build rapport by communicating warmth and enthusiasm.
	Set small goals.
	Use reinforcers such as praise, money, food, increased privileges, time with a favorite person.
	Enlist help of other staff members or family members.
	Identify obstacles to attendance.
	Consistently request person to attend.
Cognitive difficulties	Keep group time relatively short.
	Check frequently whether people are understanding.
	Simplify language and instructions.
	Allow members ample opportunity to observe and practice skills.
Responding to psychotic symptoms	For delayed response, allow extra time for people to respond or suggest that they take their turns later.
	Conduct shorter groups (30–40 minutes).
	Emphasize role plays rather than discussion.
	Give brief, clear instructions.
	Check frequently for comprehension.
	Assign active roles (such as role plays) to clients who are distracted by symptoms.
Distractibility	Keep other distractions to a minimum.
	Avoid lengthy explanations.
	Use examples, role plays to illustrate points.
	Redirect promptly to topic of group.
	Design engaging role plays that are relevant to real-life situations.
	Use a pleasant, sufficiently loud voice.
	Assign specific tasks to group members observing role plays.
Disruptions related to symptoms	Reassure people of safety of group.
	Redirect kindly and firmly to topic of group.
	When appropriate, link content of disruption to skill being taught.
	Suggest discussing person's off-topic concerns after group.
	Teach social skills designed to manage symptoms.
Withdrawal	Understand that withdrawal is not a criticism of leaders or group.
	Build rapport by communicating in a warm, low-key manner.
	Avoid excessive questioning.
	Avoid interpretations of why the person is withdrawn.

cial skills, such as forming close relationships, responding effectively to conflicts, or dealing with problematic coworkers. These clients may protest participating in a social skills training group by saying that they know all about socializing or that social skills groups are boring or that they won't learn anything new.

There are several reasons that clients with less social impairment have difficulty in acknowledging that they need social skills training. Because they are doing well as compared with others with the illness, some people feel that they do not need treatment. They may feel a need to differentiate themselves from people who have more difficulties by saying, "Those other people need social skills training, not me." They may also say that a social skills group is too easy or too repetitive. Others feel that a social skills group reminds them of the losses they have suffered because of schizophrenia, such as close friendships and the ability to interact easily with others, and they find it painful to be reminded of these losses. Still others do not see any connection between the problems they have experienced in life and the need for improved social skills.

In responding to clients who have less social impairment and object to skills training, it is important for the leaders to avoid confrontation and to focus instead on how skills training will contribute to achieving personal goals. Most people find working on goals to be a positive experience. Once goals are established, breaking them down into smaller steps will provide opportunities for the leaders to suggest how accomplishing the steps would be facilitated by developing specific social skills (see Chapter 7). For example, a person with the goal of earning a college degree may see the advantage of starting off by taking one course at a time. In thinking about what is needed to do well in the course, the person may see the advantage of using the skill of Listening to Others to make sure that he or she is understanding what the professor is saying. Once social skills have been linked to a goal, the person is usually more receptive to hearing about the benefits of social skills training.

For people who think that the group is too easy, it can be helpful for the leaders to use the analogy of learning to play the piano, in that it is essential to start with basic pieces before playing complicated ones. The leaders can explain the process of starting with the basic skills first, then building up to the more complicated skills involved in accomplishing more complicated goals. For people who protest that the group is too repetitive, the leaders can explain that practicing social skills is like practicing a musical piece over and over to make it sound smooth and automatic. It may be useful to give a title to the social skills group that reflects the learning component, such as "Social Skills Class," or "Communication Skills 101," or "Problem-Solving Workshop."

After people have started attending group sessions and show an ability to perform the basic skills, the leaders can reduce the chances of boredom by making role plays successively more challenging.

The leaders can also provide opportunities for people to practice situations that are specific to their goals. For example, when teaching Starting a Conversation with a New or Unfamiliar Person, the leaders can assign Juan, whose goal is to improve his relationships with coworkers, the role play of making brief small talk with the person at the desk next to him in the office. The leaders can encourage people to tailor their own role plays, by asking such questions as "What kinds of situations do you encounter on which you need to use this skill?" and "With whom would you like to practice this skill?"

Discomfort in Interacting with People Who are Experiencing More Difficulties

Some people who have less social impairment say that they feel uncomfortable in groups where the other members are more visibly impaired than they are. Some find it difficult to be patient with others who move at a slower pace, who take longer to perform role plays and provide feedback. They may also feel that they do not have much in common with group members who are experiencing more difficulties. Some people feel that it "brings them down" to associate with those who have the same illness as they do and who are more visibly impaired by it. People who feel this way often do not want to reveal having difficulties of any type, including problems in social situations. Being in the same group as those who have more obvious needs for better social skills may be perceived as an unpleasant reminder of their own illness.

The leaders can respond to individuals who are reluctant to be in a group whose members have mixed abilities by first reminding them of their goals and how social skills training will help them achieve those goals. If a person objects to the group format, the leaders can point out that people learn social skills best in a group because they can practice with others and get feedback from them. It is especially helpful to be able to practice social skills with a variety of people. The leaders can remind people that it is important to be able to get along with others, even those with whom they feel uncomfortable.

With some people who have less social impairment, it is helpful to acknowledge that they are more socially skilled than others in the group and to engage them in helping the other group members learn the skills through modeling or acting as the confederate in role-play rehearsals. After they are engaged in the group, the leaders must be alert to opportunities to tailor the role plays and homework to their abilities, including more challenging assignments. As mentioned earlier, people should be involved in choosing their own role plays and homework, which is stimulating and keeps them engaged.

Most people who have less social impairment can eventually be persuaded to attend groups. In rare instances, however, it may be necessary to consider one-to-one training as a preparation for joining the group. When the goal of individual training is for the person to participate in sessions of an ongoing group, the person and the group members should be simultaneously taught the same skills so that they will all be familiar with the same skills. When there are several people who have less social impairment, the leaders may consider forming a group tailored for them, with a curriculum addressing more challenging skill areas, such as forming intimate relationships, dealing with conflicts on the job, or improving family relationships.

Tendency to Engage in Excessive Discussion

Instead of following the format of the social skills training group, some clients attempt to engage the leaders or other group members in extended discussion. Even when the discussion is related in some way to the skill being taught in the group, it usually distracts other group members from the task of learning and practicing the skill. For example, a person may want to discuss at length his or her opinion that it is more difficult for men to compromise than it is for women. This may be an interesting discussion point, but it takes important time away from teaching group members actual skills that they can use in compromising.

There are a variety of reasons for engaging in excessive discussion during social skills group. Some people seem to have a strong need for expressing themselves and have few outlets for doing so. Other people are accustomed to process-oriented groups where lengthy discussion is encouraged, and they return to that format out of habit. Still others are uncomfortable with the idea that they need social skills training and turn to conversation and discussion as a way of avoiding the tasks of the group.

When people get sidetracked into discussion, the leaders can first acknowledge that the topic is interesting or that a good point is being made. However, it is important to quickly redirect the group members to the task at hand. The leaders might say, "That's an interesting example of how your father had difficulty compromising. What we're doing in this group is emphasizing the practical considerations of how we can go about compromising and negotiating." If possible, the leaders can then engage the person in an active role within the group format, such as reading the steps of the skill, role playing, or giving specific feedback.

Some group leaders find it useful to schedule time at the end of every group for unstructured socializing and discussion. For example, the group might last 45 minutes with 15 minutes at the end for conversation and coffee or snacks. Many people find it reinforcing to spend unstructured time after the group, socializing with the leaders and/or other group members. Thus, when people attempt to carry on extended conversation during the training portion of the group, leaders can direct them to continue their discussion during the scheduled socialization time. For example, if a group member wants to engage in conversation during the group, a leader might say, "We need to focus on learning how to make compromises now, but I'd like to talk about the subject you just raised at two o'clock, when we have coffee."

Table 8.4 provides a summary of strategies leaders can use for responding to problems commonly encountered when conducting social skills training groups with clients who have less social impairment.

PROBLEMS RELATED TO OLDER CLIENTS

Mobility and Transportation Problems

Although many older clients ambulate independently, others have physical problems that lead to significant difficulties with mobility. Their mobility difficulties range from mild (needing to walk slowly and deliberately) to moderate (needing a cane or walker) to severe (requiring a wheelchair at all times and needing assistance to transfer to and from the wheelchair). It is therefore very important to allow extra time for gathering older clients to attend a social skills group and to provide extra staff to assist them in making their way to the group room. Group leaders need to give older clients the feeling that there is plenty of time and that they will not be rushed. When pressured to move quickly, clients can become disoriented and angry, which detracts from their interest in participating in the group. The group room itself should be wheelchair accessible and spacious enough to accommodate wheelchairs, walkers, and canes. Extra time should also be allowed at the end of the group

TABLE 8.4. Strategies for Problems Related to Clients Who Have Less Social Impairment

General principles
1. Make a connection between group participation and achieving goals.
2. Engage in challenging role plays.
3. Encourage clients to help other group members learn targeted skills.

Specific problems	Strategies
Difficulty in accepting need for training	Avoid confrontation.
	Focus on goals.
	Provide rationale comparing social skills training to learning to play piano.
Discomfort in interacting with clients with lower-functioning clients	Remind clients of the need to get along with variety of people.
	Praise their ability to act as role models.
Engaging in excessive discussion	Acknowledge that client s topic is interesting.
	Redirect to the task at hand.
	Reserve time at the end of group for discussion.

for helping clients who need assistance with leaving the room and going to their next destination.

Transportation is an additional problem for many older clients, who usually do not have cars and/or valid driver's licenses. They do not feel comfortable or safe with public transportation and find it very tiring to take buses and trains. Many older clients prefer that social skills groups be held in their residential setting or as close to home as possible in their own community. For off-site groups, providing van transportation is essential for regular attendance. Because transportation is so time-consuming, some social skills leaders find it practical to schedule a morning and afternoon group meeting on the same day, rather than one meeting twice a week (Pratt, Bartels, Mueser, & Haddad, 2003). This is especially attractive to clients when lunch can be provided between the morning and afternoon sessions.

Visual and Hearing Impairments

Many older clients have difficulty with reading small print and seeing charts and other materials from a distance. To help alleviate this problem, the handouts containing the steps of the social skills can be made with large print (for example, a font size 36). When writing information on a flipchart, social skills group leaders must remember to write in a bold, large print and to position the chart close enough that people can easily read the material. Bright colors on the printed pages or flipcharts help to catch people's attention. Some group leaders carry a variety of reading glasses purchased over-the-counter and bring them to groups for clients to use to read handouts and charts in the group. Some clients also find magnifying glasses or magnifying plastic sheets to make a significant difference in their ability to see materials clearly (Pratt et al., 2003). Group leaders can read aloud all material for people who are blind and can make audio recordings of the steps of the skills and/or the homework assignments for them to take home.

For clients who have difficulty with hearing, it is important that group leaders speak loudly and clearly and to set up the room so that clients with hearing impairments are sitting closer to the group leaders. The group leaders should also be mindful of their tone of voice and rate of speech. A relatively low tone of voice can be heard more easily than a high tone, and a moderate rate of speech is easier to comprehend than a fast one. In addition, group leaders should avoid lengthy explanations; simple, clear, and succinct descriptions are easier for group members to hear and comprehend.

Memory and Attention Impairments

Cognitive impairments vary significantly in older adults with schizophrenia. Many experience problems with memory, attention, and information processing. Group leaders can help counteract these difficulties by frequently reviewing material and providing more practice opportunities for newly learned skills. The leaders can also adapt the curriculum to include fewer skills and a slower pace of learning. Some leaders have found it useful to print the steps of specific skills on laminated postcard-size cards that group members can take with them to use for practicing in real-life settings (Pratt et al., 2003).

Reluctance to Practice Certain Skills

In earlier generations, many people were taught that is not polite to be directly assertive or to express angry feelings. This was particularly true for women, although many men were also socialized to avoid assertive behaviors such as making direct requests or expressing anger. When these skills are introduced in group, some members are uncomfortable practicing them, saying something like "I don't have angry feelings; I never get angry" or "I wouldn't say something like that; it's not polite." One way to avoid this situation is to lead up slowly to skills related to assertiveness and anger management, helping people feel more comfortable with "easier" skills, such as Giving Compliments, before they address the more complex ones. Another way to reduce conflict is to rename skills based on terms that the clients find more acceptable. For example, some older clients will say that they do not get angry, but they freely acknowledge that they feel "upset" from time to time or "not happy" with something. Still another way to help group members begin to feel more comfortable with being assertive or expressing angry feelings is to start by asking them to participate in role plays in which they play someone else's part. For example, the group leader might say, "I would like you to play me in this role play, and show how you think I might respond if someone changed the channel on the television without asking while I was in the middle of watching my favorite show."

Generating Topics of Conversation

Because older clients are often more socially isolated and engage in fewer activities than younger clients, they may find it challenging to generate topics of conversation. However, talking about experiences from their past is often a very fruitful source of topics and may even lead to finding common interests with other group members. For example, older group members may find it easy to talk about where they were born, important relatives in their life, past jobs, past hobbies, growing up during the Depression or World War II, favorite subjects in school, and music they listened to when they were young. Group leaders may find certain packaged games and activities helpful in increasing conversation among group members, such as *Yesterdays* (Dezan, 1995), *Shake Loose a Memory* (Wheeler & Shelley, 1996), and *Penny Ante* (Freeman, 1989 and 1999). *Yesterdays* is a collection of brief read-aloud stories, large photographs, and discussion questions about everyday life in the past. *Shake Loose a Memory* and *Penny Ante* are games in which people draw cards with descriptions of life experiences (e.g., spending time on a farm, going to a parade, being in a school play) and are asked to share any memories they have of these experiences. All packaged programs should be reviewed and adapted to take into consideration the group members' comprehension level, range of life experiences, and relevant physical abilities. For example, in using the *Penny Ante* game, group leaders may want to substitute poker chips for pennies, because they are easier to handle, and may choose to remove cards that refer to experiences that are extremely rare for a particular group of clients.

Difficulty in Engaging in Group

Older adults often have a lower level of energy than younger clients and may find it more difficult to become engaged in the content of the group. They may get bored more easily and their attention may tend to wander. Many group leaders find that it helps older group members to focus on the group when the sessions are more lively and animated. One way to accomplish this is to periodically use interactive activities or games that creatively draw people into using their social skills. It is critical to link the activities with specific social skills and to avoid any juvenile games or treating the clients like children. For example, to help people become more engaged in skills involving expression of emotions, leaders can introduce the charade-style game *Name That Emotion*. In this game, the leaders write down common emotions on slips of paper, then each person takes a turn selecting a slip of paper and acting out the emotion for the other group members to guess. Some packaged activities and games can be purchased and adapted as needed, such as the following: *You Be the Judge* (Dezan, 1996), which uses brief summaries of actual news stories to start discussions about mildly controversial topics; *Let's Talk*, which uses cards with discussion questions (e.g., "Have you ever had a pet that you were very fond of?") to help people practice starting conversations; and *Shake Out the Truth* (Wheeler & Shelley, 1997), similar to the television game show *To Tell the Truth*, which can be used to encourage the use of social perception skills.

Table 8.5 lists common problems experienced by older clients.

PROBLEMS RELATED TO CLIENTS WHO HAVE MILD MENTAL RETARDATION

Low Intellectual Functioning

Clients who have low intellectual functioning have difficulty comprehending advanced vocabulary, long sentences, and abstract concepts. To increase comprehension, group leaders need to use simple language and sentence construction and must frequently repeat the important points. Frequent role-play demonstrations of the targeted skills also significantly in-

TABLE 8.5. Strategies for Problems Related to Older Clients

Problem	Strategies
Mobility impairments	Allow extra time and provide additional staff members for gathering people to attend group.
	Hold sessions in rooms that are accessible to wheelchairs and walkers.
	Provide chairs that are easy to sit in and rise from.
Transportation problems	When possible, hold groups in clients' residences or at a setting in their own community.
	Provide van transportation to off-site groups.
	Limit transportation time to off-site groups by holding two short groups in one day rather than two groups on separate days.
Visual impairments	Use extra-large print on handouts and flipcharts.
	Use bright-colored paper and markers.
	Make reading glasses and magnifying glasses available in group sessions.
	Tape record steps of skills and homework for clients who are blind.
Hearing impairments	Speak loudly and clearly.
	Avoid high-pitched tone of voice and rapid pace of speech.
	Avoid lengthy explanations.
	Arrange seating so that clients with difficulty in hearing are closer to the leader.
Memory and attention problems	Provide more opportunities to practice newly introduced skills
	Hold shorter, more frequent group sessions.
	Frequently review material that was previously learned.
	Plan curriculum to include fewer skills, covered in more depth.
	Print steps of skills on small laminated cards that people can take with them.
Reluctance to practice certain skills	Lead up slowly to skills that may be uncomfortable, such as Expressing Angry Feelings.
	Rename skills using terms that people are more comfortable with (i.e., "upset feelings" rather than "angry feelings").
	Ask people to play someone else's part in a role play.
Difficulty in generating topics of conversation	Identify topics of interest from people's past.
	Use packaged activities or games to stimulate discussion.
Difficulty in engaging in group	Keep sessions lively and animated.
	Use interactive activities or games that encourage practice of social skills.

crease group members' understanding. It may be beneficial for some group members to see the group leader demonstrate individual steps of the skills. For example, in demonstrating Making Requests, the group leader can first show some examples of "looking at the person," then examples of "saying what you would like the other person to do," and finally, examples of "telling the person how it would make you feel." Each example can be discussed, and the leader can ask questions to make sure the clients understood the components of that particular step. After each step of Making Requests has been demonstrated, the leader can put all the steps together in a role play.

Most clients with mild mental retardation have difficulty with reading, and they often respond well to pictures that represent social skills and paralinguistic elements. For example, to represent the skill of Asking for Information, a group leader might include a simple drawing of a large question mark or a person talking to a policeman. To show how close to stand to another person while talking, a simple drawing may be used to demonstrate two people standing an arm's length apart. For emotional recognition, some commercially produced posters showing a variety of facial expressions are useful, such as *Emotions Plus* (Wellness Reproductions, 2003) and *Everyone Has Feelings* (Childswork/Childsplay, 1995). The card game *Face It!* (Childswork/Childsplay, 1998) is also helpful for illustrating a range of emotions.

Impaired Social Judgment

Clients with mental retardation often have difficulty in recognizing and interpreting social cues. For example, if someone is talking on the phone, a client may not realize that it is not appropriate to start talking to that person immediately. Even if the person holds a hand over the receiver and whispers "Just a minute" or "I'm on the phone right now," some clients still have difficulty recognizing that they should wait to speak until the phone conversation is over. Or if a person is intently watching television, some clients may not realize that they should not change the channel or repeatedly attempt to engage the person in conversation. Role plays can be used to increase clients' awareness of common social cues and give them practice in responding appropriately to these cues. For example, in the skill Starting a Conversation with a New Or Unfamiliar Person, the fourth step is "Judge whether the other person is listening and wants to talk." Group leaders can spend extra time on this step, identifying and demonstrating the kinds of cues that people give when they want to talk (e.g., smiling, eye contact, making encouraging comments, animated speech) and when they don't want to talk (frowning, looking away from the person, looking at a watch, making minimal responses, speaking in a flat tone). Some skills do not include a specific step related to interpreting social cues, but the leaders can add steps as needed.

Another aspect of impaired social judgment relates to the inability to evaluate safety in interpersonal situations. For example, clients with mental retardation may respond to panhandlers by taking out a wallet and showing their money or may respond to people offering drugs for sale by starting a friendly conversation with them. When lost, they may not know whom to ask for directions and may approach strangers who will take advantage of them. It is therefore important for group leaders to include curriculum in which safety issues are directly addressed, including Refusing Requests, Asking for Information, and Refusing Unwanted Sexual Advances. There are opportunities to discuss safety issues in teaching several of the skills, such as Starting a Conversation with a New or Unfamiliar Person ("How do you tell whether someone is safe to talk to?") and Expressing Angry Feelings ("What are some examples of people that it would be dangerous to express angry feelings to?"). Group leaders can find additional curriculum in *Street Smarts: Skills for Surviving in an Urban Setting* (Center for Psychiatric Rehabilitation of the University of Chicago, 1998) and *Safe, Secure, and Street-Smart: Empowering Women with Mental Illness to Achieve Greater Independence in the Community* (Jonikas & Cook, 1993)

Many clients with mild mental retardation can learn the words to specific skills but have difficulty using them in a socially smooth manner because of problems with paralinguistic features such as volume, rate of speech, and tone of voice. Nonverbal behaviors may also be problematic, such as not respecting personal boundaries, touching other people, and picking up and examining someone's personal possessions. In addition, clients may have difficulties with conversational timing (such as beginning to speak before the other person has finished) and turn taking (not allowing the other person time to speak or respond to questions). Group leaders can help clients by addressing paralinguistic skills both as a separate subject and as part of each social skill that is taught. For example, in teaching the skill Making Complaints, the leaders can include discussions and demonstrations about the appropriate tone of voice, personal distance, and timing. Staff members and family members can also be enlisted to provide more opportunities for clients to practice interactions and to receive specific feedback about paralinguistic skills.

Memory and Attention

It can be difficult for some clients with mental retardation to stay focused on the group. If something catches their attention (e.g., an item of clothing the group leader is wearing or a bird singing in a tree outside the window) or if they think of something that happened earlier in the day, they may spontaneously start talking about it and forget the topic of the group. Even when requested to return to the topic of the group, clients may only do so for a few moments before going back to their primary interest. Group leaders should expect that it may require several attempts before clients can successfully return to the topic of the group. In addition, it is easier to hold the attention of easily distracted clients by using modalities that engage different senses. For example, group leaders can use modalities that engage the clients visually (pictures, diagrams, maps), tactilely (a ball to hold to signify that it is an individual's turn to speak), and physically (games like *Name That Emotion* that involve acting things out). Games such as bingo and charades, which encourage social interaction and turn taking, can also be used to hold clients' attention. Finally, groups that last a shorter time have a better chance of holding people's attention. In order to cover the curriculum, however, shorter group sessions should also be held more frequently.

Difficulty in Transferring Skills to a Variety of Situations

Some clients may show ability to use the social skills in the group setting, but have an especially hard time transferring what they have learned to situations that have not been practiced in the group. For example, a client may demonstrate the steps of the skill Expressing Angry Feelings in a role play with a group leader, but later the same day may impulsively push a roommate who annoys him or her. Group leaders should practice role playing as many different kinds of situations as possible, making sure to emphasize those that the clients are most likely to encounter. For example, for the skill Disagreeing with Another's Opinion without Arguing, if the group leaders learn that there have been many altercations about music, they can incorporate role plays focused on how to disagree about musical tastes without arguing. It is also helpful to support group members' practicing the skills *in vivo*, either by arranging group outings or by enlisting the assistance of staff members where the clients live or receive services.

Table 8.6 lists some strategies for clients who have mild mental retardation.

TABLE 8.6. Strategies for Problems Related to Clients Who Have Mild Mental Retardation

Problem	Strategies
Low intellectual functioning	Use simple language, uncomplicated sentence construction.
	Frequently repeat important information.
	Use pictures or diagrams to illustrate points.
	Demonstrate each step of a skill separately.
	Review skills frequently.
Impaired social judgment	Use role plays to give clients practice in recognizing social cues.
	Include curriculum with skills related to safety.
	Address paralinguistic features such as voice tone, interpersonal distance, conversational timing.
	Use role plays to give clients practice in evaluating social situations.
Memory and attention problems	Use extra-large print on handouts and flipcharts. Use bright-colored paper and markers.
	Gently but firmly redirect clients to topic.
	Use visual, tactile, and physical modalities.
	Use games that encourage use of social skills.
	Schedule shorter groups, held more frequently.
Difficulty in transferring skills to a variety of situations	Practice skills using as many situations as possible.
	Make sure to include role plays that reflect the situations clients are most likely to encounter.
	Arrange as many *in vivo* experiences for clients as possible.
	Enlist other staff members to help clients practice in additional settings.

PROBLEMS RELATED TO CLIENTS WHO HAVE CRIMINAL JUSTICE INVOLVEMENT

Difficulty in Expressing Opinions and Making Decisions

In forensics facilities, such as jails, prisons, and special units of state hospitals, clients often become accustomed to a rigid schedule and a lack of choices. Most things are decided for them, such as what to wear, what to eat, when to have meals, how often to shower, when to smoke, when to go to bed, and so on. They are not allowed to vary from the structure of the facility, and attempts to do so often result in punishment or lost privileges. Therefore, clients who are currently in forensics facilities or who have recently been discharged are often hesitant to express opinions and make their own decisions. In social skills groups it is important to emphasize skills that help clients gain more confidence in these areas, such as Getting Your Point Across, Disagreeing with Another's Opinion without Arguing, Expressing Positive Feelings, Making Requests, Making Complaints, and Solving Problems. In addition to benefiting from practicing the skills, clients will also learn from hearing other group members practice, inasmuch as they may lack experience in being on the receiving end of other people's expressing their opinions, making requests, disagreeing, and so forth.

Expressing Emotions Constructively

Hiding one's emotions is often an adaptive behavior in a forensics facility, where any sign of feelings may be seen as a weakness. For example, people who express sad or anxious feelings are often viewed as being vulnerable and easy to push around. People who compliment someone are often misunderstood as making sexual advances. However, people who look fierce and aggressively express displeasure are often respected and let alone. Therefore, clients often have very little experience in expressing a range of emotions in a constructive manner. In a social skills group, leaders need to include curriculum that helps clients develop an emotional vocabulary and allows them to practice expressing a variety of feelings. These skills include Expressing Positive Feelings, Expressing Unpleasant Feelings, Expressing Angry Feelings, Making Apologies, Giving Compliments, Accepting Compliments, and Expressing Affection. Leaders will also need to help clients identify common situations in which various feelings are likely to occur. For example, in introducing Expressing Angry Feelings, a leader might ask the group, When is the last time you felt angry? What kinds of situations tend to make you feel angry? and list the group members' answers on a flipchart.

Questioning Authority and Pushing Limits

It is not uncommon for clients to be suspicious of rules and people in positions of responsibility. They may be likely to question authority and push the limits that have been set. In some situations this is a healthy sign of clients' starting to express opinions and make decisions for themselves; in other situations it is a constant unproductive struggle that drains the energy of both clients and staff members. In social skills groups, clients may challenge the leaders and question the way the group is conducted. It is helpful for group leaders to be specific about the design and purpose of the group (see the orientation materials in Appendix A) and to spell out the guidelines of the group (see Appendix A for an example of group guidelines). When challenged, it is important for group leaders to be firm but kind in their responses and to avoid being provoked into an argument.

To help clients develop a more positive attitude toward staff members, it is helpful to talk to them about the roles of the different members of their treatment team and what each contributes. Many mental health facilities have also found it useful to include the client's parole officer in some treatment team meetings where the client is also present. This reduces misunderstandings and allows everyone to work together to support the client's return to the community. It is important, however, to educate parole officers about the goals and methods of social skills training so that they will encourage and reinforce clients in using the targeted skills.

Coping with Stigma

Clients who are currently in a forensics facility or who have spent time in a forensics facility are often prejudged by other clients, people in the community, and even mental health professionals. People may be fearful of them, may look down on them, or may suspect them of current criminal activity. Because of this stigma, clients may lack self-confidence and self-respect. In social skills groups, leaders can help by emphasizing the importance of respectful behavior and communication between group members and by frequently using opportunities to identify each group member's strengths and contributions to the group. The group should serve as a safe haven from stigma, where each member can be respected regardless of his or her background. If a group member starts to make derogatory comments about someone's having been in a forensics facility, the group leader must interrupt those comments and refer to the group guidelines that prohibit name-calling, criticizing, and making fun of each other. The group should be reminded that in social skills group, everyone is treated with politeness and respect.

When group members are experiencing significant difficulties because of stigma, the leaders may find it helpful to devote several sessions to this subject. These sessions can include a combination of education, discussion, and skill building on topics such as the following: correcting myths, identifying positive role models, becoming aware of one's legal rights, the importance of peer support, deciding whether to disclose one's history to others, fighting self-stigma, and responding to stigmatizing remarks. Books such as *Don't Call Me Nuts* (Corrigan & Lundin, 2001) are a useful source of materials about coping with the stigma of mental illness and can be adapted to address the additional stigma related to being involved with the criminal justice system.

Table 8.7 lists strategies for clients who have involvement with the criminal justice system.

TABLE 8.7. Strategies for Problems Related to Clients Who Have Involvement with the Criminal Justice System

Problem	Strategies
Difficulty in expressing opinions and making decisions	Include skills that increase confidence in expressing opinions and making decisions.
	Provide opportunities for clients to practice and observe others expressing opinions without aggression.
	Help clients identify reasonable, short-term goals.
Difficulty in expressing emotions constructively	Include curriculum to help clients develop an emotional vocabulary.
	Help clients identify situations that lead to common emotions.
Questioning authority and pushing limits	Orient clients to the purpose and structure of the group prior to their joining.
	Review and post group guidelines.
	Be firm but kind in responding to challenges.
	Avoid responding to provocation.
	Educate clients about the positive contribution of different members of their treatment team.
	When possible, include parole officer in treatment team meetings where client is present.
Stigma related to spending time in a forensic facility	Make the group a safe haven from stigma.
	Use opportunities to identify all group members' strengths and contributions to the group.
	Do not allow any group members to make critical or stigmatizing comments to others; refer to group guidelines.
	Include several sessions devoted to increasing knowledge and skills for coping with stigma.

PROBLEMS RELATED TO YOUNG CLIENTS

Difficulty in Establishing Relationships

Even in the absence of an illness like schizophrenia, young adulthood (late teens, early twenties) is a challenging period of life and a time when people are often confused about their own identity and how to establish successful relationships with others. Many questions arise for younger clients: How do you get to know someone? How do you carry on conversations? How do you find someone who shares your interests? How do you ask someone out? How do you deal with rejection? How do you progress in a relationship from being a friend to being boyfriend or girlfriend? To help clients deal with these questions, it is helpful to provide a social skills curriculum that emphasizes a developmental approach to relationships. For example, the group leader can first focus on skills for making a friend (Starting a Conversation with a New or Unfamiliar Person, Maintaining Conversations, Compromise and Negotiation, etc.) and move to skills related to dating (Finding Common Interests, Asking Someone for a Date, Expressing Affection, etc.).

As young clients learn the steps of the skills, it is important to include discussion about how to interpret social cues, such as how to tell whether the other person is interested in pursuing a conversation or is feeling comfortable in a relationship. It is also helpful to talk about strategies for dealing with negative responses. For example, what are some ways to respond when someone says that he or she does not want to go on a date? What are some ways to maintain one's self-confidence if a relationship is not working out as anticipated?

Boredom with Common Treatment Modalities

Many young clients have more physical energy than those who are older. They become restless sitting for 45 minutes or an hour and are impatient with "just talking" and "being stuck in the same old room." To prevent boredom with common treatment modalities, it is important for group leaders to explore nontraditional methods for teaching social skills, such as going to different locations (e.g., a park or museum), going out for a meal (e.g., pizza, fast food, ice cream), or sharing interests and talents (artwork, poetry, or music). The clients especially enjoy being actively involved in choosing and planning activities, which helps them build self-confidence and increases the likelihood of continued participation. When group members feel "ownership" of the group, they are much more likely to participate actively.

Young clients also enjoy group sessions that involve physical activity, such as role plays that involve moving around in the room. For example, to practice the skill Starting a Conversation with a New or Unfamiliar Person, the role play could be designed to simulate a party with several people attending (rearranging chairs and tables as appropriate and perhaps including music) and could require the client to demonstrate how he or she might walk into the room and approach someone who is listening to music or eating something. Or to practice Making Complaints, the role play could be designed to simulate the counter at a fast-food restaurant where one client plays the fast-food worker and the other plays someone who has been given the wrong order. Some clients enjoy games with physical activity, such as charades, where they can act out something related to social skills.

Challenging Authority

Young adulthood is a time when people want to separate from their parents and make their own decisions. It is natural for them to question their parents and other figures of authority, such as program directors and group leaders. They are also sensitive to being "treated like children." In a social skills group, young clients may challenge the group leaders about the purpose of the group, the logic for the group format, and the need for group guidelines. To help clients feel that they are being treated as adults rather than children, it is helpful for group leaders to include them in planning the group curriculum, solicit their opinions about group guidelines, and invite group members to rotate in co-leading the group. To give them skills in questioning authority in ways that are more likely to be effective, it is helpful to include curriculum such as Getting Your Point Across, Disagreeing with Another's Opinion without Arguing, Compromise and Negotiation, and Problem Solving.

Difficulty in Attaining Goals

Young adults are often eager to accomplish things quickly, without taking into consideration the intermediate steps that may be required. For example, a young client may want to get his or her own apartment immediately but may not recognize the steps that may be necessary for this to happen, such as stabilizing his or her psychiatric symptoms, establishing a routine for taking medications, saving money for a deposit, locating an affordable apartment, finding a compatible roommate to share expenses, and so forth. Because young adults lack life experience, they often have unrealistic expectations about how easy it will be to attain their goals. Because of their desire to be independent, however, young adults often do not want to ask for help or advice from people older than themselves who have more life experience. To help clients attain their goals, it is important for group leaders not to discourage ambitious goals, but rather to help them break down goals into a series of manageable steps. This process can be facilitated by teaching Problem Solving and Goal Achievement, which involves six steps: (1) defining the problem or goal, (2) brainstorming solutions, (3) identifying the advantages and disadvantages of each solution, (4) selecting the best solution, (5) planning how to carry out the solution, and (6) following up the plan at a later time. It usually takes several sessions to teach this skill, and it is beneficial to return to it repeatedly, as group members frequently encounter problems or have difficulty in attaining their goals.

Low Self-Esteem

Young clients often experience low self-esteem related to the difficulties described earlier: establishing relationships, boredom, conflicts with authority, and attaining goals. Consequently, group leaders who use the strategies provided for each of these difficulties will be making an important contribution to improving the group members' self-esteem. In addition, group leaders can help clients by teaching skills that provide outlets for their feelings (e.g., Expressing Unpleasant Feelings) and that encourage them to request assistance when they need it (e.g., Making a Request, Letting Someone Know That You Feel Unsafe, Asking for Information). It is also important to establish an atmosphere of respect and support in the social skills group. Group leaders should use every opportunity to identify group members' strengths and specific contributions to the group sessions. In addition, leaders need to curtail any critical or disrespectful comments group members may make to each other. Some group leaders find it helpful to end group sessions with "a round of positives," whereby each group member identifies a positive contribution made by someone else in the group. Going around the group systematically and asking each client to say something positive about the group member to his or her left ensures that everyone will hear something positive about him- or herself.

If self-esteem is especially low in a group, the leaders may find it helpful to devote several sessions to this subject. These sessions can include a combination of education, discussion, and activities related to self-esteem topics, such as those contained in the "Self-Esteem Module" developed by Lecomte et al. (1999): feeling safe, developing a positive identity, belonging to a community, pursuing personal goals, and developing a sense of competence.

Table 8.8 lists strategies for problems related to younger clients.

TABLE 8.8. Strategies for Problems Related to Young Clients

Problem	Strategies
Difficulty in establishing relationships	Use curriculum that progresses from friendship skills to dating skills.
	Include discussion about interpreting social cues.
	Help clients develop strategies for dealing with disappointment or rejection.
Boredom	Hold groups in different locations.
	Plan outings such as going out for meals or for a walk in the community.
	Explore nontraditional methods for using social skills in groups, such as sharing artwork, poetry, or music.
	Include role plays that involve moving around.
	Include games or activities that include an element of social skills and involve movement, such as charades to act out different skills.
Challenging authority	Include clients in planning group curriculum.
	Include clients in establishing group guidelines.
	Invite group members to rotate as co-leaders.
	Teach skills that increase effectiveness at questioning authority, such as Disagreeing with Another's Opinion without Arguing, Compromise and Negotiation, and Problem Solving and Goal Achievement.
Difficulty in attaining goals	Avoid discouraging ambitious goals.
	Help clients break down goals into a series of manageable short-term goals.
	Teach skill of Problem Solving and Goal Attainment.
	Return to Problem Solving and Goal Attainment when clients encounter obstacles to achieving their goals.
Low self-esteem	Include curriculum that helps clients express their feelings.
	Establish an atmosphere of respect and support within the group.
	Frequently comment on group members' strengths and contributions to the group.
	End sessions with a "round of positives" whereby group members identify each other's positive contributions.
	Include several sessions for building self-esteem.

SUMMARY

In this chapter we described clinical strategies for managing common problems encountered during social skills training. In any skills training group, it is important to set clear expectations, praise small steps toward improvement, and encourage participation from each client according to his or her ability. The leaders need to follow the structured format of the group as much as possible and model appropriate social skills in their interactions with group members, especially when making requests and redirecting clients.

Specific strategies were also provided for problems related to working with challenging clients. Some strategies involve adapting packaged activities and games to encourage social interaction. A list of resources for these activities and games is provided in Appendix A. By being alert to potential problems and applying the pertinent strategies as needed, leaders will be able to keep their groups running smoothly and effectively.

9

Working with Clients
Who Abuse Drugs and Alcohol

Drug and alcohol abuse by people with serious mental illness, including schizophrenia, is one of the most pressing problems facing the mental health system. The lifetime prevalence rate of substance abuse in schizophrenia is close to 50%, and estimates of recent or current substance abuse range from 20 to 65%. Excessive substance use by people with schizophrenia has most of the same adverse social, health, economic, and psychiatric consequences as it does for other people, but it has additional serious consequences for these individuals with multiple disabilities. It decreases adherence to treatment, serves as a source of conflict in families, and increases the risk of relapse. It also increases risk of sexual and criminal victimization and can result in unstable housing and increased rates of incarceration. Substance use also interferes with cognitive functioning, a significant problem, given that information processing is already impaired in most people with the illness. Thus, reducing substance use is a critical clinical goal for this population.

REASONS FOR SUBSTANCE ABUSE IN SCHIZOPHRENIA

It is often assumed that people with schizophrenia use substances to reduce psychotic symptoms and alleviate the sedating side effects of medication. However, the most common reasons given for use of alcohol and other drugs are to "get high" and to reduce negative affective states such as social anxiety and tension, depression, and boredom (Dixon, Haas, Weiden, Sweeney, & Frances, 1991; Spencer et al., 2002). In addition, one of the most important factors for clients whose primary substances of abuse are street drugs is a desire to be like their peers and seem *normal*. Alcohol is the most commonly abused substance in schizophrenia, but many clients abuse street drugs as well as alcohol, and others abuse only street drugs. The preference for street drugs varies over time and as a function of the demographic characteristics of the sample. For example, Mueser, Yarnold, and Bellack (1992) reported that from 1983–1986 cannabis was the most commonly abused illicit drug among clients with schizophrenia, whereas from 1986–1990 cocaine became the most popular drug, a change in pattern similar to that in the general population (Pope et al., 1990). For many clients, availability of substances appears to be more relevant than the specific central nervous system (CNS) effects.

FACTORS COMPLICATING BEHAVIOR CHANGE

An extensive body of research on substance abuse and addiction in the general population indicates that critical factors in abstinence and controlled use of addictive substances include high levels of motivation to quit, the ability to exert self-control in the face of temptation (urges), cognitive and behavioral coping skills, and social support or social pressure. Unfortunately, people with schizophrenia who abuse substances often have limitations in each of these areas. First, several factors can be expected to diminish motivation in people with schizophrenia. Many clients have some degree of negative symptoms (especially avolition and anergia) as a function of the neurobiology of the illness, medication side effects, or other social and psychological factors. Thus, they may lack the internal drive to initiate the complex behavioral routines required for abstinence. This hypothesis was supported in a recent survey of dually diagnosed people with schizophrenia, which found that about half of the clients had little motivation to reduce their substance use and only 52% were participating in substance abuse treatment. Another negative symptom, anhedonia, may reduce the experience of positive affect, thereby limiting the experience of pleasure and positive reinforcement in the absence of substance use.

A second issue is the profound and pervasive cognitive impairment that characterizes schizophrenia (Bellack, Blanchard, & Mueser, 1999). As discussed in Chapter 1, people with schizophrenia have multiple problems in information processing, including deficits in attention, memory, and higher-level cognitive processes, such as problem solving, abstract reasoning, and the ability to integrate situational context or previous experience into ongoing information processing. The higher level cognitive deficits may make it very difficult for people with schizophrenia to engage in the complex processes necessary for self-directed behavior change, the essential feature in abstaining from substances. Clients may have difficulty engaging in self-reflection or in evaluating previous experiences that contribute to the development of a sense of self-efficacy and the belief that change is possible. Deficits in the ability to draw connections between past experience and current stimuli may impede the ability to relate their substance use to negative consequences over time, and modify their behavior accordingly. Deficits in problem-solving capacity and abstract reasoning may interfere with the ability to evaluate the pros and cons of substance use or to formulate realistic goals. Problems in memory and attention may also make it difficult for clients to sustain a focus on goal-directed behavior over time.

Third, social skills deficits may impact on the ability to reduce substance use in several ways. Research indicates that a significant source of motivation to decrease drug use is positive social pressure from significant others, such as family members, friends, and employers. Unfortunately, many people with schizophrenia do not have such supportive social networks. Conversely, a major reason that they use drugs is a desire to *seem normal* and be like other people in their environment. In fact, many clients secure drugs from family members and peers and use them in the company of others. Thus, although it would be important to develop social relationships with a nonabusing peer group, these clients have difficulty developing relationships and they lack the financial resources to relocate. As a result, they often remain stuck in high-risk environments without the skills to resist social pressure to use drugs or to develop social support for abstinence from nonabusing peers.

TREATMENT OF SUBSTANCE ABUSE IN SCHIZOPHRENIA

There is, as yet, no single, well-established treatment for substance abuse by clients with schizophrenia, but there is considerable agreement in the field about the general requirements for effective treatment. First and foremost is the belief that dually diagnosed clients need a special program that integrates and coordinates elements of both psychiatric and substance abuse treatment (Carey, 1996). The typical pattern of segregating psychiatric and substance abuse treatment services is counterproductive with this population. These individuals are not able to effectively negotiate between independent treatment systems, substance use subverts psychiatric treatment, and substance abuse treatment programs are often not sensitive to the special needs and problems faced by people with schizophrenia. A related caveat is that the confrontative, highly charged style characteristic of many traditional substance abuse treatment programs (e.g., 12-Step programs) is contraindicated for people with schizophrenia. A second assumption is that treatment is best conceptualized as an ongoing process that involves a number of relatively distinct stages in which motivation to reduce substance use waxes and wanes, as elucidated by the transtheoretical model of change (TTM; Prochaska & DiClemente, 1992).

The TTM has been found to be useful for understanding the process of intentional change of problem behaviors that occurs through both interventions and self-initiated change in the natural environment. Individuals can be classified along a continuum of motivation, referred to as *stages of change*. *Precontemplation* is the first stage, in which individuals are not convinced that they have a problem or are unwilling to consider change. *Contemplation* is the stage in which individuals begin thinking about changing their behavior. They are not yet ready to change or convinced that they should change, but they can anticipate making a change within the coming 6 months to a year. During the *Preparation* stage individuals have a goal to change in the next month and can be expected to make initial plans for changing behavior. This is followed by an *Action* stage, in which individuals work at making the change. If successful, the person enters a *Maintenance* stage, where the task is to consolidate the change, integrate it into the his or her lifestyle, and prevent relapse. The course of progression through this series of stages is quite variable and rather cyclical in nature for most individuals. Motivation waxes and wanes, and relapse and regression is the norm for most behavior change (Prochaska, DiClemente, & Norcross, 1992). Over the course of time, many individuals cycle through these stages repeatedly until they are able to successfully sustain the behavior change (e.g., abstinence). Two other components of the TTM have also been found to be important in behavior change. *Decisional balance* reflects the extent to which the client believes that continued use of substances is positive (e.g., it makes the person more relaxed) versus negative (e.g., it leads to homelessness and incarceration). Change is associated with the belief that abstinence is better than continued use. The other factor is *self-efficacy*, the extent to which the person sees him- or herself as capable of resisting substance use.

The implications of the TTM for clinicians working with dually diagnosed clients are clear (Bellack & DiClemente, 1999). The client's motivation to change must be expected to vary over time, and the clinician must therefore take a long term perspective. Clinicians should not become unduly frustrated or pessimistic when a client denies the need to change or relapses after a period of success. Conversely, clinicians should be cautiously optimistic after short-term gains and continue to help clients build on their early successes. An important goal of treatment is to help change the client's decisional balance toward abstinence and to increase his or her sense of self-efficacy: to help the person believe that change is both necessary and possible.

BEHAVIORAL TREATMENT FOR SUBSTANCE ABUSE IN SCHIZOPHRENIA

A complete discussion of treatment for dually disordered clients is beyond the scope of this book, but given that many clinicians will need to address substance abuse problems with their clients we describe key features of an approach developed by Bellack and colleagues—*Behavioral Treatment for Substance Abuse in Schizophrenia* (BTSAS; Bellack, Bennett, & Gearon, 2000)—that can be incorporated into a skills training program. Readers are also referred to *Integrated Treatment for Dual Disorders: A Guide to Effective Practice*, a comprehensive guide to working with dually disordered clients by Mueser, Noordsy, Drake, and Fox (2003).

BTSAS was developed specifically to deal with illicit drug abuse by people with schizophrenia. It adapts treatment techniques used with less impaired groups to accommodate for the special disabilities imposed by schizophrenia, especially cognitive impairment and low motivation. However, we have used the program successfully with other seriously mentally ill clients as well. The literature suggests that primary reasons for drug use by many clients with serious mental illness include the desire to appear normal and be like other people, and drugs are generally used in social contexts. Hence, a major focus of BTSAS involves teaching clients how to refuse drugs and ways to interact with others that do not involve drug use. It should be noted that alcohol is the most commonly abused substance by people with schizophrenia. Moreover, the major factor in their use of alcohol is *self-medication* to reduce negative affect such as depression and boredom, rather than social factors. Alcohol use is also more likely to occur alone than in social situations, and clients generally can access alcohol on their own, rather than getting it from others. Consequently, alcohol use requires a different treatment than drug use, and skills training may be less relevant. See Mueser et al. (2003) for guidance on how to treat alcohol abuse.

BTSAS is designed as a 6-month treatment program that is administered in small-group sessions, twice a week for about 1 hour each. It is intended to be a component of a more comprehensive program of clinical care and should be integrated with other aspects of treatment.

We have previously discussed the prevalence of cognitive impairment in schizophrenia and the importance of adjusting treatment to accommodate to those aspects of schizophrenia that constrain learning and behavior change. Consistent with the approach to social skills training outlined in this book, sessions are highly structured and there is a strong emphasis on behavior rehearsal. The material taught is broken down into small units. Complex social repertoires required for refusing substances are divided into component elements, and behavior is shaped by gradually reinforcing successive approximations. Of special note, role plays around drug refusal are gradually made more and more lifelike and difficult as the client becomes increasingly skillful. The intervention emphasizes overlearning of a few specific and relatively narrow skills that can be used automatically, thereby minimizing the cognitive load for decision making during stressful interactions when the person is tempted to use drugs.

Extensive use is made of learning aids, including handouts and flipcharts, to reduce the requirements for memory and attention. Clients are prompted as many times as necessary, and there is also extensive repetition within and across sessions. Clients repeatedly rehearse behavioral skills (e.g., refusing unreasonable requests) and are given didactic information (e.g., the role of dopamine in schizophrenia and substance use) and receive social reinforcement for their efforts. Rather than teaching generic problem-solving skills and coping strategies that can be adapted to a host of diverse situations, we focus on specific skills effective for handling a few key high-risk situations (e.g., what do you do when you are offered a joint by your brother or by one specific friend, rather than what to do when *anyone* offers it to you). Although this may be viewed as placing a limit on generalization, research data clearly show that people with schizophrenia have great difficulty in abstraction and applying principles in novel situations. Hence, they are more likely to benefit from a narrow repertoire of skills to minimize demands on these higher-level processes.

Training is done in a small-group format (6–8 clients). The group format allows clients to benefit from modeling and role playing with peers. The small size provides ample opportunity for all clients to get adequate practice, while minimizing demands for sustained attention (i.e., they can rest while peers are role playing, etc.). In order to accommodate to the disorganization and life problems that are typical of these clients, makeup sessions are offered on an as-needed basis. The treatment can be adapted for either a closed-membership or open-enrollment format. The open-membership format is convenient in settings where enrollment is slow, so clients do not have to wait long to begin treatment. Groups for people with schizophrenia generally do not develop the cohesiveness that is seen in groups for less impaired clients, so new admissions are not disruptive to current members. Conversely, the modular nature of the teaching units and the highly individualized nature of the training make it easy to add new clients to the group. Units (e.g., conversational skills training) can be repeated in whole or in part as needed. Presenting previously covered units for new clients has the added benefit of giving existing members additional practice, which is always advantageous for clients with schizophrenia.

Abstinence is generally viewed as the most appropriate goal for less impaired substance abusers, and it has been suggested that it is the most appropriate goal for clients with schizophrenia as well. Nevertheless, as reflected in the TTM, abstinence is not a viable goal for all clients who enter treatment. Many will "vote with their feet" and drop out if pressured to abstain. There is also increasing evidence with populations without schizophrenia that outcomes are better when clients select their own goals than when goals are imposed by programs. Consequently, we employ a harm reduction approach and promote abstinence, but do not demand it as a precondition for participation. Moreover, our experience is that some clients with schizophrenia profit from substance abuse training and decide to reduce usage without ever formally admitting that they have a problem. As long as clients actively participate in the education and training, they can acquire skills and information that may be of use at some time in the future. In addition, we also assume that clients may become more amenable to making changes if they have first acquired some skills and developed an increased sense of efficacy for resisting social pressure and saying no to drugs. Hence, we increase social pressure on reducing drug use very gradually so as to avoid conflict or early termination. We begin goal setting for reduced substance use (via motivational interviewing) and the urinalysis contingency in the second week of treatment, but we are less proactive in setting goals for change in the early sessions than we are once clients have acquired some substantive training in social skills and coping skills.

In the following sections we describe the five components of BTSAS listed in Table 9.1 and provide examples of how they are implemented. Part II also contains sample skill sheets from the treatment. Many of the elements of the approach are similar to techniques widely used in interventions with less impaired populations of substance abusers. However, as mentioned earlier, we have systematically modified the techniques to make them suitable for clients with schizophrenia and other severe mental illnesses.

Motivational Interviewing

Motivational interviewing (MI) is a brief, client-centered intervention developed by Miller and Rollnick (2002) to stimulate people to explore their use of substances and its consequences, and to see the discrepancy between substance use and other life goals, that helps energize them to change their behavior. It has been used widely and successfully both as a stand-alone intervention and as a component of more extensive treatment programs (see Mueser et al., 2003, Ch. 7). There are a number of important differences between our approach to MI and the way it is typically employed with less impaired clients. As indicated previously, people with schizophrenia have cognitive impairments that limit their ability to deal with abstraction, to draw relationships between past, present, and future events, and to develop and pursue self-directed behavioral plans over time. Hence, the client-centered style and stimulus for self-exploration central to Miller and Rollnick's approach is not likely to be useful for most people with schizophrenia. Consequently, we adopt a more directive style, leading clients toward recognition of one or a few key factors that can serve as motivators for decreased substance use. For the most part, these focal issues involve concrete negative circumstances, such as avoiding arrest, getting back into a community resi-

---

TABLE 9.1. Components of BTSAS

1. Motivational interviewing
2. Urinalysis contingency and goal setting
3. Social skills training
4. Education and coping skills
5. Problem solving and relapse prevention

dence, or regaining custody of children. More abstract goals (e.g., taking control of one's life or regaining the respect of one's children), and lifestyle goals (e.g., pursuing one's career) are generally not relevant for our clients. Typically, the therapist is very active in reminding the client of problems identified during pretreatment assessments or other clinical contacts, rather than waiting for the client to come to his or her own realization of how substance abuse has harmed him or her.

MI sessions are used to discuss the impact that the negative consequences of substance use has had on the person's life, for the therapist to acknowledge and reinforce the client's internal motivation and any change efforts that the client has made, and to chart progress in decreasing or abstaining from substances. MI sessions are typically conducted at the beginning of treatment and periodically (e.g., every 3 months) thereafter. Each session includes several parts: an introductory discussion in which the client can tell the therapist about his or her use of drugs or progress in making changes, a discussion of the negative consequences that have occurred as a result of substance use, feedback on drug use and motivation for change from other sources (e.g., family members), and goal setting and plans for achieving the goal.

The first step of MI is to develop a relationship with the client and get the client to begin talking about drug use. This is typically accomplished by asking the client about what drugs he or she uses, whether the client has thought at all about changing his or her drug use, and what, if anything, he or she has been thinking about changing. It is vital that the therapist assume a noncritical, matter-of-fact attitude in order for the client to trust the therapist and be willing to admit to drug use. This introductory step gradually shifts to a discussion of the negative consequences of drug use, with statements such as "Now that you have told me a bit about your drug use, I want to get an idea of the things that have happened to you because of your drug use. We know that people who use drugs often experience problems that come from their use of drugs, such as problems with their families or problems with the law. Can you tell me about any problems you have had because of your drug use?"

The client is asked to elaborate on these negative consequences and suggest how they might change if he or she was no longer using drugs. For example, "You have said that one problem that you have experienced because of using drugs is that your symptoms get worse. What actually happens when you use? How do your symptoms get worse? So one good thing about not using or using less is that your symptoms would not get worse. You also said that you are not allowed to see your children because their mother won't let you come to visit when you are using drugs. It's clear from how you talk about them that you love your children very much and that you would like to see more of them. So another good thing about not using is that you might be able to see your children more."

Throughout the discussion, the therapist tries to reinforce any self-motivational statements. For example, if the client is talking about a consequence such as spending all his or her money on drugs and states that he or she would like to have money for other things, the therapist can say, "What I hear you saying is that you would like to spend your money on other things rather than drugs. What sorts of things would you buy if you didn't spend your money on drugs? It's great that you can think of things that you would do with your money other than buy drugs. That tells me that you have things that you would like to do with your money other than buy drugs."

The next segment of MI provides the client with feedback from any pretreatment assessment that was conducted, and/or information collected from other clinicians and significant others. The goal is not to catch the client in lies, but to capitalize on information about progress with avoiding drug use and evidence of the client's own motivational statements. The therapist can introduce this to the client by saying, "You may remember that you filled out a lot of forms before our meeting today. Those forms help us learn about people and what sorts of substance use issues they have. I have some information from those forms about your substance use over the last month and your responses to some questions about cutting down on your use. I want to go over this information with you."

The final section of MI is goal setting: trying to get the client to set an initial goal for reduced substance use. The therapist can introduce this section to the client by saying, "The information we just reviewed tells me that you are thinking about changing your drug use and considering being clean or cutting back on your use. That is a tough thing to think about, and I think you did a great job talking to me about it. Now I want us to do something called 'setting a goal.' This means that since we know that you are thinking about changing your drug use, we work together to come up with a goal that will get you started. We know from working with other people who have changed their drug use that setting a goal helps a person get started when he or she wants to make a change. It doesn't have to be a big goal—only something that will help you try using less and something that you think you can do." The therapist writes down the goal in the form of a contract, which both the therapist and the client sign, with each of them getting a copy to take with them.

Urinalysis Contingency and Goal Setting

People with substance use problems are notoriously unreliable in reporting their use of substances, even if they are enrolled in treatment and have a good relationship with the clinician. Thus, it is important to use urinalysis as often as possible to provide an objective measure of drug use. Breathalyzer testing for alcohol use is less useful than urinalysis for drug use as it indicates only current inebriation, whereas urine tests can signal the use of most drugs of abuse over the previous 2–3 days (up to 28 days for cannabinoids). We employ urinalysis in every session with a drug test that provides results within a few minutes. Tests that need to be sent out for analysis are better than no tests, but immediate feedback is much more clinically useful than delayed information.

Clients in our program receive between $1.50 and $3.50 for providing a clean urine sample, with the amount increasing by $.50 over successive sessions with clean samples, and resetting to $1.50 after a dirty sample or an absence. This is not a sufficiently powerful incentive to drive behavior change on its own, but the combination of money coupled with regular urine checks, social reinforcement, and public attention to drug use is intended to (1) provide a tangible consequence for (even modest) success, (2) increase the salience of goals for reduced use, and (3) circumvent fraudulent claims that the individual has not used drugs. In clinical settings where money is not available, we suggest the use of other material reinforcers that may be available, including donated items such as hygiene products, used books, food and transportation coupons, and/or a grab bag or lottery. We suspect that the monetary value of the award is less important than its use as a tangible reinforcer for achieving a goal.

Urine testing is presented as a way to help clients achieve their goals, not as a test of their being truthful. Clients are first are asked if they have been clean in regard to their target drug. If they report that they have used the drug since the last group session they are assumed to be truthful, do not have to provide a urine sample, and do not receive reinforcement. If a client claims to have been clean since the last session, he or she is asked to provide a urine sample. When the testing is complete, the results are announced in the group. Clients who have clean samples receive enthusiastic social reinforcement (e.g., "Sue, that's great. You've been clean for 3 weeks in a row now. Congratulations," "Hey, Bob, congratulations. That is the first clean one for you in a few weeks") and their money. Other group members are encouraged to be reinforcing (e.g., "Juan, what do you think about how Bob has been doing?"), and they frequently cheer and applaud for one another. Positive drug tests are followed by comments of regret and hopes for future success (e.g., "Kareem, the test shows you were using cocaine. *Sorry. Maybe you can try harder between now and our next session"*).

After each client's results have been reviewed, the therapist, in turn, questions each client who used drugs about the circumstances in which he or she used and initiates problem solving to determine what precipitated the drug use, followed by training to reduce the risk of future such events. Thus, failure is associated with proactive efforts to help the client succeed, not criticism or censure. If substance use occurred in a social situation (e.g., social pressure or temptation due to someone else using), the therapist can conduct a role-play unit on skills that may be used to avoid or cope with that situation in the future (see examples in the following section, "Social Skills Training").

If the person did not use drugs as a result of an interpersonal problem, the training unit should focus on a relevant coping skill that may circumvent the problem in the future. The emphasis is on simple behavioral plans that are rehearsed in sessions and require minimal emphasis on "willpower" or sophisticated planning and problem solving. Common problems and potential coping strategies are listed in Table 9.2.

Clients will often report that they simply had an urge to use. If avoidance/escape is not feasible or effective, the client can be taught a simple self-talk strategy, in which he or she

TABLE 9.2. Common Problems That Lead to Drug Use and Behavioral Solutions

Problem	Solutions
Being home alone and bored	Leave the house and go for a walk.
	Call a friend or significant other.
	Plan an activity in anticipation of being alone.
	Attend a 12-Step meeting.
Having money in hand (e.g., SSI paydays)	Get a representative payee or have someone hold your money.
	Bring someone with you who doesn't use when you go to get your check.
	Do not walk home past the dealer on days you get paid.
Bothered by cravings	Do something distracting, such as going for a walk or playing music with headphones.
	Call a support person.
	Visit a friend who does not use drugs.

reviews the one or two most powerful reasons for not using until the urge/craving has passed. An example of this technique is as follows.

THERAPIST: OK. Now, I want you to close your eyes. OK? Good. Now imagine you're on your sofa and you start to think about crack. You are bored, and you really feel like doing some. Can you imagine that?

MARCUS: Yeah. I can imagine that.

THERAPIST: Good. Now tell yourself why you don't want to use: Think about going back to jail and stuff.

MARCUS: If I go buy some stuff, I could get arrested and sent back to jail.

THERAPIST: OK. Now tell yourself why that would be so bad.

MARCUS: My voices get real bad when I'm locked up.

THERAPIST: So should you go out and score some crack?

MARCUS: No.

THERAPIST: Why not?

MARCUS: Because I could go back to jail.

This iterative process is repeated three or four times until the client can quickly enumerate his or her primary reasons for not using. Simultaneously, the co-therapist writes the basic question and the key responses on a 3 × 5 index card, which is then given to the client. The client is instructed to carry it in his or her wallet/pocket/purse and take it out and read it whenever he or she feels very tempted and may give in. This strategy should be rehearsed in the next few sessions, even if the client has a clean urine sample. The key is repetition of one or a few simple statements that carry considerable weight for the client and are likely to motivate restraint or to be an effective distraction until the craving subsides.

Upon completion of the urinalysis protocol and coping skills training, the next step in each group session is to review progress toward the person's goal and to work out new strategies if the client was not successful with his or her homework/goal. Each client should always have a specific goal that is reasonable and appropriate. The goal can be used as a focus point for training in sessions and for self-prompts between sessions. *Goals should be set to minimize the chances of failure.* Clients are often unrealistic in what they propose to try. Sensible but unrealistic goals (e.g., "I don't want to use cocaine anymore") should not be rejected. Rather, the therapist should frame an intermediate goal that can be achieved and that moves the client toward the more superordinate goal (e.g., "How about if this week you try to use only on weekends?"). Of course, the therapist must use his or her knowledge of the client, the specific situation, and what he or she knows about behavior change in general in order to determine what is realistic and what is not. The general rule of thumb is to be conservative. If the client keeps failing to achieve session or weekly goals, it may be wise to generate an intermediate-level goal that is more attainable (e.g., if the client can't avoid using crack all week, perhaps he or she can try to restrict use to 1 or 2 days). It is critical to remember that behavior change is difficult and must be shaped by gradual approximations to the desired goal.

An important part of the process of setting goals is a review of the reasons for the goal: why the person wants to change. When discussing members' motivation to remain clean, reasons should be framed in "I" statements that reflect concrete consequences of behavior. Clients are more likely to refrain from using when their motivation is to avoid something negative (e.g., "I will go back to jail if I use") or achieve something positive ("I will be able to get my own apartment if I stay clean."), as opposed to a more abstract reason (e.g., "I want the respect of my family"). Whenever possible, the client should be encouraged to make an explicit statement to a significant other (parent, case manager, sibling, etc) about the plan. The person, time, and place in which the commitment will be made should be identified, and the client should role play what he or she will say to the person.

Depending on group size and how well clients are doing in reducing substance use, the urinalysis contingency and goal setting at the beginning of each session may consume 15 minutes to 60 minutes (e.g., if several group members test positive and require considerable rehearsal for coping techniques). Skills training, education, or other segments of treatment are carried out in the rest of each session. Consequently, it is impossible to specify precisely how many sessions each component will require.

Social Skills Training

Skills training is a major component of BTSAS, occupying upwards of half the sessions. As discussed earlier in this chapter, drugs are typically consumed in a social context. Certain people and the places where drugs have frequently been used become conditioned cues for drug use, generating urges to use and weakening resolve to abstain. In many cases peers or family members actively attempt to persuade the person to use so as not to use alone. It is not unusual for peers and family members to enlist people with schizophrenia to purchase drugs for them with offers to share. Neighborhood drug pushers see people with mental illness as "easy marks" and can be very forceful in trying to make sales. The primary goal of skills training is to teach clients how to effectively cope with these high-risk social situations by refusing drugs and alcohol, avoiding situations that pose a risk, or escaping when drug refusal is not successful. There are three interconnected skills required for success: (1) the ability to say *no* firmly and repeatedly, (2) the ability to anticipate and/or identify high-risk situations, and (3) a sense of self-efficacy for success that develops with practice and social reinforcement in the training sessions.

The basic strategy for skills training is identical to the approach we have described earlier for teaching other social skills. Training typically begins with a few sessions on conversation skills to orient clients to the training process, followed by a few sessions on assertion skills (e.g., Refusing Requests, Making Requests) unrelated to drug use. The literature indicates that people with schizophrenia who abuse drugs often have better social competence than those who do not use drugs, so this initial training can often be completed within three to four sessions. The focus then shifts to drug situations.

Although the basic structure of training remains the same (e.g., modeling, role play, feedback, etc.), skills training for drug use has some important differences from other training. Most important, the trainer must be very familiar with the drug culture in which the clients live, and able to reflect the language of drug use and the interpersonal style of drug interactions. For example, inner-city residents refusing drugs from pushers cannot employ the same social niceties that a typical trainer will employ with a clerk in a store. In a similar vein, role plays around drug use are generally much more confrontative than those employed for training other skills. Most clients have an easy time saying no to one or two semipolite requests from a role-play partner. To make the situation realistic, and thereby increase the likelihood that the person will acquire skills that will generalize to the community, the trainer must be very persistent and demanding. We have suggested in earlier chapters that role plays should not be stressful, and that is true here as well. However, the therapist must be forceful and persistent if the situation is to reflect the client's experience in the community. Of course, role plays should always end with the client successfully avoiding drugs, whether or not the client gets the confederate to change his or her behavior. Frequently this means the client turns around and physically leaves the interaction as the only effective way to end the social pressure and avoid drugs. Repeated success at resisting high levels of pressure in the clinic will gradually increase the client's sense of self-efficacy and make it more likely that he or she will try to resist real pressure to use drugs in the community.

We have included several skill sheets for teaching refusal skills in Part II. The following paragraphs provide some additional hints and guidelines for effective treatment.

It is particularly important to make the role-play situations very personally relevant for group members. Clients should each be requested to identify *specific* partners and situations where drug use is likely and to indicate the *specific* language that would be used by the partner. Information from the motivational interview will be especially useful here. After the first two sessions, and as the level of difficulty and pressure of the role plays in this section increase, therapists may want to include various props (e.g., bottles of beer/liquor, crack pipe, or other appropriate paraphernalia) to increase realism. Props can help to make the role plays more realistic as well as increase their level of difficulty.

A standard gambit taught to clients for turning down requests in situations that do not involve drugs, is to suggest an alternative. For example, in refusing a request from someone suggesting that the client accompany him to a movie, the client may suggest that they go out to eat instead. In a drug situation the client might be asked if she wants to go get some crack cocaine and party. An alternative may be going to a movie—if the person is not already holding cocaine. However, suggesting an alternative would not be a suitable response if the other person has cocaine on him at the time. Being around drugs increases temptation and the risk of drug use. Clients working toward abstinence should *always* avoid being around drugs. The appropriate response is simply to refuse the invitation or to suggest that the client would be glad to accompany the person another time when he doesn't have any drugs with him.

The therapist should try to get group members to identify potential role-play situations that will be highly relevant for them before the next session. For example, "Who will you be seeing in the next few days that you have used drugs with in the past?" "What risky situation will you be in before our next session?" As clients achieve success in becoming abstinent, they face fewer risky situations on a daily basis and they can be asked to anticipate situations further in the future, or recall them from the past. For example, "Might you run into someone whom you used to use with?" Table 9.3 provides a list of some appropriate situations to suggest to clients who are having difficulty in thinking of risky situations.

TABLE 9.3. Common High-Risk Situations

1. Having money/pay day. This is a *very* relevant situation for many people who receive, or interact with people who receive, large monthly disability or biweekly welfare checks. There is an increased likelihood that the client may either treat a peer or be treated to drugs or alcohol at those times.
2. Running into or being approached by a dealer on the street.
3. Attending a social get together around holiday times.
4. Being asked to use by a family member with whom the group member frequently uses drugs or alcohol.
5. Having a phone conversation with someone who calls asking for drugs or offering to share.
6. Being asked to use drugs by another client at the treatment/mental health center.

Two very common situations requiring somewhat different drug refusal skills are situations in which clients need to refuse to use drugs with family members or friends (i.e., people that they know) and situations in which they need to refuse offers of drugs from drug dealers or people they don't know or don't know well. Some clients experience both situations (i.e., a family member or friend frequently pressures them to use, and they often encounter drug dealers who offer them drugs to buy or free samples). Others experience only one or the other. Clients have reported that they can use all of the steps outlined in the curriculum with people that they know, but that making eye contact or giving a reason are often irrelevant to interactions with strangers (especially dealers). Therapists need to discuss this with clients during the drug refusal skills sessions and help them create plans for encounters with strangers and drug dealers if these situations are relevant to them. For example, one client told us that he would have to be polite and respectful to the drug dealer in refusing offers and he could not turn his back on the dealer and walk away unless he wanted to risk getting beaten up or shot. This client was helped to develop a plan in which he came up with a reason that he felt could be used with the drug dealer ("I'm not using today because I have a urine test tomorrow, and if I come up positive I'll have to go to jail") and role played the way he thought he would have to interact with the dealer in order to get out of the situation safely. The overall message here is to be aware of the need to tailor plans and role plays to the different situations clients face.

Tailoring Training for New Group Members in Open Enrollment Groups

Tailoring is particularly important for new group members. They should be *faded* into the group so that expectations and demands are gradually increased. They should be included as participant observers during the first week as they learn about the group by observing existing members. It is helpful to have a new member sit next to one of the therapists, who can quietly explain or describe what is going on. New members should be invited to provide feedback to role plays and to engage in role plays if they choose. In the latter case, the scenarios should be kept briefer than those presented for experienced group members and performance criteria should be simpler. Expectations for participation in all aspects of treatment should be increased beginning in the second week of attendance. Like all other members starting in a group, they should begin to participate in the urinalysis contingency and goal setting in the second week as well. References to specific material from earlier sessions should be briefly explained to new members as needed until units are formally repeated. It is often helpful to have experienced members explain important points to new members in their own words, as this process reinforces the material for the "teacher" and clarifies it for the new member.

In most cases, new members should be well acclimated to the group process within 2 weeks and should be functioning as full members within 3–4 weeks. There is one constraint on adding new members: When all existing members started together and are due to graduate in the following 4–5 weeks, it is very difficult for a new member to catch up, and it is better to have the client wait until a new group can be formed.

Education and Coping Skills

The education and coping skills section of BTSAS is intended to present members with information that will increase their motivation to avoid drugs and to teach coping skills that will increase their chances of success. Members are given a basic explanation of the neurochemistry of schizophrenia and how alcohol and illicit substances can counteract the effects of antipsychotic medications and increase symptoms of schizophrenia. They learn how habits and cravings affect their use of drugs and alcohol. They are encouraged to identify people, places, and things that may trigger drug and alcohol use, as well as situations that present high risks for using when someone is trying to stay clean or reduce his or her use. Members are assisted in developing their own coping strategies and working toward their own substance use reduction goals with the use of personalized information about triggers and high-risk situations. Although it is necessary to use a didactic format to present this information, participants will *not* respond well to a lecture. The therapist should not speak for more than about 5 minutes without involving one of the participants. Some useful strategies for making this presentation seem less like a classroom lecture are included in Table 9.4.

TABLE 9.4. Strategies for Presenting Didactic Material

- Ask a member to summarize or repeat a segment: The more clients express the material in their own words, the more they will incorporate the key points (e.g., "So, Susan, can you tell us what dopamine is?" "That's right. It's a brain chemical that is a problem in schizophrenia.").
- Ask for a *personally relevant experience* (e.g., "Rafael, can you think of a time when your voices got worse after you scored some crack?") In doing so, therapists are seeking an example with which the group member will closely identify, perhaps even identify what specifically about his or her *own* drug and alcohol use *scares* that group member.
- Relate the material to information previously provided by group members (e.g., refer to material from motivational interviewing [MI] sessions or from goal setting).
- Do not ask questions that yield yes/no or one-word answers (e.g., "Is that clear?" "Do you all understand that?" "Are there any questions about that?").
- Ask leading questions that get clients to explain points in their own words (e.g., "So, Maurice, can you tell us why cocaine makes your schizophrenia worse?" "Juan, can you show us on this diagram what happens when you take your medicine? OK, now what happens if you smoke a joint?")

The problems clients encounter in achieving their goals often inform the development of coping strategies. When we talk about group members' cravings and their attempts to avoid using, we explain to them that we will work with them to develop avoidance and re-fusal strategies that will help them avoid drugs and achieve their goals. We also help them to revise goals that appear to be too ambitious and to develop goals that are more attain-able. Whenever possible we role play coping skills that will help a client deal with high-risk situations.

It is important for the therapists to *generalize individual high risk situations* to commonly experienced categories of high-risk situations. For example:

CLIENT: No, I didn't meet my goal of not using for 3 days.

THERAPIST: What made it difficult for you?

CLIENT: Danny came by and offered me a blast and I was really bored.

Despite the fact that the client describes a personal high-risk situation, the content of the situation can be framed as a general high-risk category: being bored.

This generalization of individual high-risk situations is important for *three reasons*:

1. It keeps information relevant for all group members and thus will help keep every-one engaged.
2. The limited cognitive ability of people with schizophrenia makes it essential to keep information to a limited number of key themes and problems that are repeated again and again to increase learning.
3. Because this is a group intervention, and in light of the participants' possible cogni-tive deficits, it is impossible to cover every idiosyncratic problem faced by group members.

It is important to keep in mind that participants should not be expected to remember everything that is presented. The goal is to have them learn and retain any of several key points that will help motivate and sustain reduced substance use. For example, one client may learn to use dopamine as a buzzword or prompt for the negative effects of cocaine, whereas another may simply remember that her antipsychotic medications won't work as well if she smokes crack. Another important strategy is to make extensive use of graphic materials and handouts. All didactic material should be prepared in advance on flipcharts and handouts. We generally give clients goal sheets, homework sheets, and handouts of di-dactic materials in every session. It is helpful to give group members loose-leaf binders when they begin treatment, in which they can keep handouts for easy reference. The binder also serves as a palpable cue that they are engaged in a special program.

The education and coping section of BTSAS includes eight units: (1) positive and nega-tive aspects of using substances, (2) biological basis of schizophrenia and antipsychotics, (3) how drugs and alcohol affect the illness and its treatment, (4) habits, cravings, triggers, and high-risk situations, (5) avoidance strategies, (6) escape and refusal, (7) HIV and drug use, and (8) hepatitis and drug use. The unit on the positive and negative aspects of substance use is designed to underscore why members are at risk and why they have elected to reduce drug use. The units on biological factors explain that one of the most critical reasons for abstinence is that all drugs act by increasing dopaminergic activity in the brain, whereas antipsychotics work, in part, by blocking dopamine. Thus, drugs reduce the effects of medications and increase the risk of relapse. This can serve as a powerful, easy-to-remember motivating factor for members to use in risk situations. The next three units (habits, avoidance, and escape) teach clients why reducing drug use is so hard, and why will power is not as effective as anticipating risk and escaping or avoiding it. The final two units reflect the fact that HIV and hepatitis are at virtual plague levels among people with serious mental illness who abuse drugs. Table 9.5 presents a representative section from the unit on high-risk situations, which can be used to guide the development of teaching programs for other topics. The regular text is the actual trainer responses, and text in italics is instructions/ suggestions for the trainer.

Problem Solving and Relapse Prevention

Achieving abstinence from drugs is a process that unfolds over time. Motivation waxes and wanes as a function of a host of neurobiological, psychological, and environmental factors. Success may breed complacency that increases exposure to high-risk situations. Stresses and life events produce negative emotional states that rekindle memories of drug use, increase urges, and decrease willpower to resist drug use. Cues that were associated with drug use in the past may be encountered unexpectedly and rekindle urges to use. Lapses are common and present a risk of becoming full-blown relapses. These various risks are of concern for anyone attempting to eliminate drug use, but they are particularly problematic for people with schizophrenia, given their decreased ability to exert self-control, to conduct effective problem solving, and to see the continuity of events over time. In addition, the prevalence of polydrug abuse is common in this population and different substances must be targeted sequentially for most clients. In that regard, skills and motivational factors relevant for one substance will not automatically generalize to abstinence from other substances. Consequently, treatment must be extended over time so that training in skills and coping strategies can be applied across substances, to high-risk events that occur intermittently, and in periods of decreased motivation.

As in earlier segments of treatment, each session during the problem solving and relapse prevention (PS/RP) unit begins with urinalysis and reinforcement and goal setting. The PS/RP sessions then include introducing clients to a range of high-risk situations and having them practice coping in these situations by using the skills that have already been taught (refusal, escape, avoidance) or others that are discussed in the course of the group. Many sessions include problem solving in high-risk situations that the participants have encountered or will encounter in the near future, as well as others that participants may not have previously considered. Other sessions vary according to the needs of individual group members. The primary emphasis is on (1) developing goals for secondary drugs that are abused, for clients who make continued progress with their primary drugs, (2) continued problem solving, support, and motivation enhancement for clients having difficulty in meeting goals, and (3) relapse prevention skills for clients who have achieved periods of

TABLE 9.5. Training Clients to Handle High-Risk Situations

We said that triggers are the people, places, or things that you connect with using drugs or alcohol. Because triggers are associated with the pleasurable feelings you had when you were using, they can cause you to crave drugs or alcohol. So, when you are in a situation where your triggers are present, you are in a *High-risk situation* (HRS). These situations are called high-risk situations because there is a high risk that you will use when you are in them. Where there is a trigger, there is a high risk for you to use.

What we want to do now is to help you identify some of these situations in your own lives so that we can help you to cope with them and avoid using at these times when you don't want to use.

We talked about the *negative consequences of your use* a few days ago. Each of you came up with some negative consequences during that group session. [*Therapist uses flipchart to review meaningful personal consequences that members generated in prior sessions.*]

You have all given lots of negative consequences that come from your use of certain drugs or alcohol. _____, what is a situation in which you find yourself almost always using?

1. *Solicit an example from a group member and go through the triggers that make up his or her HRS.*
2. *Refer to the type of HRS that the example represents and further describe the multiple/single trigger HRSs.*

HRSs occur where there may be:

- *More than one trigger.* HRSs can occur when *more than one trigger* act at the same time. For example, Alex, can you tell us about a time when you didn't want to use, but some or all of the triggers you just told me about were there, and you ended up using?

  [*Insert an example given by a member using the list of triggers he or she previously identified.*]

  In that situation, there were several triggers acting at the same time that *increased* the chance that you would use the drug/alcohol automatically.

  What negative consequences might happen as a result of using drugs in that situation? [*Get members to identify possible negative consequences and prompt as necessary. Also refer to goals from the Motivational Interview.*] A situation where you are facing more than one trigger may lead to a craving for the drug, which will make it more difficult for you to say "no" to it.

- *One trigger.* Another example of an HRS could be when there is *one trigger* that is so *strong*, you will use almost automatically. For example, if there is one person whom you use with *each time* you see him or her, that may be enough to cause you to use automatically. Or it could be *one trigger that is very hard for you to avoid.* For example, the person you live with is a strong trigger for you if you use with that person every day, because it would be really hard for you to avoid that person. So for you, this would be a high-risk situation. What negative consequences might happen if you used with that roommate who is a trigger for you?

  [*Get members to identify potential risks and prompt as needed. Have participants identify their own HRSs.*]

Everyone who has a problem with drugs and alcohol has at least a few HRSs. When people try to cut down or quit, they usually have some success in easy situations. For example, when someone runs out of money to buy drugs or alcohol, or goes to the hospital to receive treatment for his or her mental illness, it can be *easier* to stop using in those situations because the person doesn't have the money to get the alcohol or the ability to get out onto the street to buy the drugs. Being on conditional release can also make it easier to stay clean. Has anyone here been on conditional release? What was it like keeping clean when you knew you would go back to jail if you used/drank? [*Probe for information from participants who were able to stay clean for a certain amount of time when they were in jail, on conditional release, or on probation or parole.*]

(continued)

TABLE 9.5. *(continued)*

When you have problems with drugs and/or alcohol, it's very hard to stay clean when you are in an HRS. You may automatically drink or drug at certain times or in certain places or with certain people. _____, you said that you automatically drink with _____. So, if you know what your triggers are, then you can make a plan to *avoid* them. A plan will give you something you can do to prevent yourself from getting into a situation where you would automatically use. _____, for you, that might be staying off the corner when you know that _____ will be there.

Let's find out what some HRSs may be for each of you. _____, think of a time when you didn't want to use, but you did. Tell us about it.

[*Help members identify HRSs by asking leading questions similar to those from the session on triggers regarding person, place, feeling, sensation (smell, sight). Try to concretize a time period for the person by asking him or her to think about a period of time when he or she was not using; for example: "Think of a time in the last week/between now and this past Christmas/between now and your last birthday, etc." Then ask, "So, why is that an HRS for you? And what were the negative consequences that you could face if you did end up using?" If no group member is able to think of a time, the trainer should make use of information gathered from the motivational interviews at this point.*

List on board each HRS and trigger components of that HRS, followed by the possible negative consequences for each group member. If a client has difficulty answering, ask other members to help. It is important to help participants focus on what they were feeling, doing, where were they, etc. BEFORE they actually used, as they may have trouble distinguishing what they were doing, feeling, etc., when they were actually using from what they were experiencing before using.]

abstinence. The basic training strategies (e.g., rehearsal, extensive use of prompts, having participants repeat information in their own words) employed in earlier training sessions continue to be used throughout. In addition, material covered in earlier sessions is systematically reviewed and related to current experience when the core curriculum is completed (typically by the end of the 4th month). Entire units (e.g., refusal skills training, education about dopamine and schizophrenia) are repeated as needed for new members.

Therapists should note that the PS/RP unit is not as structured as previous units. The content of the PS/RP unit varies somewhat according to the needs of individual clients. Several topics are considered integral to the unit and should be covered in all groups. Other modules have been developed for use with certain groups, depending on the members in the group and the issues being presented. The standard modules are presented in Table 9.6.

Additional topics related to coping with high-risk situations that may also be helpful in some groups include:

1. Medication management
2. Dealing with partners who use drugs
3. Creating a drug-free social support network (how to meet people who don't use drugs)
4. General assertiveness training (e.g., how to refuse unreasonable requests, asking someone to change his or her behavior)

TABLE 9.6. Training Units in Problem Solving/Relapse Prevention

- *Relapse prevention.* The aim is to teach clients about the persistence of high-risk situations, to help identify situations that will be risky in the near future, and to devise coping strategies for each. Once the general framework of PS/RP is presented, subsequent sessions will involve identifying high-risk situations (either those that clients come up with or those that therapists suggest) and applying the principles of PS/RP to each (i.e., planning for each high-risk situation).

- *Addressing other substances of abuse.* Research shows that clients with a history of polysubstance abuse who use one drug are at substantially increased risk to relapse for another. Thus, continued use of a secondary substance is a high-risk situation for relapse. Clients who have addressed a primary drug (i.e., cocaine) but are still using a secondary drug (e.g., alcohol) are at higher risk for relapsing to cocaine as long as they are drinking.

- *Coping with lapses (slips).* Lapses (isolated occasions of use) can easily become relapses (full-blown return to use). Thus, a lapse is a high-risk situation. The primary focus is to make clients aware of the distinction between lapses and relapses and the danger of moving from the former to the latter. Given that most people with schizophrenia have difficulty with abstraction, the focus is very specific.

- *Coping with negative affect, including boredom, stress, depression, and symptoms.* Research shows that negative affective states are the most common reasons for relapse. In addition, studies on reasons for substance use among clients with schizophrenia find that one of the most commonly stated reasons for use is coping with negative affect, especially boredom. Thus, negative affect is a high-risk situation. The goal here is to help clients plan for negative affect and to discuss other coping strategies other than substance use.

- *Dealing with decreases in motivation.* Motivation to maintain abstinence waxes and wanes over time. Periods of low motivation are high-risk situations for drug use. Clients often say that they never want to use drugs again, with little understanding that there will be temptations and periods of time when they are less motivated to maintain abstinence.

- *Money management.* Money is a continuous source of risk for many clients. This unit covers practical strategies for controlling that risk by minimizing a person's access to money. Tactics include formally establishing representative payees, giving benefit checks to case managers or significant others for deposit before cashing them, establishing concrete goals for savings (e.g., to move to a better apartment, to buy kids' Christmas presents), and not carrying money unless going directly to a store for a specific purchase.

5. Specific assertiveness training (dealing with an aggressive partner or family member)

6. Employment skills (connecting with job training, how to prepare for a job interview, etc.)

It is important to note that the topics to be raised in the PS/RP unit require ongoing monitoring, discussion, and intervention. These modules are designed to give therapists a starting point for addressing these topics, but these are not topics that can be covered in a single session. Each topic needs to be repeatedly discussed, and client progress toward goals needs to be continuously monitored. For example, addressing secondary substances of abuse is an important part of the PS/RP unit. This is a topic that cannot be adequately addressed in one session. The session can serve as the mechanism for approaching the topic both generally in the group and more specifically for individual clients. However, the use of other substances should be continually monitored and client progress toward reducing or abstaining from a secondary substance must be repeatedly addressed. An example is a client who has successfully abstained from a goal drug who then changes his or her designated goal drug to a secondary substance (e.g., from cocaine to marijuana). For many clients, the secondary drug of abuse is alcohol. Efforts to reduce or abstain from alcohol need to be reinforced and addressed. Other PS/RP sessions involve helping clients create plans for coping with some high-risk situation. Those topics and the plans that were generated need to be frequently revisited; a plan may have to be updated or completely changed in the event that the client has found that plan unworkable. For example, a PS/RP session on money management involves therapists helping clients develop plans for managing their money. This is not a one-session type of topic—therapists need to determine whether a client has designated a payee, opened a bank account, arranged for direct deposits, or otherwise followed through on plans that were established during the session.

Table 9.7 provides an example of how to teach clients to deal with *lapses*.

STRATEGIES FOR SPECIAL PROBLEMS

Ambivalence about Attending Group

At times, some group members may want to stop coming to group, or have difficulty committing themselves to reducing substance use. This is to be expected for anyone with a substance use problem and may be accentuated by the ambivalence that is often characteristic of schizophrenia.

This situation should be addressed without confrontation. The therapist should indicate that shifts in motivation are common, that they are not an indication of failure, and that it is important to continue learning skills so they are in the person's repertoire when he or she does decide to try to reduce substance use. The following is an example of the supportive, but directive approach to be employed:

> "We are glad that you have been part of this group with us. You may not feel like talking about drugs and alcohol today, but you are an important part of this group. The other members learn from what you have to say and the things you contribute by being here. You don't have to role play today if you don't feel up to it. We can take it session by session for a while and work with you on staying in the group. People sometimes have a hard time with group meetings about drugs and alcohol, and we'll work hard to help you.
>
> "I understand that this is not a good time for you to get off crack, but you were motivated to use less when you started treatment, and you will probably become motivated again somewhere down the line. This is still a good time to learn strategies that will be helpful when you do want to quit or cut back, so we can increase your chance of being successful."

Issues and Problems That Extend Beyond the Skills Group

As mentioned earlier, many clients who abuse substances have legal and financial problems related to the abuse. They may also have impaired relationships with family members, no steady address, and poor physical health. These problems can be very distracting to clients and can make it difficult for them to concentrate on social skills training. In addition, crises related to domestic problems may interfere with group attendance, especially for clients

TABLE 9.7. Teaching Clients How to Deal with Lapses

One of the things we know about giving up drugs is that most people have a bad day sooner or later. They may think they have it licked and decide they can do just a little. Or maybe they are having a bad day and lose self-control. Lots of people who give up drugs talk about how hard it is not to do drugs when they are feeling stressed out or depressed, and that these bad feelings lead them to want to use. Sometimes they just have a weak moment and forget why it is so important for them to stay clean. Lots of people tell us that peer pressure sometimes gets so bad that they have trouble saying "no." Whatever the case, most people who are giving up drugs make a slip at one time or another and use. We call these times slips or *lapses*.

The big problem with lapses is that they can become full-blown *relapses,* or a return to regular drug use. Sometimes lapses make people feel as though they have failed, so they just give up and start using again. Or sometimes they feel as though they can control it and continue to do a little, but they gradually get caught up again. So a lapse is a high-risk situation, because a little bit of drug use can quickly turn into a full-blown relapse.

The most important thing for you to remember is that a lapse does not have to become a relapse. You need to just get back to your hard work the next day. We have found that it is easier to keep a lapse from becoming a full-blown relapse if we talk about it in group and figure out what to do if a lapse happens. So it's better when there is a plan—some sort of idea of what you could do if you experience a lapse. Why do you think it's better to have a plan? That's right—if you have a plan, you will already know what to do, and you will be able to quickly get back on track again instead of letting the lapse turn into a full-blown relapse.

Many people who don't have a plan don't know what to do if they have a lapse, so they just throw in the towel and go back to using. That is very common when people are trying to change a really tough behavior like drug use. A person will have a lapse, feel really bad about it, and just say, "I screwed up, I'm no good and I can't do this. I'm just going to forget about being clean and go use." Has that ever happened to anyone here—you had stopped using for a while, then had a lapse and then said, "Just forget it," and you went back to using? What we do in this group is talk about what *else* you could do if a lapse happens instead of going back to using, so that you have a plan to get back to after the lapse occurs.

Planning for lapses

OK, so let's figure out what each of us can do if we have a lapse. Right after the lapse occurs is the most difficult time to know what to do and a time that you are at very high risk to have a lapse become a full-blown relapse. There are three steps for you to use right after a lapse:

Step 1: Keep calm. Most people who have a lapse feel really bad afterward—guilty, as though they have failed. This reaction is normal and will pass with a little time. You might feel bad for a while, but the bad feelings will pass if you let them. Remind yourself that the lapse was a one-time thing, a mistake, and one that you will learn from and plan for so that you will be able to cope with it next time. It is *not* a sign of failure—everyone makes mistakes.

Step 2: Implement a plan. The more quickly you can get back on track after a lapse, the better off you will be and the more likely that a lapse won't turn into a full-blown relapse. First, get rid of all drugs or alcohol that are around, as well as any other triggers that are present. Second, escape the high-risk situation. Third, do something else that will take up your time and that will get you involved in something other than using drugs. For example, you can go to an AA/NA meeting, go to a group, meet a friend who doesn't use drugs, go for a walk, etc.

Step 3: Ask for help. Other people can help you cope with a lapse so that it doesn't turn into a full-blown relapse. Talk to your therapist, your counselor or doctor, to other group members, to family members, or anyone else who is helpful to you. There are also treatment and crisis centers that you can call in times of need. We have some listed on the handout.

(continued)

TABLE 9.7. *(continued)*

[*Note to therapist: Write steps on the board and give group members handouts and wallet cards before explaining each step. Get group members' thoughts on each step: Have they done such a thing before? Would they add anything to that step? etc.*]

Making a lapse plan for each group member

Now we want to talk about high-risk situations that could involve a lapse and then plan for what to do if a lapse occurs. Who would like to start? How about you, John? What's a high-risk situation for you that could lead to a lapse if you don't plan ahead?

[*Give the client time to come up with a high-risk situation. If the client has trouble thinking of one, present a situation to the client based on what you know about him or her and his or her use, such as the following:*] I know it can be tough to think of one. You know, you always used to use with your ex-wife, right? Let's imagine you run into her this Saturday night at a party, and she persuades you to smoke a joint, just like old times. You say no, you don't do that any more, but she talks and talks and you finally give in and decide to just do one. The next day you're feeling really rotten for having given in and feel as if all your hard work is down the drain. That's an example of a lapse.

OK, let's apply the lapse steps to this situation. The first step is *Stop*. What would you do?

[*Go through each step with the group member and write his or her plan on the board under each step. Be as concrete as possible. Incorporate role plays where appropriate. Role plays may be particularly useful for Step 3 (asking for help). For example, if the group member is in a situation with other people and he or she needs to leave the situation, the role play can center on the group member telling the other people that he or she is not going to use drugs any more and that he or she needs to leave the situation. Write the escape steps on the board and then do the role play.*]

---

living in the community. See Mueser et al. (2003) for guidance on issues such as housing, vocational rehabilitation, and medication compliance.

Obviously, social skills training cannot address all the problems of clients with substance abuse. Leaders working with this population will find it advantageous to work closely with other agencies and professionals who can address the multiple problems involved. Appropriate agencies include community mental health centers, health clinics, emergency housing agencies, detox centers, legal assistance offices, supported employment programs, job clubs, Alcoholics Anonymous (AA), and Narcotics Anonymous (NA). It is important to note that although some dually diagnosed clients benefit from AA and NA, they may need some help to develop skills to participate in such meetings. Social skills training can include communication skills that teach how to participate in meetings. Conducting a mock meeting is also helpful to give clients a chance to practice what they might say in an actual meeting. Clients should be encouraged to investigate different meetings to determine which of them feel more comfortable.

It is also important to be aware of how different professionals contribute to the treatment of a dually diagnosed client. For example, social workers can determine which services the client is entitled to, and intensive case managers can coordinate appointments and services and, in some cases, arrange transportation. It is important for all involved professionals to plan treatment together, to address as many of the client's problems as possible, to communicate frequently, and to avoid duplication of effort. If the client's problems are being addressed, he or she will be less distracted by them, more likely to attend group regularly, and better able to concentrate on social skills training while in the group.

Because many clients have unstable living situations, it is a good idea for the leaders to identify a contact person in case there is a need to communicate concerning absences or changes in the schedule of the group. The contact person may be a relative, friend, or a professional whom the client trusts and sees frequently. The contact person can also be helpful in providing encouragement to the client to attend the group.

There are several social skills in the curriculum that can be used to help clients solve problems related to substance abuse. Examples of these include Making Requests, Refusing Requests, Disagreeing with Another's Opinion without Arguing, Getting Your Point Across, Compromise and Negotiation, Listening to Others, and Solving Problems. When clients feel they are learning skills that help them improve their situation, they are both more motivated and more focused on the group.

Attending Group While Intoxicated or High

The course of reducing substance abuse is not a smooth one. Clients go back and forth in the stages of commitment to change and fluctuate in their ability to follow through on their resolve to curb substance abuse. Even when progress has been made in both commitment and ability to follow through, there are frequent setbacks when clients resume abusing substances. Clients in inpatient settings usually do not have access to substances. However, clients living in the community continue to have access and may even attend group intoxicated or high. Although this situation is actually rare, it can be very frustrating to leaders, because such clients may concentrate poorly, behave inappropriately, and set a negative example for other group members.

It is helpful for the leaders to keep in mind that difficulty in avoiding substance use is one of the major reasons that clients cannot treat the problem themselves and that setbacks are inevitable in treating substance abuse. However, because it is nearly impossible to conduct social skills groups with clients who are intoxicated or high, precautions must be taken to reduce the incidence of such situations. When the leaders are orienting the clients to the group, they must clearly state that group members may not attend the group if they have used substances before coming to the group that day. This rule can be included in written orientation materials and may also be included in a list of basic rules that is posted in the group room.

Leaders must be aware of the signs of substance abuse and able to assess its severity. Signs vary by the specific drug being used, although common signs of drug abuse include dilated pupils (sometimes disguised by dark glasses), agitation, drowsiness, euphoria, nervousness, and slowed reflexes. Alcohol abuse tends to result in drowsiness, slurred speech, loss of motor coordination, slowed reaction time, and feelings of depression. Leaders need to become familiar with the signs for the specific substances abused by the clients in their social skills group.

There is a range of severity of the effects of substance abuse. In some situations the client may have abused a small amount of alcohol that morning and be only mildly impaired and able to behave appropriately in the group. In other situations the client may have abused cocaine just prior to attending group and may be hyperalert, highly energetic, more symptomatic, and unable to concentrate on the group. Different responses are of course, used in these different situations and depend on the policy of the facility housing the group.

Leaders need to plan in advance what they will do if a client arrives at the group showing signs of using drugs or alcohol. It is important not to wait until such a situation actually occurs. Having a clear plan of action will minimize confusion and cause the least disruption to the group. Leaders must, however, first determine their policy concerning substance use and the presence of intoxicated people on the premises. Some facilities forbid substance use on their property but allow a nondisruptive person to remain if he or she used the substance before arriving. Other facilities require immediate expulsion of anyone with evidence of substance abuse. There are also different policies concerning how people who are expelled from the group may be transported away from the premises. For example, an agency would be at risk for liability if its staff members allowed an intoxicated person to drive. The leaders need to be prepared with lists of relatives who can transport the client, taxi companies to call, and funding sources for paying for transportation. In addition, the leaders must decide where the client can go if he or she is expelled from group: home? the community? a detox center? another treatment facility? Information should be obtained concerning security personnel available to the leaders if a client refuses to cooperate.

In making policies about how to handle group members who use substances prior to attendance, it is important to keep in mind that these clients are often those who need the treatment most. If the client's behavior is manageable, it is preferable to keep him or her in the group. Moreover, it is important *not* to tell these clients to "come back when you've dealt with your substance use." The goal of integrated treatment programs is to avoid fragmentation of services to dually diagnosed clients; therefore, integrated programs should provide easily available treatment resources for clients to turn to when they need help in returning to sobriety. The decision to exclude clients who use substances from group sessions or from the treatment facility should be made reluctantly.

When a client attends the group high or intoxicated, the leaders should respond to the situation immediately by using the following kinds of planned actions. Depending on the severity of the situation, the leaders can gently but firmly inform the client that they are aware of the substance abuse and repeat the rule forbidding this behavior. The leaders may prefer to speak to the client outside the group room, especially if he or she is likely to become agitated. If the leaders determine that the situation is severe enough to warrant expelling the client from the session, the client must be informed that he or she cannot continue in the session, although he or she is welcome to return to the next session if sober. Depending on the action plan, the leaders then direct the client to the appropriate type of transportation and destination.

In addition, the leaders should refer the client to a specific member of the treatment team (preferably available on-site) to talk about the current substance abuse to help him or her return to sobriety before the next group meeting. It is best if the client can meet with the appropriate staff member immediately or within a few hours. When the leaders of the social skills training group are members of the client's integrated treatment team and have time available after the group session, they may be the most appropriate persons to work with the client.

Before the next scheduled session of the group, the leaders can call the client to encourage sobriety for the next group meeting and to express that both leaders and group members look forward to seeing him or her again soon. The next time the client attends a group meeting and is not intoxicated, the leaders should praise him or her for this accomplishment.

SUMMARY

Substance abuse by people with schizophrenia and other severe and persistent mental illnesses substantially increases their risk for a variety of serious health, psychiatric, and environmental consequences and is a major problem for the public mental health system. In this chapter we discussed some of the issues involved in substance abuse and substance abuse treatment and described a treatment approach that can be implemented in the context of skills training groups. Clinicians working with dually diagnosed clients must be sensitive to the fact that motivation to reduce substance use waxes and wanes, and treatment requires a long-term perspective. Abstinence should be encouraged and efforts to change should be reinforced, but many clients will function best with a program that emphasizes harm reduction. Behavioral Treatment for Substance Abuse in Schizophrenia (BTSAS) is an innovative program that uses skills training techniques to teach clients critical skills needed to reduce substance use. Conducted in small groups, BTSAS teaches clients how to refuse drugs and alcohol from significant others and increases their sense of self-efficacy in their ability to resist social pressure. Each session begins with a urinalysis to detect substance use, and clients receive social and material reinforcement for success. Evidence of drug use is followed by problem solving rather than censure. Short-term goals that the client has a reasonable chance to achieve are set in each session. Clients are taught how to anticipate risky situations and are encouraged to avoid or escape from these situations, rather than relying on willpower to resist substance use. Strategies were described for dealing with special problems, such as ambivalence about attending group, coming to group intoxicated, and the need for help outside their group.

10

Reducing Relapse by Creating
a Supportive Environment

Stress is major factor in precipitating relapse in clients with schizophrenia. Even when it does not lead to relapse, stress can interfere significantly with clients' ability to learn or practice new skills. Stress exists in many different forms, including life events, daily hassles, boredom, conflict, overdemanding environments, and critical, negative communication. One way to reduce stress for clients is to increase the usual support and structure available in their immediate environment. This chapter focuses on specific strategies for creating a supportive environment that will both facilitate the learning of social skills and reduce the risk for symptom relapse. The strategies are applicable to family members as well as staff members.

RECOGNIZING A STRESSFUL ENVIRONMENT

What determines whether an environment is stressful to someone with schizophrenia? First, the way people communicate is very important. Clients find yelling and arguments to be stressful even when they are not directly involved. It is particularly distressing, however, when staff members or family members criticize them (e.g., "You're too lazy to get out of bed") or order them around (e.g., "Get over here right now for your medication").

Second, the atmosphere of the physical setting is significant. Clients find it stressful when the setting is crowded and noisy and there are no comfortable places to sit quietly. Third, the level of structure affects the client's stress level. Clients experience stress if the environment is overdemanding (e.g., if clients are required to be involved in highly organized activities all day). Stress also results when the environment does not provide mean-ingful structure (e.g., if clients are not expected to do chores or be involved in any activi-ties). A setting that is unpredictable or confusing may be upsetting to clients, such as if there are several competing activities going on at the same time or if meals are served at widely different times each day. Table 10.1 contains a summary of factors that contribute to a stressful environment.

Clients, like everyone else, are faced with daily stressors, which are often referred to as *hassles*. These stressors are usually minor, but they can add up if they occur regularly. For example, messy roommates, unpleasant chores, frequent criticism, and being around argu-ments or conflicts are all hassles that can wear people down. The negative effects of ongo-ing daily hassles can be as stressful as major life events, and they should be recognized as such.

In addition, research shows that most people experience life events (major life occur-rences, such as moving, losing a job, being ill, and experiencing a loss) as stressful. Even events that are the source of happiness, such as getting married or starting a new job, can be the source of stress. Recognizing when the client experiences a life event that is likely to be stressful is helpful for staff members and family members. For example, when a client living in a community residence gets a new roommate or experiences a death in the family, staff members can anticipate that this might be stressful and can prepare themselves to pro-vide more support.

TABLE 10.1. Elements of a Stressful Environment

Patterns of communication
- Loud voices
- Giving orders/making demands
- Frequent criticism and expression of anger
- Heated arguments
- Name calling

Physical setting
- Distracting amount of noise
- Crowding
- Poor housing conditions
- Unsafe neighborhood
- Poor access to public transportation
- Lack of privacy
- Unappetizing food

Level of structure
- Demanding, rigid schedule
- Unpredictable schedule
- Lack of stimulation and meaningful activities

THE IMPORTANCE OF FAMILY MEMBERS AND STAFF MEMBERS IN CREATING A SUPPORTIVE ENVIRONMENT

As stated in earlier chapters, leaders need to create an environment conducive to learning within the group. This includes providing a comfortable setting, avoiding criticism and negativity, encouraging the efforts of the group members, and giving generous amounts of positive feedback. However, the group takes place for only a few hours per week. The clients' remaining time involves contact with people who are not group leaders. The total amount of time the clients spend in the skills training group is minimal as compared with that spent outside the group. Thus, although the group leaders are important, family members and other staff members often have far more contact with clients and provide more ongoing support. If family members and staff members are not supportive, and if they contribute to a high-stress environment, it works *against* the progress made in the social skills group. A critical or demanding environment provides few opportunities for clients to practice skills and receive positive feedback. Even if the group leaders conduct an effective social skills group, their work can be undone by the environment. Yet a supportive environment both inside and outside the group contributes to optimal acquisition and generalization of skills.

CHARACTERISTICS OF SUPPORTIVE STAFF MEMBERS AND FAMILY MEMBERS

Knowledge of Schizophrenia, Behavioral Management, and Social Skills Training

It is very important for family members and staff members to be well informed about the illness of schizophrenia, especially in regard to symptoms and how they affect behavior. Understanding the illness-related reasons for clients' difficulties can help staff members and family members respond more empathically and equip them to develop more effective strategies for overcoming the difficulties. For example, recognizing that the cognitive impairments due to the illness can make it difficult for the client to understand complex language gives family members the necessary insight to reword requests more simply and repeat important information. Understanding that the positive symptoms of the illness (such as auditory hallucinations) can be very distracting helps staff members to think of strategies for increasing clients' concentration in groups. Finally, knowing that the negative symptoms of schizophrenia include decreased motivation helps family members to be more patient and supportive with their relative who is starting a new activity.

The supplemental reading list in Appendix A contains several publications that staff members and family members can read to learn about the illness.

It is useful to keep some basic texts, such as *Understanding Schizophrenia* (Keefe & Harvey, 1994), *Coping with Schizophrenia: A Guide for Families* (Mueser & Gingerich, in press), and *Surviving Schizophrenia* (Torrey, 2001), easily available as references. Chapter 1 of this book also contains specific information that can be helpful to staff members and family members about how schizophrenia contributes to difficulties in social skills.

It is also helpful when all staff members are well informed about the basic principles of behavioral management and the philosophy of social skills training. *Behavior Modification: What It Is and How to Do It* (Martin & Pear, 1996) contains useful chapters about defining behavior, getting a behavior to occur more often with positive reinforcement, decreasing a behavior with extinction, and getting a new behavior to occur by shaping.

Chapter 4 of this book contains definitions and examples of social learning principles, including modeling, reinforcement, shaping, overlearning, and generalization, as well as the techniques for conducting social skills training.

Behavioral Family Therapy for Psychiatric Disorders (Mueser & Glynn, 1999) describes the methods for using social skills training with families that include a mentally ill member and provides educational handouts about several mental illnesses, including schizophrenia and schizoaffective disorder. "Social Skills Orientation for Professionals," a handout in Appendix A, provides a short overview of social skills training. In addition to reading about the aforementioned topics, staff members should be kept informed about specific social skills training groups that are being conducted at their facility by attending ongoing staff training meetings (addressed in more detail later in this chapter).

Use of Good Communication Skills

It is important for staff members to use good communication and problem-solving skills themselves. There are two main reasons for this. First, staff members and family members who use good communication skills serve as positive role models for clients. The more opportunities clients have to observe effective social skills in others, the better they can learn the skills. Second, using good social skills helps staff members and family members communicate with clients in a clear, direct manner, with less probability of misunderstanding or causing conflict. When staff members and family members use good communication skills with each other, it contributes to better working relationships and promotes teamwork. Part II of this book contains an extensive curriculum of social skills that can be used to improve communication. In addition, Table 10.2 provides suggestions for skills that are especially useful in communicating with clients: getting to the point, expressing feelings directly, using praise effectively, checking out what the client thinks or feels, and being clear and specific.

It is also important to avoid certain types of communication that commonly lead to stress and tension with clients who have schizophrenia. Table 10.3 lists some examples of pitfalls to supportive communication; staff members and family members who avoid these pitfalls will be rewarded by fewer arguments and a calmer atmosphere for all concerned.

Staff members and family members who can manage conflict effectively contribute greatly to a less stressful environment. Conflicts that stem from disagreements and misunderstandings are frequent sources of stress to clients with schizophrenia. Using the communication skills provided in Table 10.2 and avoiding the pitfalls in Table 10.3 can help prevent some conflicts. To resolve a conflict, however, it is usually best to address it as soon as possible, staying calm, speaking clearly, and paying attention to both sides of the conflict. In addition, it is helpful to avoid blame or criticism, to use short, clear statements, to highlight the main points, and to focus on specific behaviors rather than on

TABLE 10.2. Guidelines for Communicating with Clients

Get to the point
- Clearly state your topic or concern.
- Use direct, simple language.
- Keep it brief.

Express feelings directly.
- Use "I" statements.
- Make verbal feeling statements.
- Speak in a calm voice.
- Don't assume the client will know how you feel if you don't tell him or her.

Use praise effectively.
- Make eye contact.
- Tell the client specifically what he or she did that pleased you.
- Use an "I" statement to say how it makes you feel.

Check out what the client thinks or feels.
- Listen carefully; don't rush the client.
- Ask questions when you don't understand.
- Repeat what you heard and ask whether that is what the client meant.
- Ask more questions, if necessary.

Be clear and specific.
- Avoid long sentences and introductions to topics.
- Make direct requests that specify exactly what you would like the client to do.
- Concentrate on one topic at a time.

TABLE 10.3. Pitfalls to Supportive Communication

Communication problem	Example of nonsupportive statement	Alternative statement
Coercive statements ("shoulds")	"You *should* know when lunch is served."	"I would appreciate it if you would come to lunch at 12:30."
Mind reading	"You're angry because your friends forgot to visit."	"You look angry. Are you feeling that way?"
Making "always" or "never" statements	"You never take your medicine as you're supposed to."	"I'm concerned that you did not take your medication this morning."
Giving orders	"Pick up your clothes right this minute."	"I would appreciate it if you could pick up your clothes from the floor before breakfast."
Put-downs, sarcasm	"You re so lazy."	"I was disappointed that you did not take out the garbage last night."
Mixing positive and negative	"You're dressed OK, but your hair is a mess."	"I like your new outfit today."

Note. Adapted from Mueser and Gingerich (in press). Copyright Guilford Publications. Adapted by permission.

personality or attitudes. Using the skills of Making Requests, Compromise and Negotiation, Leaving Stressful Situations, and Solving Problems (see curriculum in Part II) can help staff and family members resolve conflicts in some instances. Informal problem solving, using the basic principles but not necessarily the specific steps of the Solving Problems skill, can also be helpful.

Ability to Prompt and Reinforce Use of Skills

Members of a social skills group are better able to generalize skills they have learned in the group to other settings when they receive support and encouragement from people outside the group. The most important support is provided by staff members or family members who prompt clients to use specific social skills in situations that arise in their natural surroundings and who praise them for using a skill or attempting to use one. An instance of prompting occurs when a staff member notices a client who is starting to get into an argument and reminds him, "This would be a good time to practice Expressing Angry Feelings the way you've been learning in social skills group." If the client does not remember how to express an angry feeling, the staff member can review the steps of that skill. If the client attempts to use the skill, the staff member can reinforce the effort by saying something such as "I like the way you stayed calm in expressing your feelings, and how you were specific about what Sam did that upset you." The more often clients are encouraged to practice the skills they are learning in group, the more likely they will be able to use them spontaneously in real-life situations. Helping clients complete their homework assignments is a structured way of helping them use their skills in situations outside the group.

Working as a Team

Teamwork and sharing responsibility are very important in minimizing stress in the environment. Schizophrenia is a very complex and confusing illness, whose symptoms can lead to unpredictable and even alarming behavior. If most of the responsibility for managing clients falls on too few people, it will become burdensome and stressful for those few. When family members or staff members are under significant stress, clients are aware of it and find it distressing. However, when the responsibility is shared and when people know that they can count on each other's help, it is less burdensome and stressful. In community residences, inpatient programs, and day treatment centers it is helpful to explicitly divide the tasks among staff members in each shift and rotate tasks that are particularly difficult (for example, waking up clients who prefer to keep sleeping). In promoting teamwork, it is also useful to have clear guidelines to follow in certain key situations, such as responding to aggressive behavior. When guidelines are well known in the residential or treatment setting, staff members can minimize confusion about what to do and can concentrate instead on dealing with the situation. In the home setting, it is also useful for family members to divide responsibilities and to have a plan of action about what to do in situations such as symptom exacerbation (Falloon et al., 1984; Falloon, Laporta, Fadden, & Graham-Hole, 1993; Mueser & Glynn, 1999).

CHARACTERISTICS OF A SUPPORTIVE LIVING SITUATION

Structured but Not Overtaxing Routine

Because the symptoms of schizophrenia may result in a client's internal experience of the world being quite confusing, it is helpful if the client's external environment is organized and predictable. A daily routine that strikes a balance between understimulation and overstimulation is important in preventing both excessive withdrawal and overexcitement. Therefore, it is beneficial to have periods of organized activities interspersed with unstructured time for clients to relax and unwind. The amount of time spent on organized activities should be adapted to clients' cognitive capacities to avoid overtaxing them. For example, many clients are able to work several hours per week, but not more than 2 hours at a stretch. It is also critical to monitor the client's symptoms and functioning over time so that scheduled or structured activities can be flexible and responsive to clinical changes. For example, if a client who usually enjoys trips to the zoo has an increase in hallucinations one day, it would be important to explore with the client whether a trip to the zoo would be helpful or whether it might exacerbate this symptom.

Reasonable House Rules

The presence of realistic house rules at home or at a residential setting contributes to reducing stress in the environment. Research has shown that people with schizophrenia often lack an understanding of the unwritten rules that govern much social behavior (Penn, Corrigan, Bentall, Racenstein, & Neman, 1997). Explicit household rules can help compensate for clients' lack of social judgment by making clear what is expected and what is not allowed. If there is a lack of clarity about expectations, it can result in unpredictable behavior, frequent arguments, and high levels of stress. Because all settings are different, the house rules should be tailored to individual needs and requirements and should be kept to a minimum so that it is not an effort for clients to remember them. However, there are certain fundamental rules related to ensuring the safety of people and property and preventing disruptive, socially unacceptable, or illegal behavior. An example of six basic house rules is included in Table 10.4.

TABLE 10.4. Basic House Rules

- No violence to people or property.
- No inappropriate touching.
- Smoking is permitted only in designated areas.
- Bathe and shower regularly.
- No illegal drug use.
- Everyone must do some chore(s) to help in the running of the house.

Note. Adapted from Mueser and Gingerich (in press). Copyright Guilford Publications. Adapted by permission.

IMPROVING STRESS MANAGEMENT
IN THE CLIENT'S ENVIRONMENT

Recognizing the Signs of Stress

Recognizing the sources of stress, as described earlier, helps staff members and family members to take preventive action. However, it is also important to recognize the signs indicating that stress is already affecting the client. These can include changes in *physical state* (headaches, muscular tension, indigestion), *thinking* (difficulty in concentrating or paying attention), *mood* (irritability, anxiety) and *behavior* (pacing, nail biting). In addition, clients with schizophrenia may experience an increase in the symptoms of their illness, such as more hallucinations or delusions, when they are under stress. Most clients show a combination of signs in response to stress. When staff members and family members recognize the stress response pattern of the individual client, they can begin to help him or her to manage the stress. Many clients are unaware of their own patterns and benefit greatly from the feedback of others.

Reducing the Sources of Stress

When staff members and family members are familiar with what clients find stressful and the signs of stress, they can help the clients to reduce the stress to which they are exposed. To help clients avoid unnecessary stress, it may be useful to consider situations that have been stressful in the past. Although it is undesirable to avoid *all* stress, inasmuch as this would interfere with taking on new roles and activities, some situations that have caused excessive stress in the past can be avoided or modified. For example, if a client became tense and agitated when he or she went home for 4 days at Thanksgiving, staff and family members may suggest abbreviating the next holiday visit to make it more manageable. Or if living with a messy roommate consistently irritates an orderly client, a change of roommates may be advised.

A common source of stress that can often be reduced are expectations that are too high. If a client finds volunteering five mornings a week to be too much of a strain, perhaps the activity can be reduced to two or three mornings per week. Another common source of tension that can be addressed is an understimulating environment. Doing nothing all day, and having no activities to look forward to and that provide meaning in life, can be just as stressful as having too much to do and being exposed to too many demands.

Working with a client to increase his or her scheduled activities can reduce a client's experience of stress due to understimulation. Getting a part-time job, going to a local peer support program, joining a local club in the community, attending a day program, taking a class, or scheduling regular physical exercise (such as taking a walk, swimming, or bowling) can decrease stress, increase a sense of well-being, and give the client something to look forward to. Some clients also enjoy activities such as going to the movies, taking a van ride, doing arts and crafts, or eating out.

Communicating Directly

As mentioned earlier in this chapter, it is very important for staff members and family members to communicate clearly and directly with clients. This is especially important when the client is under stress. For example, if a client is experiencing stress in beginning a new job, it is helpful for a staff member to express direct interest in the responsibilities of the job, to ask questions about which aspects the client finds stressful, and to help the client engage in problem solving to reduce any stress he or she may experience.

In addition, it is helpful to encourage clients to communicate directly about stressful situations, which often provides some immediate relief. The longer clients keep feelings to themselves, the more likely it is that their emotions will be released in an inappropriate way, such as through social withdrawal, arguments, aggressive behavior, or self-destructive behavior. When clients talk about their feelings as they arise, the process itself can prevent stress from building up.

Direct discussions also give staff members and family members an opportunity to suggest ideas for dealing with a stressful situation. For example, if a client is able to express that he or she is experiencing stress from increased auditory hallucinations, a staff member or relative can suggest some coping strategies, such as increasing distraction from the voices and consulting with the physician regarding a medication evaluation. Not all clients volunteer information about their feelings; it is important to inquire gently about what they are experiencing. For example, a staff member might say, "I noticed that you missed 3 days of your program this week; how have you been feeling?" However, if the client prefers not to talk about feelings, he or she should not be pressured to do so.

Sometimes talking to a single staff member or family member is not sufficient to help a client reduce his or her stress level. If the client is experiencing a severe amount of stress, it may be helpful to get together with others who are familiar with the client to discuss the situation and explore possible solutions to the problem that is causing the stress. This meeting should include the client, when possible, as well as relatives and staff members from other agencies who are well acquainted with the client and/or may have the resources to implement certain solutions. For example, residential staff members often find it useful to include a client's case manager in such meetings because he or she coordinates several aspects of the client's care and knows what resources might be available. It is important that such meetings use the basic principles of problem solving (see Appendix A) and focus on solutions. Family members often benefit from holding family meetings in which they and the client work together on solving problems (Falloon et al., 1984; Mueser & Glynn, 1999).

Helping Clients Reframe Their Thoughts

Some clients are able to reduce stress by reframing their thoughts about a situation. The more negatively clients view particular situations, the more stress they experience. When they respond with negative, self-defeating thoughts such as "This is awful, I can't stand it," or "I'm going to crack under this pressure," it tends to make the situation worse. However, they may be better able to deal effectively with the situation when they can replace self-defeating thoughts with more positive self-talk, which includes making coping-oriented statements to themselves, such as "I'll do my best," "I can deal with this," and "I am strong enough to handle this." Staff members and family members can coach clients explicitly on using positive self-talk and can help develop simple phrases that work well for them. They can then remind the clients of the phrases when they note that the clients are showing signs of stress. For example, a family member might tell a client, "It seems like the voices are bothering you more today; try saying, 'These voices are annoying, but I can ignore them,' as we talked about last week."

Using Relaxation Techniques

Learning simple relaxation techniques such as deep breathing exercises and progressive muscle relaxation is helpful to some clients. These methods of stress reduction require a staff member or family member to teach the steps of the skill to the client and to encourage him or her to practice the technique regularly. Relaxation techniques are best taught when the client is relatively calm; they are generally not effective if they are introduced in the middle of a crisis. Although there are many books and classes available for learning relaxation techniques, some are too complicated to use with clients. It is preferable to choose techniques that have clear instructions, are not too time-consuming to practice, and can be used in a variety of settings (Davis, Eshelman, & McKay, 1995; McKay & Fanning, 1987). Clients are often receptive to learning a deep breathing exercise, such as the one in Table 10.5.

Clients may also be encouraged to develop their own approach to relaxation, including choosing relaxing images or selecting music or recordings of nature sounds to accompany their imagery. The specific technique used to relax is not important. Rather, the point of relaxation is for the client to set aside time to calm down and relax in a way that works best for him or her.

Managing the Stress Level of Staff Members and Family Members

Finally, it is important for staff members and family members to be aware of their own stress levels. Working with people with schizophrenia can be quite stressful; it is very common for staff members and family members to feel overwhelmed. Stress in staff or family

---

TABLE 10.5. Deep Breathing Exercise

1. Make yourself comfortable, sitting in a chair or on a couch with good back support.
2. Breathe deeply through your nose and out from your mouth, approximately 10 times.
3. Notice the way your chest fills with air as you inhale, then empties when you exhale.
4. As you breathe deeply, silently repeat a calming word or short phrase such as "Relax," "Unwind," or "At ease" as you exhale. Do this about 30 times, but do not worry about exact counting.
5. Think of standing under a waterfall or shower; imagine the water washing away feelings of tension.
6. Begin to breathe normally again. Concentrate on your breathing.
7. Sit quietly for a minute or two before returning to activity.

Note. Adapted from Mueser and Gingerich (in press). Copyright Guilford Publications. Adapted by permission.

members may be reflected by negative communication patterns, such as criticism, hostility, speaking in a loud voice, or in other ways, such as tension, body language, facial expression, or frequent worrying. The experience of tension or stress in staff or family members can be passed on to clients, either directly (via communication) or indirectly. The techniques described earlier for clients (communicating directly, reframing thoughts, using relaxation techniques) can also help others in contact with a client to cope more effectively with tension and stress. In addition, it is helpful for them to give each other a break when the pressure becomes too great. Taking a little time away from the situation can be relaxing and can give people new perspectives and renewed energy for dealing with their responsibilities.

DEVELOPING A SOCIAL LEARNING MILIEU IN A RESIDENTIAL OR INPATIENT PROGRAM

Rationale

Some inpatient and residential settings have succeeded in creating a milieu in which social learning and skills training are strong components of the philosophy of treatment and are woven into nearly every aspect of the staff members' interaction with clients. Two factors are vital to the success of such a milieu.

First, support from the administrative, departmental, and supervisory levels of the setting is critical (Corrigan, 1995). Without the backing of professionals at the upper levels, it is very difficult to schedule social skills groups, to encourage the cooperation of staff members, and to free up time for staff members to attend social skills groups and training sessions. However, if the administrators and supervisors provide strong backing for a social skills program, there is a high likelihood of success. One of the best ways to ensure such backing is for group leaders to arrange regular meetings with administrators and supervisors to discuss clients' progress in skills training and to report any problems that have been encountered. Some form of written monthly or bimonthly report containing information about the number of groups held, attendance, homework compliance, and skills acquisition can help staff members and administrators to appreciate the scope of the skills training groups and to track clients' progress in these groups.

Second, the participation of all staff members is crucial. The social skills training group sessions provide a good beginning for clients to learn skills, but, as we have previously emphasized, most of the work of putting those skills into practice goes on outside the group. On-line staff members, who usually have the most contact with clients, need to be familiar with the skills being taught, to recognize opportunities for clients to use the skills, and to help clients with their homework assignments. Social skills programs without the support of on-line staff members are unlikely to succeed.

Training On-Line Staff Members

One of the first steps for bringing a social learning focus into the general milieu is to teach all staff members the general principles of social skills training: social learning theory, modeling, practice, positive and corrective feedback, and generalization to the natural environment. It is helpful for the group leaders to conduct a workshop (or series of workshops) explaining and demonstrating social skills training for all staff members who have contact with clients. After the introductory training, group leaders should continue staff training on a regular basis. An effective model of ongoing training involves weekly meetings with staff members who represent each shift. Each representative staff member is expected to report back to others on his or her shift about what was discussed at the meeting and to return with feedback and questions from coworkers. In this model of staff training, all of the meetings follow a similar format, as shown in Table 10.6.

At staff training meetings, it is important for staff members to understand that they are learning something that will help them to do their jobs more effectively and with less stress. The agenda must be flexible enough to respond to staff members' concerns about other clinical issues related to their work with clients. Staff members often have questions about how to respond effectively when clients are delusional, noncompliant, verbally abusive, or difficult to motivate. The group leaders who conduct staff training can give suggestions about which skills the staff members can encourage the clients to use and which skills staff members themselves can use in specific problematic situations. For example, when staff members report that clients blame them for things they did not do, the staff members could be directed to use the skill of Responding to Untrue Accusations. When clients are reluctant to do their household chores, staff members can be advised to try Making a Request, followed by Expressing Positive Feelings when clients do even a portion of their tasks. When clients curse the staff members, they can be directed to use the skill of Ex-

---

TABLE 10.6. Format of Staff Training Meetings

1. Review last week's homework assignment.
   - Thank staff members for their assistance.
   - Engage in problem solving to help clients who did not complete their assignments.

2. Discuss the social skill that was taught at the last group.
   - Hand out copies of the steps of the skill.
   - If it is a new skill, model an example of how it can be used.
   - Ask staff members to engage in brief role plays of the skill.

3. Hand out homework assignments for practicing the current skill in the clients' environment.
   - Review instructions.
   - Answer questions about assignment.

4. Discuss opportunities for clients to practice the new skill.
   - Elicit ideas from staff members about situations in which the clients could use the skill.
   - Suggest how staff can prompt clients.
   - Remind staff members of the importance of providing positive feedback for any efforts.
   - If necessary, role play examples of prompting and providing feedback.
   - Anticipate any difficulties in completing the homework.

5. Discuss general problems that staff members experience in managing clients.
   - Suggest ways that the social skills model can be used to address the problems.
   - Provide information about schizophrenia and other behavioral techniques as needed.

6. Elicit ideas for social skills that clients would benefit from learning in future groups, including skills not yet developed.

pressing Unpleasant Feelings. When necessary, new skills can be designed specifically for staff members, using the principles described in Chapter 6.

When staff members attend training on a regular basis, they become familiar with the social skills perspective and terminology and begin to approach problems with the question "What skills would be most effective to use in this situation?" As staff members begin to speak the same language as the social skills leaders, the clients receive a consistent message and have multiple sources of prompting and positive feedback for using their social skills. Staff members also find that by using social skills themselves and by prompting clients to use skills, they are better equipped to deal with difficult situations, which helps them do their jobs more effectively and with less stress.

Displaying Social Skill Materials

As part of creating a social learning milieu, it is helpful to post copies of the skills being taught in the group. For example, staff members can post copies of the current skill on the central bulletin board. Copies of skills that are relevant to ongoing issues (e.g., Eating and Drinking Politely) can be permanently posted in the appropriate areas. Copies of all the social skills contained in the curriculum in Part II should also be available to all staff members.

Some residences also find it useful to post attendance charts in the room where the group is held so that clients and staff members can see at a glance who has been attending.

Encouraging Client Attendance at Social Skills Training Groups

As mentioned in Chapter 5, it is important to schedule social skills training groups at a time when clients are most likely to attend. Having the group be a fixed part of the week's schedule is very helpful. In addition, staff members need to reduce the chances that the group will conflict with another activity that the clients want to attend or are required to attend.

For example, if outings, medical appointments, or cigarette breaks are scheduled at the same time as the social skills group, there may be a disincentive to attend the group. Clients benefit from regular attendance; missing even occasional group sessions causes them to lose momentum and to get out of the habit of attending.

To ensure the continuity of the skills training group, it is also important that groups are not canceled when a leader is sick or on vacation. It is very useful to have a backup leader or to have another staff member act as co-leader when one of the leaders is unable to attend.

Providing Consistent Positive Feedback and Constructive Suggestions in Day-to-Day Interactions

Positive feedback is one of the most powerful tools for shaping the behavior of clients. Sometimes staff members think that praising the clients will spoil them or that it is unnecessary because people should know when they've done something right. Some staff members think that their responsibility is to point out incorrect or inappropriate behavior, rather than to help clients learn more appropriate alternatives. Helping staff members understand that positive feedback is more potent in changing behavior than negative feedback is an important goal for social skills leaders. When clients are praised for something they have done, it not only boosts their self-esteem, it also increases the probability that the behavior will be repeated. Staff members and family members need to be adept at the skills of Expressing Positive Feelings and Giving Compliments (see Part II). It is especially important to be specific, by telling the client exactly what he or she did that was pleasing. For example, a staff member might tell a client, "I really liked the way you cleared the table without being asked. I was very pleased." Staff members need to be alert to instances when the client does something well and should be generous with positive feedback.

Of course, clients may also behave in ways that are inappropriate or offensive. In such cases, staff members and family members need to provide constructive feedback (see guidelines in Appendix A). First, it is important to find something to praise, even if it is a small aspect of the client's behavior. For example, if a client loudly demands his or her hourly cigarette instead of requesting it politely, a staff member might still be able to give positive feedback for asking at the appropriate time. Clients appreciate hearing that they haven't done *everything* wrong. Second, focus on only *one* aspect of the client's behavior that needs improving, even if he or she has done several things incorrectly. If more than one error is pointed out, clients often begin to tune out or have difficulty pinpointing what they did wrong. Be specific and brief about the actual behavior that was a problem. Third, avoid critical language (e.g., "You know that's the wrong way to ask for a cigarette"). Finally, make a brief suggestion for how the client can improve his or her behavior. For example, a staff member might say, "I liked the way you asked for your cigarette at the time we agreed on; I would appreciate it if you could ask me for your cigarette in a quiet voice, though." The most effective suggestions for improvement avoid the word *should* and use simple, direct language that does not require the client to guess what he or she is expected to do.

SPECIAL CONSIDERATIONS FOR FAMILY MEMBERS

Research has shown that family members can be very helpful in creating a supportive environment for their ill relative (Dixon et al., 2001; Gingerich & Bellack, 1995; McFarlane, 2002), especially if they receive support and accurate education about the illness. Family members often have a special rapport and strong relationship with the client that professionals cannot hope to duplicate. However, family members also experience additional pressures. For example, family members who provide care for an ill relative cannot leave at the end of their shift, unlike the staff of a residential program. Schizophrenia is an illness that is poorly understood by the general public, and for this reason many family members feel isolated and stigmatized by having an ill relative. It may be hard to find people who understand their situation and the problems they are dealing with. Family members often feel that they have little time for friends or other activities because all their time is taken up with managing the illness (Lefley, 1996; Marsh, 1996). It is difficult to provide a supportive environment for the client when they are under such stress.

Before family members can provide support to their ill relative, they must take care of their own needs and get adequate support for themselves. One way for family members to receive more support is to share responsibilities for caring for their ill relative. One family member cannot do everything; teamwork is very important. When several family members are involved, it is easier to take breaks and to pursue friendships and hobbies that they all enjoyed before their relative developed schizophrenia. Another way for families to get support is to seek out community resources and services, such as psychosocial clubhouses, consumer-run drop-in centers, vocational programs, or day programs for their ill relative. Clients may need to be encouraged to attend community programs, both for their own socialization needs and for their family members' needs.

Many family members benefit greatly from the support offered by organizations such as the National Alliance for the Mentally Ill (NAMI), which is the largest self-help and advocacy organization in the United States for relatives of persons with a psychiatric disorder (2101 Wilson Boulevard, Suite 302, Arlington, VA 22201, 703-524-7600; it also has a Help Line at 800-950-6264). Each state has a chapter, and many communities also have their own chapters. NAMI is an excellent source of up-to-date information about the illness of schizophrenia and current treatment strategies. It also provides a very good way to meet other family members who have similar experiences, both at the monthly meetings of the local chapters and at the annual conventions of the national organization. One of the greatest stresses that family members report is feeling that they are all alone, that they are isolated in their experience. Belonging to an organization such as NAMI helps people to realize that there are many others who are in a similar situation, who understand what they are going through, and who might be able to offer suggestions for each other's problems.

SUMMARY

A supportive environment, both inside and outside the social skills training group, is essential for clients to learn and generalize new skills. The most important factors in a supportive environment are staff members and family members, the physical setting, the level of structure, and stress management.

The presence of supportive staff members and family members who are knowledgeable about schizophrenia and its treatment, who use good communication skills themselves, and who prompt and reinforce appropriate social skills, is extremely beneficial to clients. The manner of communication is especially important; staff members and family members should avoid giving orders, making critical or hostile comments, and speaking in ways that are indirect or confusing to clients.

The physical setting also contributes to the climate of support; it should be safe, provide adequate privacy, be relatively quiet, and be in good condition. In the setting, reasonable house rules, a structured but not overtaxing routine, and a predictable schedule help to reduce sources of stress for the client. When stressors do occur, they should be handled in a supportive manner, using strategies such as empathic listening, problem solving, and encouraging clients to use relaxation techniques or participate in recreational activities.

In addition to helping clients deal with stress, residential settings can develop a social learning milieu where social skills training is a strong component of the rehabilitation philosophy of treatment and is woven into nearly all aspects of the staff members' interaction with clients. The milieu is most effective when all staff members receive ongoing training in the principles of social learning, when written materials about social skills are available and on display in the living environment, when clients are encouraged to attend the skills groups, and when staff members provide consistent positive feedback and constructive suggestions to clients regarding their use of social skills.

11

Parting Tips for Social Skills Training

In the preceding chapters we have provided an extensive explanation and description of social skills training and provided instructions and materials for conducting skills groups. The technique is fairly straightforward, and a clinician who has some facility at working with people with schizophrenia should have little difficulty mastering the intervention. However, some points need to be reiterated, and a few others need to be considered in order to maximize results.

1. *Teaching social skills is teaching, not group psychotherapy.* Most people working in mental health became interested in the field because they wanted to help people, and it is generally assumed that the way to help is through some form of verbal psychotherapy. Regardless of the specific brand, these approaches all assume that conversation about emotionally important issues is a central ingredient for change. That is absolutely *not* the case with social skills training. This is an educational, skill-building procedure. Conversation is a vehicle to transmit information and make people feel comfortable with one another, not to teach behavioral skills. As previously indicated, a piano or tennis instructor does not bring a group of students together to *talk* about striking the piano keys or the tennis ball and discuss how the students *feel* about it. The participants in social skills training are often willing to discuss their problems; sometimes they prefer talking to working at learning. Nevertheless, talking and self-exploration are issues for other groups. The leader must make up his or her mind before beginning as to whether he or she will be conducting a social skills group or doing a little social skills training in the course of a more open-ended verbal psychotherapy. The former is the only way to really develop complex new behaviors. We suggest that the leader bring a check sheet with him or her to each session, in which the lesson plan is outlined, and that at least 45 minutes of each 60-minute session be devoted explicitly to the plan (i.e., role playing and modeling). We have found that using this type of imposed structure is the only way to achieve the goals of social skills training. The remaining time at the end, after the work is done, can be used for discussion, coffee and cookies, medication

checks, or any other clinically or socially useful activity. However, learning is work, and work is done first or it tends not to be done at all.

The level of planning and organization implied in Point 1 is particularly important for effective teaching. Prepare written materials (handouts and poster boards) in advance, come to sessions with a set of role-play scenarios already prepared, and stick as closely as possible to the script. When we suggest doing two to three role plays with each member we *mean* two to three brief role plays with each member—not one or two, sprinkled with conversation and differing wildly in content or length. Keep in mind that role plays are not vehicles to stimulate discussion *about* social situations or to rehearse a single, long-winded, idiosyncratic dialogue. Think of learning to serve in tennis by serving once, hitting a few volleys, talking about your grip, volleying a little, and then trying another serve, versus hitting 10 serves in a row and getting corrective feedback after each shot. Finally, keep in mind that every group is a little different. Learning to be an effective leader requires that you practice implementing the structure with different groups whose members present somewhat different challenges.

2. *Learn to do social skills training.* Doing social skills training effectively is a skill. Consequently, the leader must learn how to do it in the same way that participants learn their new social skills. That means starting slowly, practicing, and securing feedback. Where possible, it is very helpful to observe a skills group conducted by experienced skills trainers, or to watch videotapes of the process. Short of that, skill can be bootstrapped by soliciting feedback from co-leaders or supervisors who are familiar with the goals. As with all new skills, it is important to start slowly. Select easy skills to teach, work with a co-leader, and set very minimal goals. Practice *doing* skills training, and don't worry too much about the outcome. Get used to role playing and to running a structured group. Become comfortable with the role of teacher and with keeping a group on task. Keep in mind that the structure (how you teach) is much more important than the content (what you teach). Most neophyte leaders function as if the opposite were true and spend too much time talking.

3. *Don't work in isolation.* In all likelihood, each of the participants in your groups will be receiving antipsychotic medication, have a case manager, and (potentially) one or more therapists, in addition to the group leaders. Keep in touch with your colleagues. Find out when the client has been put on a new medication or has received a major change in dosage. Learn how he or she is doing in other settings—Is this a particularly bad time for the client? Is he or she showing prodromal signs of relapse? Of special note is the issue of whether the member is giving you a hard time, which he or she is not giving others, or vice versa. Similarly, what is going on in the person's life outside the treatment center? Are there conflicts at home? Do you need to be in touch with family members or residence managers to ensure that the member's new skills are being reinforced, or to teach a specific skill needed to avoid conflict in the home (e.g., the member is fighting with a sibling or housemate, and you can teach a skill to alleviate the conflict). As a general rule, generalization of the effects of training will be enhanced to the extent that the skills you teach are (a) relevant to the person's immediate environment and (b) reinforced by the environment.

4. *Never, never underestimate the cognitive deficits of your members.* We have previously highlighted the problems people with schizophrenia face in memory, attention, and higher-

level problem solving. This is one of the most important and most difficult points for most clinicians to understand. Clients with schizophrenia who are asymptomatic can appear to maintain lucid conversations, seem to learn and understand well, and respond affirmatively to questions about whether they understand. We have regularly observed such apparently well-functioning clients nod appropriately to instructions, parrot the leader's role-played responses, and yet be totally unable to generate an appropriate response when the situation is slightly changed. Whether they don't remember, are easily distracted, or are so concrete that they can't transpose ideas from situation A to situation B, they often lack the capacity to learn from continuities across situations. The only solutions to this dilemma that we have found to be effective are (a) to impose as much structure as possible and minimize demands on abstraction (use prompts and handouts, identify simple commonalities across situations for the person to focus on, and keep instructions very, very simple and straightforward); and (b) to practice, practice, practice (the more automatic the response is in situation X, the less the demand on working memory and analysis). Finally, do not ask your participants whether they understand: Have them demonstrate! Similarly, do not preach or lecture. Keep your instructions brief, and always use visuals (handouts, posters) for *anything* you want them to remember. Finally, keep role plays brief and narrowly relevant to what you are trying to teach. It is typical of new leaders to get caught up in role playing, staying in a role too long and leading the interaction far from the few specific points the participant is supposed to practice. The longer the role play lasts, the greater the likelihood that the participants will forget what they are supposed to be focusing on.

5. *Although the subject is not directly related to social skills training, keep in mind that your members will be at high risk for HIV and AIDS.* The techniques used for teaching safe sex and low-risk behaviors are very similar to the techniques described in this book for social skills training. We advise all social skills training leaders to consider including an HIV unit if members are not already learning the material elsewhere. Moreover, given the learning and motivational problems faced by individuals with schizophrenia, a refresher course would be appropriate even if they have had prior instruction. Training materials are readily available from the National Institutes of Health, the National Institute on Drug Abuse, the Centers for Disease Control and Prevention, and other federal agencies. Useful Internet sources include www.nih.gov and www.nida.gov.

6. *Be positively reinforcing.* It is natural for most of us to tell others what they have not done or what they have done wrong when we are giving instructions. A key to making this intervention work well is to be consistently positive and reinforcing. Some new skills trainers interpret this caveat to mean that they must be bubbly and effusive and praise everything. To the contrary; a laid-back style will work fine as long as participants hear that they doing OK and that you and the other group members approve. Most people with schizophrenia have long histories of failure and frustration. Social skills training is one place that they can be assured of success because (a) the level of demand is geared to their capacity, not some abstract or unreachable standard, and (b) communications are always positive, emphasizing what they have done well, not what they have done poorly.

Even difficult group members (and some are difficult) can be controlled without much negativity and censure if the leader can focus on rules and the situation, rather than the person's bad behavior. The following brief examples illustrate how a group leader can phrase comments to help a client reduce unwanted behavior: (a) "It is important that we don't make fun of one another here. Fred, if you are having trouble not laughing when Jon tries to talk, maybe you would like to take a brief break"; (b) "Steve, Susan may find it distracting when you touch her during group; why don't you come over here and sit next to me. Then it will be easier for you not to touch her." Remember, you can't lose your temper, be sarcastic, or speak in an angry tone of voice and still be an effective teacher. Group members will turn off or, if they are really testing you, will be reinforced for their inappropriate behavior. Of course, everyone must feel safe, including the leaders. If a member is really posing a threat, he or she should be asked to leave, and the overall positive tone must be temporarily suspended.

7. *Be persistent.* We believe that this manual provides all of the information needed for you to conduct effective skills training groups. However, we have not said it is easy. The leaders must do more homework for skills training than for other treatments in order to be adequately prepared. The intervention can be fun for both leaders and participants, but everyone works hard. There is no sitting back and letting others do all the work. It may often seem easier to just talk about something or move on to a new topic, rather than repeat the same role play for what seems like the umpteenth time. Nevertheless, remember our tennis and music analogies. It's like the old joke: How do you get to Carnegie Hall? Practice, practice, practice.

Part II

STEPS FOR TEACHING SPECIFIC SOCIAL SKILLS: CURRICULAR SKILL SHEETS

OVERVIEW OF SOCIAL SKILLS CURRICULAR SKILL SHEETS

FOUR BASIC SOCIAL SKILLS

Core social skills are the basic building blocks on which effective communication is based. These social skills include the ability to listen to other people (and to let them know you are listening), to make requests of others in a positive and diplomatic fashion, and to express feelings to other people, including both positive and negative feelings. Because these skills are important for a wide variety of social situations and are not limited to close personal relationships, all clients who participate in social skills training benefit from learning and reviewing core social skills. With some individuals, extensive practice of core social skills is critical to helping them achieve their personal goals.

<u>SKILL</u>: Listening to Others

<u>RATIONALE</u>: Whenever you are in a conversation, it is important to show the other person that you are listening, that you are paying attention. When the other person can tell you are listening, he or she is more likely to want to continue talking to you. There are some specific things you can do to show your interest to the other person.

<u>STEPS OF THE SKILL</u>:

1. Look at the person.
2. Let him or her know that you are listening by either nodding your head OR saying something like "Uh-huh" or "OK" or "I see."
3. Repeat back what you heard the other person saying.

<u>SCENES TO USE IN ROLE PLAYS</u>:

1. Listening to someone who is talking about a favorite hobby.
2. Listening to someone who is talking about a favorite TV show.
3. Listening to a staff member who is talking about the rules at the community residence.
4. Listening to your doctor telling you about your medication.
5. Listening to a friend talk about a recent outing.

<u>SPECIAL CONSIDERATIONS WHEN TEACHING THIS SKILL</u>:

1. Role plays should be set up using two people: One person talks about a topic, while the person who is practicing the skill follows the steps.
2. Clients often have difficulty paying attention when someone is speaking to them. It is important to keep the role plays short (30 seconds or less) and simple when first practicing the skill.

SKILL: Making Requests

RATIONALE: In anyone's life, situations come up where it is necessary to ask another person to do something or to change his or her behavior. A request that is heard as a demand or as nagging usually does not make the other person want to follow through with the request. Making a request in a positive way, however, is usually less stressful and is more likely to lead to the request being met. There are no guarantees, of course, but a request usually goes better if you keep in mind the following points.

STEPS OF THE SKILL:

1. Look at the person.
2. Say exactly what you would like the person to do.
3. Tell the person how it would make you feel.
   In making your request, use phrases like:
   "I would like you to _____."
   "I would really appreciate it if you would do _____."
   "It's very important to me that you help me with _____."

SCENES TO USE IN ROLE PLAYS:

1. Ask someone to go to lunch with you.
2. Ask someone to help you with a chore or an errand.
3. Request a counselor to talk about a problem.
4. Ask your friend to borrow his or her music tape.
5. Ask someone at the day program to turn down his or her radio.

SPECIAL CONSIDERATIONS WHEN TEACHING THIS SKILL:

1. It is important to tailor this skill so that the higher-functioning clients do not get bored. Therefore, it is helpful to elicit specific situations in which a client may have wanted to make a request but was unable to.
2. For lower-functioning clients, it is helpful to suggest just one phrase, such as "I would appreciate it if you would _____," to use when making a request.
3. Remind clients that although a request made in this manner is most likely to lead to receiving the request, it does not guarantee that the request will be granted.

<u>SKILL</u>: Expressing Positive Feelings

<u>RATIONALE</u>: When people have encountered a series of difficulties, they tend to focus on the problems around them and forget to notice the positive things that other people do. Noticing positive things helps to increase a person's sense of belonging and sense of being able to do things well. Moreover, a person who knows he or she is doing something well is more likely to repeat what he or she has done to please others.

<u>STEPS OF THE SKILL</u>:

1. Look at the person.
2. Tell the person exactly what it was that pleased you.
3. Tell him or her how it made you feel.

<u>SCENES TO USE IN ROLE PLAYS</u>:

1. A staff member at the community residence cooked a meal you enjoyed.
2. A friend helped you out with a problem.
3. A counselor woke you up so that you would be on time for an appointment.
4. A family member gave you a ride to an outside appointment.
5. A coworker at your new job ate lunch with you.

<u>SPECIAL CONSIDERATIONS WHEN TEACHING THIS SKILL</u>: Sometimes clients may protest that it is not necessary to say positive things because people already know when they are doing something nice. Group leaders can remind clients that *everyone* likes it when someone has appreciated something that he or she has done.

SKILL: Expressing Unpleasant Feelings

RATIONALE: Even when people do their best to please each other, there will be times when things are displeasing or unpleasant. It is only natural in the course of living with other people and going to programs with other people that unpleasant feelings arise. Examples of unpleasant feelings are anger, sadness, anxiety, concern, and worry. How people express their feelings can help to prevent arguments and more bad feelings. It is helpful to keep certain things in mind when expressing an unpleasant feeling.

STEPS OF THE SKILL:

1. Look at the person. Speak calmly and firmly.
2. Say exactly what the other person did that upset you.
3. Tell the person how it made you feel.
4. Suggest how the person might prevent this from happening in the future.

SCENES TO USE IN ROLE PLAYS:

1. Your roommate left dirty clothes in the living room.
2. Your case manager missed an appointment with you.
3. You are worried when your roommate is out later than expected.
4. Your family canceled a weekend visit.
5. Your friend was late meeting you for lunch.

SPECIAL CONSIDERATIONS WHEN TEACHING THIS SKILL: This skill requires that group members identify an unpleasant feeling (Step 3). However, not all members will be able to do this. It is helpful in the first session of teaching this skill to generate a list of unpleasant feelings. The list can be written on a flipchart and placed where it can be seen when group members are role playing.

CONVERSATION SKILLS

Conversational skills involve the ability to initiate, maintain, and end conversations with others in a friendly, rewarding, and socially appropriate fashion. Human beings are social creatures, and the ability to converse easily and without anxiety is crucial to well-being and a sense of social connection with others. People with schizophrenia often lack adequate conversational skills, in part because of slower information-processing speed and difficulties in identifying interesting topics, resulting in social interactions with others that are frequently awkward. Good conversational skills are critical for establishing friendships and other close relationships, as well as for getting along with coworkers in the workplace. For many people with schizophrenia, training in conversation skills is aimed both at increasing the frequency of interactions with others and improving the quality of those interactions. Because good conversational skills require the ability to track and spontaneously respond to the other person, including changes in topics and nonverbal hints, competence at conversational skills often requires many months of training. Although extensive practice is needed for many people to become comfortable in conversing with others, there are many opportunities to practice conversational skills with a wide variety of people.

SKILL: Starting a Conversation with a New or Unfamiliar Person

RATIONALE: There are many situations in which you want to start a conversation with another person. This may be someone you don't know well or someone you have never met but would like to get to know. Sometimes people feel shy about starting a conversation. We find that things go more smoothly when you keep specific steps in mind.

STEPS OF THE SKILL:

1. Choose the right time and place.
2. If you do not know the person, introduce yourself. If you know the person, say "Hi."
3. Choose a topic that you would like to talk about OR ask a question.
4. Judge whether the other person is listening and wants to talk.

SCENES TO USE IN ROLE PLAYS:

1. A new person is starting at the day program.
2. People are waiting for an activity to begin at the community residence or the day program.
3. You are at a family gathering.
4. You are sitting with another person at lunch.
5. You are meeting your new case manager for the first time.

SPECIAL CONSIDERATIONS WHEN TEACHING THIS SKILL:

1. Steps 1 and 4 require the client to make judgments regarding the appropriate time and place to begin a discussion, as well as whether the person being addressed is interested in participating. Therefore, it is important for group leaders to spend time assisting clients with the identification of social cues they can look for when making such judgments.
2. Clients may need assistance in identifying topics of conversation. Group leaders may want to generate a list of topics with the group that can be used for starting a conversation.

SKILL: Maintaining Conversations by Asking Questions

RATIONALE: Sometimes you may want to go further than a brief conversation; you may want to talk longer with someone because you like the person or are interested in what is being said. Often, people don't know how to keep a conversation going, or they feel uncomfortable. One way to keep a conversation going is by asking questions.

STEPS OF THE SKILL:

1. Greet the person.
2. Ask a question about something you would like to know about.
3. Judge whether the person is listening and is interested in pursuing the conversation.

SCENES TO USE IN ROLE PLAYS:

1. Watching a TV program with another person who also seems to enjoy the program.
2. Seeing your roommate after he or she has spent a day with his or her family.
3. Having a cup of coffee with a friend at the day program.
4. Sharing a chore (such as cleaning up after dinner) with someone.
5. Talking to a counselor about a supported employment program.

SPECIAL CONSIDERATIONS WHEN TEACHING THIS SKILL:

1. Clients may have difficulty in determining what kinds of questions are socially appropriate to ask in different situations. Group leaders can use the role-play scenes to help clients identify socially appropriate questions to ask in various situations. For example, group leaders can ask clients to generate a list of questions that would be appropriate to ask a friend with whom they are having coffee *before* role playing the scene so that they have some options to choose from.
2. Group leaders need to distinguish "general" questions from those that are more specific. Providing the group with examples of the two types of questions will be useful.
3. Group leaders may need to assist members with the identification of social cues required in Step 3.

SKILL: Maintaining Conversations by Giving Factual Information

RATIONALE: Asking questions is one way to keep a conversation going. Another way is to give factual information to the other person. This allows people to learn more about each other and the kinds of things they might have in common. Factual information is the kind of information that tells someone who, what, where, when, and how.

STEPS OF THE SKILL:

1. Greet the person.
2. Share some information about a topic you would like to discuss.
3. Judge whether the other person is listening and is interested in pursuing the conversation.

SCENES TO USE IN ROLE PLAYS:

1. Telling someone at the community residence about an outing planned for the weekend.
2. Telling a friend about a movie or TV show you saw recently.
3. Telling a counselor or a staff member about what you discussed in group.
4. Telling someone about an article you read in the newspaper.
5. Telling a staff person about a meal you liked at a restaurant.

SPECIAL CONSIDERATIONS WHEN TEACHING THIS SKILL:

1. Group leaders should use the role-play scenes to help members identify information that is appropriate to give in each situation used. Group leaders can discuss with members the importance of being discriminating with the type of information they provide in a given situation. For example, personal information that would be appropriate to provide to a counselor during a therapy session would not be appropriate to discuss with an acquaintance in a social setting.
2. Group leaders may need to assist members with the identification of social cues required in Step 3.

<u>SKILL</u>: Maintaining Conversations by Expressing Feelings

<u>RATIONALE</u>: Giving factual information is one way to keep a conversation going. Another way is to tell someone how something makes you feel. This allows people to learn more about each other's feelings and whether they may have more in common to talk about. Examples of feelings that might be expressed are happy, sad, excited, disappointed, pleased, upset, and irritated.

<u>STEPS OF THE SKILL</u>:

1. Greet the person.
2. Make a brief statement about how something makes you feel.
3. Judge whether the other person is listening and is interested in pursuing the conversation.

<u>SCENES TO USE IN ROLE PLAYS</u>:

1. Telling a staff member that you don't like your assigned chore at the community residence.
2. Telling your case manager that you enjoyed the last group.
3. Telling a family member that you are excited about going to the movie this weekend.
4. Telling a staff member that you are disappointed that a day program party was canceled.
5. Telling a friend that you liked a TV program last night.

<u>SPECIAL CONSIDERATIONS WHEN TEACHING THIS SKILL</u>:

1. Group leaders should assist members with generating a list of different feelings that people might want to express to each other.
2. Group leaders should also assist members with identifying situations that they are likely to encounter when expressing feelings would be appropriate.
3. Group leaders may need to assist members with the identification of social cues required in Step 3.

SKILL: Ending Conversations

RATIONALE: Conversations don't go on forever. Sooner or later someone must end a conversation. Many times it may be up to you to end the conversation. There are many reasons for ending a conversation, including running out of time, needing to go somewhere else, or running out of things to say. You can end conversations more smoothly if you keep certain steps in mind.

STEPS OF THE SKILL:
1. Wait until the other person has finished speaking.
2. Use a nonverbal gesture such as glancing away or looking at your watch.
3. Make a closing comment such as "Well, I really must be going now."
4. Say, "Good-bye."

SCENES TO USE IN ROLE PLAYS:
1. Talking about a TV show with someone at the community residence, but it becomes time for the evening group.
2. Finishing lunch with another person at the day program, but it becomes time to meet with your counselor.
3. Talking with a friend before group starts.
4. Talking with a new person at your drop-in center, and you run out of things to say.
5. Talking with a friend during breakfast, and it's time to go to work.

SPECIAL CONSIDERATIONS WHEN TEACHING THIS SKILL: Clients may not be aware of how the use of nonverbal gestures can either help make a social interaction run more smoothly or make it more awkward. A brief group discussion regarding how to utilize nonverbal gestures can be quite helpful. If a client still does not understand how to use nonverbal gestures, skip Step 2 and go to Step 3.

SKILL: Entering into an Ongoing Conversation

RATIONALE: There are times when everyone wants to enter into a conversation that is in progress. There may be interesting topics people are discussing or a desire to share an opinion or perhaps just a need to be part of a group. We have found that many people have difficulty knowing exactly how to do this in a way that will not interrupt the "flow" of the conversation. We have found that using the following steps is helpful when attempting to enter into a conversation that is in progress.

STEPS OF THE SKILL:

1. Wait for a break in the flow of the conversation.
2. Say something like "May I join you?"
3. Decide whether the people engaged in the conversation are OK with your joining in.
4. Say things related to the subject of the conversation.

SCENES TO USE IN ROLE PLAYS:

1. You are at a party and are interested in joining in on an ongoing conversation.
2. You are at your day program and overhear several people talking about last night's baseball game. You also saw the game and want to join their conversation.
3. At your clinical case conference it seems as though everyone but you is discussing your goals. You want to share your ideas about new goals.
4. You are having dinner with your family members, and they are discussing different options for a summer vacation. You have some ideas and would like to share them.
5. Friends are deciding what movie to see, and you want to make a suggestion.

SPECIAL CONSIDERATIONS WHEN TEACHING THIS SKILL:

1. This skill requires that clients be able to read body language so as to make judgments about when it is appropriate to enter into an ongoing conversation. Before teaching this skill, it will be helpful for group leaders to review the importance of body language as well as practice reading body language. Group leaders can model different types of body language while having a conversation and encourage group members to decide whether it would be appropriate to join in. For example, it would not be appropriate to enter into a conversation if the people talking look serious or upset.
2. This skill also requires that clients make decisions about when to enter into a conversation. Some group members will have difficulty judging when there is a break or pause in the conversation. Therefore, it will be useful for one group leader to spend time engaging one or two clients in a conversation while the rest decide when there is a pause or break in the conversation.

SKILL: Staying on the Topic Set by Another Person

RATIONALE: Whenever you are in a conversation with another person, it is important to show that you are paying attention to what is being said. Being able to stay focused on the topic being discussed demonstrates to the person that you are listening and are interested in what is being said.

STEPS OF THE SKILL:

1. Decide what the topic is by listening to the person who is speaking.
2. If you do not understand what the topic is after listening, ask the person.
3. Say things related to the topic.

SCENES TO USE IN ROLE PLAYS:

1. A staff member at the community residence talks to you about the new chore list.
2. A counselor at the day program is talking to you about a new group that has started.
3. A friend talks to you about a movie he or she has seen.
4. Your roommate talks to you about painting your room a new color.
5. Your doctor is talking to you about eating healthful foods.

SPECIAL CONSIDERATIONS WHEN TEACHING THIS SKILL:

1. This skill has two specific tasks: identifying the topic and saying things related to the topic. Group leaders may need to focus on only one of the tasks per role play when working with clients who have difficulty concentrating.
2. Group leaders should begin each role play by clearly stating what the topic is. For example, they should begin by saying something like "I want to talk to you about _____," and then repeat key words throughout the role play.

SKILL: What to Do When Someone Goes Off the Topic

RATIONALE: Having a conversation with another person requires that both people understand what the topic is. Understanding the topic allows both people to contribute to the discussion, which then makes it more meaningful for both of them. Sometimes, however, we find ourselves in a situation in which the other person suddenly has gone off the topic being discussed, leaving us feeling confused. When this occurs, it is best to immediately let the other person know that we are confused and then to try to get back to the original topic.

STEPS OF THE SKILL:

1. Say something like "That's interesting; can we talk about that after we finish this discussion?"
2. If the person has forgotten what the topic is, politely remind him or her.
3. Judge whether the other person is still interested in the original topic.
4. If the other person is interested, continue the discussion. If he or she is not interested, politely end the conversation or talk about something new.

SCENES TO USE IN ROLE PLAYS:

1. You are in the middle of a discussion with a friend about a movie you both saw, when your friend suddenly starts talking about the weather.
2. You are telling your mother about the new job you just started, when your mother starts to tell you about your cousin who just enlisted in the army.
3. Your case manager is discussing with you the progress you have made at the supported employment program, when she is interrupted by a phone call. After the call, she returns to the conversation with you and starts discussing when you and she can go shopping for a coat for you.
4. Your roommate asks you for directions to the museum. As you start to tell him the directions, he suddenly changes the topic to shopping.
5. You are having lunch with a friend who is telling you about a TV program she saw last night, when, in the middle of her description, she starts to tell you about a new person she just met.

SPECIAL CONSIDERATIONS WHEN TEACHING THIS SKILL:

1. Some clients may find it difficult to tell the other person that they do not understand because they feel as though they are being rude. Group leaders can help clients practice polite ways to interrupt a conversation.
2. This skill is very useful when dealing with a person who is symptomatic and is having difficulty concentrating.

SKILL: Getting Your Point Across

RATIONALE: There are times when we all have something we want to talk about or explain to others. Being able to get your point across in a clear and concise manner is an important component of effective communication. It makes it easier for others to understand and respond to what you are saying.

STEPS OF THE SKILL:

1. Decide on the main point you want to get across.
2. Speak in short sentences and stay on the topic.
3. Pause to let the other person speak or ask questions.
4. Answer any questions.

SCENES TO USE IN ROLE PLAYS:

1. You tell a friend the best place to buy a pair of sneakers.
2. You tell a staff member that you want to start to hold your own cigarettes.
3. You tell your new roommate at the community residence how the chore assignments work.
4. You suggest to a family member a place you would like to go on an outing.
5. You explain to your case manager that you are bored at the day program.

SPECIAL CONSIDERATIONS WHEN TEACHING THIS SKILL: Group leaders can discuss with clients the importance of staying calm and speaking in a clear voice that is not too loud or too soft when trying to make a point. For example, group leaders can discuss how it is more likely that a person will not be listened to when he or she is yelling and agitated. Therefore, in order to be understood, it is important to be in reasonable control of one's feelings.

SKILL: What to Do When You Do Not Understand What a Person Is Saying

RATIONALE: Situations often come up in which we do not understand what someone has said to us. Maybe the person was speaking too quickly, or used words that we didn't understand, or even said too many things at once. There are also are times when we may be distracted and find it hard to concentrate on what the person is saying. Whatever the reason, it is better not to pretend that we understand when we really don't understand. Using the steps of this skill will help you to clear up any misunderstandings you may have about what has been said.

STEPS OF THE SKILL:

1. Tell the person that you are confused or that you did not understand what was said.
2. Ask the person to repeat or explain what was just said.
3. Ask further questions if you still do not understand.

SCENES TO USE IN ROLE PLAYS:

1. Your job coach has described some new tasks you will be expected to do. You are not sure that you understand everything your job coach has said.
2. You have asked a staff member to give you directions to go downtown, but have difficulty understanding the directions because the staff person talked very quickly.
3. Your doctor has prescribed new medication for you and explained how it will help to make you feel better. You are not sure you understand.
4. Your case manager at the day program has explained to you about a new group she will be conducting. She has an accent and speaks very quickly, so you missed a lot of what she was saying.
5. Your teacher at the vocational rehabilitation center is giving a lecture on improving interviewing skills and is using words you do not understand.

SPECIAL CONSIDERATIONS WHEN TEACHING THIS SKILL:

1. This skill can be used to help clients who are symptomatic and are finding it difficult to follow conversations.
2. Group leaders can help clients generate a list of strategies to improve understanding, including asking the other person to slow down or to speak more loudly.

ASSERTIVENESS SKILLS

Assertiveness is the ability to forthrightly state what one wants, express one's feelings directly (especially negative feelings), and to resist the efforts of others to get one to do something that one does not want to do. Most people find that being assertive (or "sticking up for one's rights") is challenging in at least some situations, but people with schizophrenia experience even greater difficulties with these skills. Some of these problems may be due to a desire to please others, to avoid conflict, not being sure of what one really wants, or just not knowing how to say "no." Thus, part of teaching assertiveness skills involves helping clients recognize what they do and what they do not want in particular social situations.

Clients with schizophrenia often require extensive practice in assertiveness skills before they become comfortable expressing themselves to others. Common situations that clients encounter that require good assertiveness skills include interacting with friends, family members, doctors (and other members of the treatment team), coworkers, and supervisors. When learning assertiveness skills, clients often benefit from discussing what are realistic expectations or demands of other people and what are not. Clients who have difficulty determining when it is appropriate to be assertive benefit from discussing common social situations and getting feedback from other group members. Finally, it may be desirable to inform some other people who interact with the clients, such as treatment team members or family members, about work on assertiveness skills so that these individuals can support appropriately assertive social skills, rather than discourage these efforts.

SKILL: Refusing Requests

RATIONALE: We can't always do what other people ask us to do. We may be too busy, or not feel capable, or may believe that what is being asked is unreasonable. If we refuse in a rude or gruff manner, it can make for hurt feelings or anger. Yet if we are not clear about refusing or if we speak in a hesitant way, it may lead to a misunderstanding or argument.

STEPS OF THE SKILL:

1. Look at the person. Speak firmly and calmly.
2. Tell the person you cannot do what he or she asked. Use a phrase such as "I'm sorry but I cannot _____."
3. Give a reason if it seems necessary.

SCENES TO USE IN ROLE PLAYS:

1. Your case manager asks to meet with you at 3:00 P.M., but you already have an appointment.
2. A friend asks you to go to a basketball game, but you don't like basketball.
3. Your roommate asks you to pick up some groceries, but you're feeling tired.
4. A friend asks you to lend him or her money, but you are broke.
5. Your counselor asks you to help prepare dinner, but you have plans to watch a special TV show.

SPECIAL CONSIDERATIONS WHEN TEACHING THIS SKILL:

1. It is important for the group leaders to remind clients that there are some situations in which a request is made of them when refusing would be inappropriate, such as when a staff person asks the client to complete his or her assigned chore or follow a safety rule.
2. There are also instances when refusing a request may result in some harm to the client. Situations such as the client's refusing to take medication or go to the doctor need to be handled delicately, because the consequences can be severe. In these instances, it may be helpful to encourage clients to use the skill Compromise and Negotiation instead of Refusing Requests.

<u>SKILL</u>: Making Complaints

<u>RATIONALE</u>: A number of unpleasant situations can be avoided by expressing yourself clearly and making requests in a positive way. However, situations often arise in which something displeasing does happen. At those times you need to make a complaint. Making a complaint usually works best if you can also suggest a solution.

<u>STEPS OF THE SKILL</u>:

1. Look at the person. Speak firmly and calmly.
2. State your complaint. Be specific about what the situation is.
3. Tell the person how the problem might be solved.

<u>SCENES TO USE IN ROLE PLAYS</u>:

1. You lose money in a vending machine.
2. Someone interrupts you when you are speaking.
3. You order a cheeseburger, but the waitress brings a plain hamburger.
4. You buy a bus pass, and the clerk gives you the wrong change.
5. Someone in a nonsmoking area lights up a cigarette.

<u>SPECIAL CONSIDERATIONS WHEN TEACHING THIS SKILL</u>:

1. This skill requires that a group member be able to identify possible solutions *before* stating a complaint. Group leaders should encourage group members to brainstorm possible solutions before a role play is practiced so that the participants have an idea of what solution they will propose ahead of time.
2. Group leaders can remind members that this is the best way to make a complaint, but there are no guarantees that the solution they suggest will be carried out.

<u>SKILL</u>: Responding to Complaints

<u>RATIONALE</u>: As careful and considerate as you might try to be, there will be times when someone has to make a complaint to you. For instance, you accidentally bump into someone or you forget an appointment. If you get upset when someone complains to you, it only makes the situation worse. Following the steps of the skill will help you respond in a calm manner.

<u>STEPS OF THE SKILL</u>:

1. Look at the person and remain calm.
2. Listen to the complaint, keeping an open mind.
3. Repeat back what the person said.
4. Accept responsibility and apologize if necessary.

<u>SCENES TO USE IN ROLE PLAYS</u>:

1. Someone complains to you that you interrupted him or her.
2. Someone complains to you that you lit up a cigarette on the bus.
3. Your case manager complains that you are late for your appointment.
4. Your counselor at the community residence complains that you have not done your weekly chores.
5. Your roommate complains that your music is too loud.

<u>SPECIAL CONSIDERATIONS WHEN TEACHING THIS SKILL</u>: There may be some group members who have a difficult time remaining calm while listening to a complaint being lodged against them. Therefore, it may be helpful for group leaders to discuss strategies for managing angry feelings. For example, taking a time-out or counting to 10 may be a useful strategy to employ in certain situations.

SKILL: Expressing Angry Feelings

RATIONALE: A type of feeling that many people have special difficulty expressing is anger. At times everyone gets angry. This does not have to lead to shouting or hitting or cutting off friendships or relationships. It is usually helpful to relieve feelings of anger by expressing yourself in a direct, honest way. Sometimes you might want to wait until you have "cooled off" a little and are feeling calm.

STEPS OF THE SKILL:

1. Look at the person; speak firmly and *calmly*.
2. Tell the person specifically what he or she did that made you angry. Be brief.
3. Tell the person about your angry feelings. Be brief.
4. Suggest how the person might prevent the situation from happening in the future.

SCENES TO USE IN ROLE PLAYS:

1. Dinner is late every night for a week.
2. Your roommate smokes in the room, which is against house rules.
3. Your relative promises to cash your check by Friday but does not do so.
4. Someone spills coffee on your new white slacks without apologizing.
5. Someone borrows your radio without asking and breaks it.

SPECIAL CONSIDERATIONS WHEN TEACHING THIS SKILL:

1. Many group members have a particularly difficult time expressing angry feelings, even in the context of a controlled role play. It is therefore important to devote some time "preparing" group members for this skill. Spending one or two sessions helping members identify common "early warning signs" of anger (such as feeling tense, heart racing, etc.), as well as strategies for managing angry feelings (one of those strategies being the skill at hand), will be extremely useful.

2. Depending on the composition of the group, it may be helpful to divide this skill into three parts and practice each part as a separate role play. The first part would encompass Steps 1 and 2; the second part would encompass Step 3; and the third part would encompass Step 4. Not all members will need the skill divided in this way, but for those who are having some difficulty, this allows them to have positive role-play experiences while practicing the skill.

From *Social Skills Training for Schizophrenia* (2nd ed.) by Alan S. Bellack, Kim T. Mueser, Susan Gingerich, and Julie Agresta. Copyright 2004 by The Guilford Press. Permission to photocopy this skill sheet is granted to purchasers of this book for personal use only (see copyright page for details).

SKILL: Asking for Information

RATIONALE: There are many times when people need to ask others for information. People ask for information about directions, how to do certain tasks, to explain something that they just read. The list of things to inquire about is endless. Often people feel awkward or apologetic about asking for information and therefore choose not to ask. It has been our experience that things go much better when we have all the information we need and that in most cases people are more than happy to share with you what they know.

STEPS OF THE SKILL:

1. Use a calm and clear voice.
2. Ask the person for the information you need. Be specific.
3. Listen carefully to what the person says.
4. Repeat back what he or she says so that you understand what has been said.

SCENES TO USE IN ROLE PLAYS:

1. Asking a staff member about what public transportation to take downtown.
2. Asking your counselor about how to use the washing machine.
3. Asking a sales clerk at a clothing store about where the jeans are.
4. Asking your case manager about applying for a work training program.
5. Asking your doctor about side effects of your medication.

SPECIAL CONSIDERATIONS WHEN TEACHING THIS SKILL:

1. This skill requires that the client make a judgment about who might be an appropriate person to approach for information. Not all clients will be able to do this. Therefore, it may be helpful for the group leaders to get clients to identify an appropriate person to approach *before* they role play.
2. Group leaders can point out that this skill is especially useful when clients find themselves in situations in which they need assistance or information.

<u>SKILL</u>: Letting Someone Know That You Feel Unsafe

<u>RATIONALE</u>: All of us at some time in our lives feel unsafe. Sharing our fears with someone we trust usually makes things feel less scary. That person may have suggestions that will help you cope with feeling unsafe or that will help you change the situation you are afraid of.

<u>STEPS OF THE SKILL</u>:

1. Choose a person you trust to speak to.
2. Tell that person what is making you feel unsafe. Try to be *specific* about your fears.
3. Ask the person for advice.

<u>SCENES TO USE IN ROLE PLAYS</u>:

1. You tell your case manager that you feel unsafe at the day program.
2. You tell your staff member that you feel unsafe in large crowds and do not want to go on the planned outing.
3. You tell your roommate that you feel unsafe walking in the neighborhood at night.
4. You tell your family member that you feel unsafe around a new person who has come to live at your residence.
5. You tell your doctor that you feel unsafe taking the new medication prescribed.

<u>SPECIAL CONSIDERATIONS WHEN TEACHING THIS SKILL</u>: This skill requires that the client make a judgment about who might be an appropriate person to trust. Not all clients will be able to identify people whom they trust. Therefore, it may be helpful for group leaders to get clients to identify people they might be able to trust in different situations *before* role playing.

SKILL: Asking for Help

RATIONALE: Most people, at one time or another, find themselves in situations they cannot handle on their own, situations in which they need to ask for help from others. Often people feel uncomfortable or shy about asking for help. It has been our experience that in most cases people are more than willing to provide help when asked.

STEPS OF THE SKILL:

1. Choose a person whom you feel you can trust.
2. Use a calm and clear voice.
3. Tell the person what you need help with. Be specific.
4. Listen carefully to what the person suggests.
5. Thank the person for his or her help.

SCENES TO USE IN ROLE PLAYS:

1. You are having trouble completing an application for a volunteer job.
2. You just bought an item for your room and realize that it is too heavy to carry on your own.
3. You have taken the subway downtown and suddenly realize that you have gotten off at the wrong stop and now you are lost.
4. You are walking down the street, and someone steals your wallet or purse.
5. You are taking a walk and you trip and sprain your ankle. You realize that you will not be able to walk all the way home.

SPECIAL CONSIDERATIONS WHEN TEACHING THIS SKILL:

1. This skill requires that a client make a judgment about who might be an appropriate person to approach for help. Not all clients will be able to make this judgment.. Therefore, it may be helpful for the group leaders to elicit from clients who (e.g., friend, staff member) or what groups of people (e.g., police, local store owners) are safe to ask for help.
2. It may be helpful for group leaders to identify situations in which clients have needed help in the past and/or may need help with in the future. Making a list of these situations on a flipchart is often useful.

SKILL: Responding to Unwanted Advice

RATIONALE: There are times when we find ourselves in the uncomfortable position of receiving unwanted advice. This advice usually comes from a person who knows you well (e.g., a good friend or family member), who believes he or she has your best interest at heart. Unwanted advice can also come from a person you don't know very well, such as an acquaintance at your day program or even a stranger. Many people are uncomfortable with responding to this type of advice, especially when it comes from a friend or family member. We have found that there are some specific steps you can keep in mind that can be helpful when you are faced with unwanted advice.

STEPS OF THE SKILL:

1. Politely acknowledge the advice given.
2. Express appreciation for the person's concern.
3. Tell the person that you will think about it, and then change the subject.
4. If the person persists, let him or her know that you are not interested in the advice.

SCENES TO USE IN ROLE PLAYS:

1. A friend tells you to stop taking your medication.
2. A family member tells you not to look for a job.
3. A friend tells you that using a little marijuana won't hurt you.
4. Your roommate tells you that the shirt you are wearing looks bad on you and suggests another shirt to wear.
5. A housemate tells you that it is OK to skip your assigned chores.

SPECIAL CONSIDERATIONS WHEN TEACHING THIS SKILL:

1. This skill may be especially difficult for two sets of clients: those who are used to "going along" with things just to keep the peace and avoid conflict and those who receive the advice from a friend or family member and do not want to upset that person or hurt his or her feelings. It is therefore important to spend some time discussing what specific concerns clients have, and then address those concerns.
2. It may also be helpful to review the skill Disagreeing with Another's Opinion without Arguing to help clients remember that they can disagree with another person while not hurting that person's feelings.

CONFLICT MANAGEMENT SKILLS

The ability to handle conflict with other people is a complex and critical skill for most aspects of successful living, including enjoying close relationships with others and being effective at the workplace. Conflict management skills, which overlap with assertiveness skills, are helpful for people with schizophrenia, who often have difficulty in handling interpersonal conflict. Common reactions to conflict include withdrawing from the situation or simply denying that the conflict exists. Such coping strategies may provide temporary relief, but often worsen the situation in the long run, as the conflict remains unresolved.

An important part of teaching conflict resolution skills is teaching clients how to understand and respond to the other person's viewpoint, as well as how to give their own. Showing another person that you understand his or her perspective demonstrates understanding and regard for that person and can reduce anger and hostility on both sides. Active listening skills, such as rephrasing what the other person has said, are extremely helpful in resolving conflict and can be learned with frequent practice. There are many social situations clients face that involve potential conflict, which can be a focus of skills training. Common situations include relationships with family members and friends, negotiating treatment decisions with one's psychiatrist or other treatment team member, dealing with problems with coworkers or supervisors at the workplace, and dealing with inpatient or residential staff members. In addition to soliciting possible conflict situations from clients themselves, information from other people with whom clients have regular contact may be valuable as to what conflict situations clients experience.

<u>SKILL</u>: Compromise and Negotiation

<u>RATIONALE</u>: Often, people find that they disagree with each other, even when they want to do something together. At these times it is helpful to work out a compromise. In a compromise, each person generally gets some of what he or she wants, but usually has to give up something. The goal is to reach a solution that is acceptable to all involved.

<u>STEPS OF THE SKILL</u>:

1. Explain your viewpoint briefly.
2. Listen to the other person's viewpoint.
3. Repeat the other person's viewpoint.
4. Suggest a compromise.

<u>SCENES TO USE IN ROLE PLAYS</u>:

1. You want to go to lunch with your friend at the pizza parlor. He or she does not want pizza that day.
2. Your case manager asks you to schedule an appointment for 2:00 P.M. on Wednesday. You have plans to go on a day program outing at that time.
3. You and your friend want to go see a movie. You want to see an action movie, and your friend wants to see a comedy.
4. In planning an outing for the Community Residence, the counselors suggest bowling. You would rather go out for ice cream.
5. You want to visit your family next weekend. They have other plans.

<u>SPECIAL CONSIDERATIONS WHEN TEACHING THIS SKILL</u>: Not all clients will understand what it means to negotiate and come to a compromise. Therefore, it is important that the group leaders spend time explaining these concepts *before* beginning a role play. For example, to negotiate something, both parties have to state what it is that they want to get out of the interaction. Once all the wishes have been listed, both parties must review the list and decide upon a compromise. A compromise usually occurs when both parties get *some* of what they wanted.

SKILL: Leaving Stressful Situations

RATIONALE: There are times when we find ourselves in situations that we consider stressful. For instance, when others criticize us or when we do something that another does not like. Often, remaining in situations that are stressful only makes us feel worse and at times may even aggravate the situation. It often happens that leaving until you have calmed down and then dealing with it afterward is the most productive way of managing a stressful situation.

STEPS OF THE SKILL:

1. Determine whether the situation is stressful (i.e., tune in to your thoughts, feelings, and physical sensations).
2. Tell the other person that the situation is stressful and that you must leave.
3. If there is a conflict, tell the person that you will discuss it with him or her at another time.
4. Leave the situation.

SCENES TO USE IN ROLE PLAYS:

1. A relative has falsely accused you of stealing $10.00.
2. A friend is angry because you won't go to a bar with her.
3. A relative is upset because he found drugs in your room.
4. A staff member at the community residence is upset because you came home late and forgot to call and let her know.
5. Your roommate is angry because you wore his shirt without asking to borrow it.

SPECIAL CONSIDERATIONS WHEN TEACHING THIS SKILL:

1. Group leaders should assist the group in understanding Step 1 by generating a list of ways a person can tell whether he or she is feeling stressed. This is important, because many clients are not in touch with what may be stressful to them.
2. It is important to emphasize that this skill is to be used only with people whom the clients know and want to maintain a relationship with. This skill should not be used with "strangers out on the street," as it could have dangerous repercussions. For example, it would be very dangerous to use this skill if you have been approached on the street by someone who wants to rob you. In situations such as that, giving the person what he or she asks for and going for help after the person leaves is probably safer than using the skill.

SKILL: Disagreeing with Another's Opinion without Arguing

RATIONALE: Not all people with whom we come in contact will agree with all of our ideas or opinions, just as we do not agree with all of theirs. Disagreeing with another person's opinion does not have to lead to bad feelings or an argument. In fact, life would be boring if everyone had the same ideas. When you disagree with another person's opinion, things often go more smoothly if you keep certain things in mind.

STEPS OF THE SKILL:

1. Briefly state your point of view.
2. Listen to the other person's opinion without interrupting.
3. If you do not agree with the other person's opinion, simply say that it is OK to disagree.
4. End the conversation or move on to another topic.

SCENES TO USE IN ROLE PLAYS:

1. You and a friend have different opinions about a movie you just saw.
2. You and your roommate have different opinions about which musical group is better.
3. You and a staff member at the community residence have different opinions about what type of clothing looks best on you.
4. You and a family member have a different opinions about how to celebrate your birthday.
5. You and a counselor disagree about what has been the most helpful thing in getting you a job.

SPECIAL CONSIDERATIONS WHEN TEACHING THIS SKILL: It is important to emphasize that this skill is designed to be used in situations in which there are no significant consequences for having a different opinion. In situations in which there may be more serious consequences, such as disagreeing with a doctor's opinion about using medication, the skill Compromise and Negotiation should be employed. There may also be situations in which any kind of disagreement may cause a strong or even violent reaction, such as when encountering a political or religious extremist. In these situations, Leaving Stressful Situations may be a more appropriate skill to use.

SKILL: Responding to Untrue Accusations

RATIONALE: Most of us have found ourselves in situations in which we have been accused of doing something that we have not done. Usually when this happens, the person making the accusation truly believes that we have committed the act and is not able to listen to reason. It is therefore important to remain calm and not get into a fight or argument when this occurs. We have found that there are some specific things you can do to help stay calm when you are falsely accused of something.

STEPS OF THE SKILL:

1. Using a *calm* voice, simply deny the accusation.
2. If the other person continues to accuse you, ask the person to stop.
3. If the person does not stop accusing you, tell him or her that you are going to ask a staff member to assist with the situation.
4. Walk away and get assistance if necessary.

SCENES TO USE IN ROLE PLAYS:

1. A housemate accuses you of stealing his or her clothes from the communal dryer.
2. A housemate accuses you of not doing your assigned chores.
3. A person at the day program accuses you of listening in on his or her conversations.
4. A staff member at the community residence accuses you of starting a fight with another resident.
5. A relative accuses you of stealing money during your last visit.

SPECIAL CONSIDERATIONS WHEN TEACHING THIS SKILL:

1. Group leaders can point out that some untrue accusations occur when someone simply has made an error, whereas other accusations are the results of symptoms of an illness. In both instances, it is important to stay calm and not get into an argument.
2. It is important to note that clients may not have access to a staff member, as referred to in Step 3. Group leaders can work with clients to generate a list of other helpful people to turn to if no staff member is available. The skill Leaving Stressful Situations may also be useful when staff members are not around.

<u>SKILL</u>: Making Apologies

<u>RATIONALE</u>: Even when people are very careful, they sometimes do things that bother or inconvenience others. Rather than ignore the situation or get into an argument over it, we have found it generally makes things go more smoothly if the person apologizes for his or her behavior as soon as possible. This is true no matter whose fault it was.

<u>STEPS OF THE SKILL</u>:

1. Look at the person.
2. State your apology: "I'm sorry for _____."
3. If realistic, assure the person that it won't happen in the future.

<u>SCENES TO USE IN ROLE PLAYS</u>:

1. Being late to group because of talking to a friend.
2. Bumping into someone while using the vending machines.
3. Interrupting someone who is talking during dinner.
4. Borrowing a CD without asking the owner.
5. Shouting at someone when you're in a bad mood.

<u>SPECIAL CONSIDERATIONS WHEN TEACHING THIS SKILL</u>: It is important to point out that apologies are appropriate even when the client did not intend to upset the other person ("I didn't know it was his CD") or when the situation was not his or her fault ("But I only bumped into him because Sandy pushed me"). Remind clients that the person who is upset will usually feel better because of receiving an apology.

COMMUNAL LIVING SKILLS

People with schizophrenia often live in close proximity to other people with severe mental illness in inpatient psychiatric settings (either short term or long term), transitional housing arrangements (as clients transition from inpatient to outpatient settings), supervised residences in the community, or even at times with family members. The close proximity to other people in these communal living arrangements can provide special challenges to people who have severe psychotic symptoms or substantial cognitive impairment. Clients can benefit from learning social skills for dealing with these common situations.

The communal living skills in this section are oriented toward helping people deal with challenging social situations encountered in living environments that include multiple people with severe mental illness, including supervised living arrangements. These skills address common situations such as being concerned that someone else has stolen something from one's room, being falsely accused by others of doing something that one did not do, responding to poor eating and drinking manners, and responding to concerns about spreading germs. Although clients may be able to articulate some of these problem situations, input from staff members is also critical. Repeated practice of communal living skills and posting the steps of the skills in common living areas can minimize the stress and tension of communal living for clients and staff members alike.

SKILL: Locating Your Missing Belongings

RATIONALE: Everyone has times when he or she cannot locate something that belongs to him or her. Sometimes we have lost the item altogether either because of carelessness on our part or because someone else has taken it. Most of the time, however, when we cannot find an item of ours, it is because we have simply misplaced it. Following certain steps can help us to search for the missing item in a systematic way that, it is hoped, will lead us to find it.

STEPS OF THE SKILL:

1. Ask yourself these questions:
   a. When did I have it last?
   b. Was there anyone around me at that time?
2. Take some time to look carefully for the item you cannot find.
3. If you still have not found the item, ask someone for help. Say something like "Have you seen my _____? I am looking for it."

SCENES TO USE IN ROLE PLAYS: Refer to item 2 under "Special Considerations When Teaching This Skill."

SPECIAL CONSIDERATIONS WHEN TEACHING THIS SKILL:

1. It is helpful if this skill is taught in conjunction with the skill What to Do If You Think Somebody Has Something of Yours, as the two usually go hand in hand. Group leaders can explain that before a person decides that someone else has his or her belonging, it is important to first follow the steps of this skill to make sure it hasn't been misplaced.
2. Group leaders can have members practice this skill by having them tell another person how they are planning to go about looking for a particular missing item.

<u>SKILL</u>: What to Do If You Think Somebody Has Something of Yours

<u>RATIONALE</u>: If you think that a person has something of yours and you would like to get it back, it is important to remain calm and talk to the person. It is not usually helpful to accuse someone, because the person will try to defend him- or herself, which makes it harder for you to get the person's cooperation. Besides, you may be mistaken about the person, and accusing him or her will undoubtedly cause bad feelings.

<u>STEPS OF THE SKILL</u>:

1. Using a calm voice, ask the person if he or she has the item. *Do not accuse the person.*
2. Listen to the person's answer.
3. If you are not satisfied with his or her answer, ask a staff person or someone you trust for help.

<u>SCENES TO USE IN ROLE PLAYS</u>:

1. Your favorite T-shirt is missing, and you think your roommate may have it because he has a habit of borrowing things without asking.
2. A friend has often told you that she loves your necklace. Recently you discover that it is missing and wonder if she has it.
3. You were sitting in the kitchen drinking a soda. You left the room briefly to use the bathroom. When you returned, you noticed that your soda was missing. There was only one other person in the room with you, so you decide to ask that person if he has the soda.
4. The wallet you left on your dresser is missing. You think a certain person living in the house who has a reputation for stealing may have taken it, and you confront him about it.
5. You think that a staff member has been keeping your mail from you and ask about it.

<u>SPECIAL CONSIDERATIONS WHEN TEACHING THIS SKILL</u>:

1. This skill should be taught after clients have practiced the skill Locating Your Missing Belongings. Clients may need to be reminded about looking carefully for their items before asking people if they have them.
2. It may be helpful for group leaders to point out that it is better not to ask someone if he or she has your item while in front of other people.

SKILL: Asking for Privacy

RATIONALE: Everyone needs privacy at some time or another. When you live with other people, it is often difficult to ask for privacy. This is especially true if you are sharing a room with another person. Therefore, it is important to learn how to ask for privacy in a respectful way.

STEPS OF THE SKILL:

1. Identify the person you need to talk to about getting privacy.
2. Choose the right time and place.
3. Explain to the person that you need some private time.
4. Tell the person of a time period when you will need privacy.

SCENES TO USE IN ROLE PLAYS:

1. You tell your roommate that you need some time alone.
2. You have come back to the residence with a friend and would like to have a private conversation. You ask staff members for some options.
3. Your case manager comes to visit, and you ask her if you can go to a coffee shop to have a private conversation.
4. You ask a staff member to meet with you privately to discuss your progress on goals.
5. You are home visiting with family and need some privacy, so you ask a family member where you can go to have time alone.

SPECIAL CONSIDERATIONS WHEN TEACHING THIS SKILL:

1. This skill may require that the person has mastered the skill of Compromise and Negotiation.
2. Group leaders should be aware that, given the space limitations at community residences, it may not always be possible for a request for privacy to be granted. Group leaders need to have in mind an alternate option for getting privacy (i.e. temporarily using another space at the residence, such as a staff office or the kitchen).
3. It is important to convey to group members that their request may not granted if staff members do not think that the person would be safe (e.g., if an individual has recently expressed feeling suicidal).

SKILL: Checking Out Your Beliefs

RATIONALE: Sometimes we think something may be true, but others disagree. It helps to check out our beliefs by talking to someone we trust. Hearing that person's point of view can be helpful. We may not change our minds, but at least we know that there is another way people might see the situation.

STEPS OF THE SKILL:

1. Choose a person you trust to talk to.
2. Tell the person what your belief is.
3. Ask the person what his or her opinion is.
4. Repeat back the opinion, and thank the person for his or her point of view.

SCENES TO USE IN ROLE PLAYS:

1. You believe that the owner of the corner store mocks you every time you buy something from him.
2. You believe that a person from the day program wants to harm you.
3. You believe that your supervisor at work does not like you.
4. You believe that one of the staff members at the community residence is angry with you.
5. You believe that you are being followed every time you leave the community mental health center.

SPECIAL CONSIDERATIONS WHEN TEACHING THIS SKILL:

1. This skill requires that the client make a judgment about who might be an appropriate person to trust. Not all clients will be able to do this. Therefore, it may be helpful for the group leaders to get clients to identify people whom they trust *before* they role play.
2. This skill can be extremely helpful to clients who are symptomatic and are experiencing disturbing delusions. It is a skill that might be most appropriate to teach when a situation arises in which a client is having delusions and is confronting other people with them.

SKILL: Reminding Someone Not to Spread Germs

RATIONALE: When people live together, it is important to be careful not to spread germs. Although people usually try to be careful about not spreading germs, sometimes they forget or they don't realize that something they are doing is likely to spread germs. When you notice that someone is doing something that is spreading germs, you can point it out by using the steps of this skill.

STEPS OF THE SKILL:

1. Look at the person.
2. Tell the person how he or she is spreading germs: *Be specific.*
3. Suggest what the person can do differently.
4. Thank the person if he or she follows your suggestion. If your suggestion is not followed, tell someone in charge.

SCENES TO USE IN ROLE PLAYS:

1. You are talking to a friend who begins to cough without covering his or her mouth.
2. You notice that your roommate seems to be leaving his or her used tissues around the bedroom.
3. The last few times you have entered the bathroom at the Community Residence, you have noticed that the toilet has not been flushed. You decide to mention this during a house meeting.
4. You are having dinner at the community residence, and another person uses your fork.

SPECIAL CONSIDERATIONS WHEN TEACHING THIS SKILL:

1. It is helpful for group leaders to spend a session having members generate a list of situations that promote the spread of germs, and another that addresses how to prevent the spread of germs, before beginning to role play.
2. Some members may be reticent to use this skill outside the group because of a concern that they may cause an argument or fight. Group leaders need to emphasize that using this skill is to be done in a polite and calm manner. It is helpful when practicing this skill to frequently remind clients that "reminding" is not the same as "yelling" or "being angry."

SKILL: Eating and Drinking Politely

RATIONALE: Many social situations involve eating and drinking. People will enjoy including us in these situations when we eat and drink politely. Many people know how to do this already, but it always helps to review the main points.

STEPS OF THE SKILL:

1. Take your time and check the temperature of the food or drink.
2. Take small bites or sips, and chew all food thoroughly.
3. Swallow what is in your mouth before speaking.
4. Use a napkin to wipe hands and mouth.

SCENES TO USE IN ROLE PLAYS: See item 2 under "Special Considerations When Teaching This Skill."

SPECIAL CONSIDERATIONS WHEN TEACHING THIS SKILL:

1. Group leaders should remind group members that the steps listed in the skill are just "main points" and should then assist them in generating a list of other components that are involved in eating and drinking politely.
2. This skill needs to be practiced with actual food and drink. If the group session already includes snacks, it is preferable to bring in special food (e.g., pie, pizza, or ice cream) to use when practicing. Group leaders provide feedback on how well the group members followed the four steps of the skill, as well as on any other component that the group identified as being important.

FRIENDSHIP AND DATING SKILLS

Close interpersonal relationships are crucial to a good quality of life for most people, as they bring human connection, acceptance, social validation, meaning, and love. However, people with schizophrenia often experience significant difficulties in establishing and maintaining close relationships with others. At the same time, increasing and improving interpersonal relationships is a common goal for many people with schizophrenia, which can improve the quality of their lives and may have positive effects on the course of their illness. Thus, many clients are highly motivated to learn these skills.

The friendship and dating skills included here require at least basic competence with conversational skills. Without some ability to initiate, maintain, and end appropriate conversations, taking the next steps toward developing friendships and dating is close to impossible. Additional work on conversational skills can also be conducted in the context of training friendship and dating skills. Although conversational skills are important for developing close relationships with others, two other skill areas may be critical for improving the quality of close relationships and maintaining those relationships over time: assertiveness skills and conflict resolution skills. Therefore, these may be important skill areas to cover either before or after teaching friendship and dating skills.

SKILL: Giving Compliments

RATIONALE: Giving specific compliments is a good way to express positive feelings. Compliments are usually given about something that can be seen, such as an article of clothing, a haircut, or a pair of shoes. Giving and receiving compliments make people feel good about each other.

STEPS OF THE SKILL:

1. Look at the person.
2. Use a positive, sincere tone.
3. Be specific about what it is that you like.

SCENES TO USE IN ROLE PLAYS:

1. Liking someone's new pair of shoes.
2. Liking the color of someone's sweater or shirt.
3. Noticing someone's new pair of jeans.
4. Noticing someone's recent haircut.
5. Liking the way someone is combing his or her hair.

SPECIAL CONSIDERATIONS WHEN TEACHING THIS SKILL: This is a good skill to review frequently. Clients usually enjoy it, and it can be a welcome break from more difficult skills, such as Expressing Angry Feelings and Compromise and Negotiation.

SKILL: Accepting Compliments

RATIONALE: In addition to being able to give compliments, it is important to be able to receive or accept compliments from others. If you accept a compliment well, people are more likely to compliment you again in the future. It is important not to minimize or undo a compliment.

STEPS OF THE SKILL:

1. Look at the person.
2. Thank the person.
3. Acknowledge the compliment by
   a. Saying how it made you feel *or*
   b. Stating your feeling about the item that was complimented.

SCENES TO USE IN ROLE PLAYS:

1. Person A tells Person B he or she likes that person's shoes. Person B accepts the compliment.
2. Person B tells person C he or she likes the color of that person's shirt. Person C accepts the compliment.
3. Person C tells person D that he or she likes that person's jeans. Person D accepts the compliment.
4. Person D tells person E that he or she likes that person's haircut. Person E accepts the compliment.
5. Person E tells person A that he or she likes that person's hair style. Person A accepts the compliment.

SPECIAL CONSIDERATIONS WHEN TEACHING THIS SKILL: This skill is best practiced in conjunction with the skill Giving Compliments. After group members have had an opportunity to practice giving compliments to the group leaders, it usually works well to go around the room and have each group member give a compliment to the person sitting next to him or her. The person receiving the compliment then has the opportunity to practice the steps for Accepting Compliments.

<u>SKILL</u>: Finding Common Interests

<u>RATIONALE</u>: One of the best ways to meet new people or develop friendships is to learn something about others. At the same time, sharing something about yourself also encourages the development of new relationships. Talking to another person about common interests that you may have is an easy and enjoyable way to learn more about each other.

<u>STEPS OF THE SKILL</u>:

1. Introduce yourself or greet the person you want to talk with.
2. Ask the person about what activities or hobbies he or she enjoys doing.
3. Tell the person about what activities or hobbies you enjoy doing.
4. Try to find a common interest.

<u>SCENES TO USE IN ROLE PLAYS</u>:

1. You want to get to know the new person at the day program.
2. You and your roommate want to do some activity together, but you do not know what each other likes.
3. You are interested in getting reacquainted with a family member who has just moved back into the area.
4. You are having lunch with a person you just met on your new job.
5. You are at a party and meet someone you would like to get to know better.

<u>SPECIAL CONSIDERATIONS WHEN TEACHING THIS SKILL</u>: After group members have spent several sessions role playing this skill and feel relatively comfortable with it, group leaders can change the format of the group to one that is less structured. Group leaders can choose a topic to discuss relating to common interests and then facilitate the discussion. Members seem better able to talk about subjects that are related to things that happened before the onset of their illness. Topics that are particularly popular include favorite TV programs watched as a child, games that you played as a child, and music that you used to listen to when you were younger.

<u>SKILL</u>: Asking Someone for a Date

<u>RATIONALE</u>: There are times when you may find yourself attracted to another person; it could be someone you have just met or perhaps someone you already know. In either case, you may want to pursue dating that person. We have found that it is a little easier to ask someone for a date if you follow the steps listed here.

<u>STEPS OF THE SKILL</u>:

1. Choose an appropriate person to ask.
2. Suggest an activity to do together.
3. Listen to the person's response and do one of the following:
   a. If the person responds positively to your suggestion, choose a day and time to get together. Be willing to compromise.
   b. If the person indicates that he or she is not interested in going out on a date, thank the person for being honest with you.

<u>SCENES TO USE IN ROLE PLAYS</u>:

1. There is a new person at your day program whom you would like to get to know.
2. You discover that you have a lot in common with a person at work and decide to ask him or her out.
3. There is a person with whom you volunteer whom you would like to get to know.
4. You are at a party at a friend's house, and you meet someone whom you would like to ask out.
5. You decide to ask your new neighbor out on a date.

<u>SPECIAL CONSIDERATIONS WHEN TEACHING THIS SKILL</u>:

1. Some clients may have difficulty identifying appropriate people to date. Group leaders should spend time before practicing the skill helping clients identify some important factors to consider when choosing a potential date. For instance, clients can ask themselves questions such as "How well do I know the person?" "Is this person available to date, or is he or she involved in a relationship?" "Is this someone who is not allowed to date me" (e.g., a staff member is off-limits)? "What things do I have in common with this person?"
2. Group leaders need to remind clients that there is always a chance that the person they are asking may refuse their invitation. It is therefore important to be prepared for that possibility. Strategies for handling a possible rejection should be identified, such as remaining calm and not getting angry at the person. Moreover, clients can always talk to a friend or someone they trust afterward and share their feelings about the incident.

SKILL: Ending a Date

RATIONALE: Dates don't last forever. Sooner or later it comes time to say, "Good-bye." There are many reasons it may be time to end a date, including completing the activity you had planned, running out of things to say, and sometimes even because you are having a bad time. Ending a date may feel awkward, but we have found that by keeping certain steps in mind, you can end a date more smoothly.

STEPS OF THE SKILL:
1. Thank the person for spending time with you.
2. If you enjoyed the date, tell the person that you would like to get together again.
3. Say, "Good-bye."

SCENES TO USE IN ROLE PLAYS:
1. It is time to end a date with a person from work. This was your first date with this person, and you had a very nice time.
2. It is time to end a date with a person whom you like very much. This has been your third date, and you are wondering how the person feels about you.
3. It is time to end a date with a person your friend fixed you up with. This was a blind date, and you did not have a very good time.
4. It is time to end a date with a person whom you like very much. You want to let the person know you had a great time, but you are not yet comfortable with kissing.
5. It is time to end a date with a person whom you have been dating exclusively for several months.

SPECIAL CONSIDERATIONS WHEN TEACHING THIS SKILL: It is customary for many people to end a date with a good-bye kiss when a good time has been had. Not everybody wants to end a date with a kiss, however. Some people prefer to just shake hands, and others are not comfortable with any physical contact. Clients will need to decide whether they want to give or receive a kiss or a handshake and then judge whether the other person is feeling similarly. Group leaders can help clients recognize clues that will help them determine how the other person is feeling so that they can make a decision as to what to do. Group leaders can also remind clients that if they are having a difficult time figuring out what the other person is feeling, they can always ask the person directly. For example, a person might say, "I had a very nice time today and would like to kiss you good-bye. Is that OK with you?"

SKILL: Expressing Affection

RATIONALE: There are times when you may find that you like someone very much and want to let that person know how you feel. Letting someone know that you care about him or her can seem awkward or even a little scary. We have found that following these few steps can help to make expressing affection go a little more smoothly.

STEPS OF THE SKILL:

1. Choose a person whom you are fond of.
2. Pick a time and place where you can be with the person in private.
3. Express affection using a warm and caring voice tone and/or by offering a warm physical gesture.
4. Tell the person why you feel this way.

SCENES TO USE IN ROLE PLAYS:

1. You have just finished a date with a person whom you like very much.
2. You have been dating this person exclusively for the past 4 months.
3. It is your grandmother's birthday, and you want to let her know how important she is to you.
4. It is Valentine's Day, and you have just received flowers from a person you have dated a few times.
5. You want to let a friend know how much he or she means to you.

SPECIAL CONSIDERATIONS WHEN TEACHING THIS SKILL:

1. Group leaders should point out at the beginning of group that this skill focuses on the verbal expression of affection. However, group leaders should use this skill as an opportunity to have a frank discussion about the physical expression of affection as well. Step 3 offers an opportunity to have this discussion.
2. This skill requires that a group member be able to identify the people to whom it is appropriate to express affection. It will be helpful for group leaders to discuss with members how to decide who is and is not an appropriate choice to express affection to.
3. Group leaders should remind group members that even when they choose an appropriate person to express affection to, their gesture may not be well received. It will be useful for group leaders to help members identify clues to look for that may indicate that the other person is uncomfortable and to know how to respond in such instances.

<u>SKILL</u>: Refusing Unwanted Sexual Advances

<u>RATIONALE</u>: Nobody should ever feel pressured into having sex when he or she does not want to. Sometimes people may feel pressured by someone they have just met, or perhaps by someone they know well or are currently dating. It is important to be able to make your feelings clearly known in a firm and direct manner.

<u>STEPS OF THE SKILL</u>:

1. Using a firm voice, tell the person that you are not interested in having sex.
2. Depending on your relationship with that person, explain why you feel that way.
3. If the person does not listen and continues to pressure you, leave the situation.

<u>SCENES TO USE IN ROLE PLAYS</u>:

1. A person you have just met wants to have sex with you.
2. A person you have been dating for the last month pressures you to have sex. You like this person a lot but are not yet comfortable with the idea of becoming sexually involved.
3. A person at the day program who frequently gives you money and cigarettes now demands that you repay him or her by having sex.
4. Your partner whom you are living with wants to have sex, but you are not feeling the same way at the moment.
5. A person with whom you work has helped you out and now tells you that you owe him or her. He or she starts pressuring you to have sex.

<u>SPECIAL CONSIDERATIONS WHEN TEACHING THIS SKILL</u>:

1. Before practicing this skill, group leaders should have a discussion with group members about the importance of never being pressured into doing something they do not want to do. Group leaders can remind group members, "If a person truly cares about you, that person will respect your decision without putting you down."
2. Some group members have a difficult time distinguishing between what is real and what is not real. It is very important for group leaders to frequently remind members that this is just a role play and then talk about why it is important to practice this skill. If a group member seems to have a difficult time distinguishing between the two, then the role play should be stopped and replaced by a general discussion about strategies for handling pressure to engage in sexual activity.

SKILL: Requesting That Your Partner Use a Condom

RATIONALE: When engaging in sexual activity, it is important to protect yourself from contracting sexually transmitted diseases. Requesting that your partner use a condom is one way to significantly reduce your risk of contracting a sexually transmitted disease. For women, it is also one important way to reduce your chances of having an unwanted pregnancy.

STEPS OF THE SKILL:

1. Choose a time and place where you and your partner can talk in private.
2. Tell your partner that you would like him to wear a condom.
3. Explain your reasons for making the request.
4. If he refuses, tell him that you will not engage in any sexual activity with him until he uses one.

SCENES TO USE IN ROLE PLAYS:

1. You want to have sex with a person you just met.
2. You want to have sex with a person whom you have been dating for the last month.
3. You want to have sex with a person whom you have been dating regularly for the last year.

SPECIAL CONSIDERATIONS WHEN TEACHING THIS SKILL:

1. It will be useful for group leaders to remind members that this request is best made before engaging in sexual activity. It is also better not to wait until the *moment* before they are about to engage in intercourse to make the request.
2. Some group members have a difficult time distinguishing between what is real and what is not real. It is very important for group leaders to frequently remind members that it is just a role play and then talk about why it is important to practice this skill. If a member seems to have a difficult time distinguishing between the two, then the role play should be stopped and replaced by a general discussion about strategies for requesting that a partner wear a condom.

<u>SKILL</u>: Refusing Pressure to Engage in High-Risk Sexual Behavior

<u>RATIONALE</u>: Engaging in high-risk sexual behavior can have serious consequences. High-risk sexual activity greatly increases your chances of contracting sexually transmitted diseases (STDs), including AIDS. Knowing how to refuse pressure to engage in high-risk sexual activities is one important step toward taking care of yourself and your health.

<u>STEPS OF THE SKILL</u>:

1. Tell your partner that you will not engage in the high-risk sexual activity.
2. Explain your reason for refusing to do so.
3. If you still want to engage in sex, suggest a different sexual activity that is safer.
4. If the person continues to pressure you, tell him or her that you need to leave.

<u>SCENES TO USE IN ROLE PLAYS</u>:

1. A person you have just met wants you to engage in a high-risk sexual activity.
2. A person you have been dating for about a month and like a lot pressures you to engage in a high-risk sexual activity. You want to have sex with this person but are not willing to put yourself at risk by giving in to his or her request.
3. Your partner, whom you have been involved with for more than a year, thinks it might be fun try something new to spice up your sex lives. Unfortunately, what he or she has in mind is considered to be a high-risk sexual activity.

<u>SPECIAL CONSIDERATIONS WHEN TEACHING THIS SKILL</u>:

1. Before practicing this skill, group leaders should have the group generate a list of sexual behaviors that are considered to carry a high risk for contracting STDs, especially AIDS. Group leaders will also need to have a discussion about how people contract AIDS and other STDs. They may also need to dispel any myths surrounding the transmission of these diseases, as well as myths about who is likely to carry these diseases.
2. Some clients have a difficult time distinguishing between what is real and what is not real. It is very important for group leaders to frequently remind group members that this is just a role play and then talk about why it is important to practice this skill. If a member seems to have a difficult time distinguishing between the two, then the role play should be stopped and replaced by a general discussion about high-risk sexual behaviors.

HEALTH MAINTENANCE SKILLS

The ability to manage one's health care involves a complex set of skills. It requires that individuals have an understanding of their illness and the medication that they are taking as well as the ability to advocate for themselves in a setting that is often viewed as intimidating. Advocating for oneself involves the ability to use a combination of skills including assertiveness skills, communication skills, and conflict management skills (e.g. compromise and negotiation). Not surprisingly, most people find that the combination of understanding their own illness and advocating for themselves in medical settings is challenging at best and overwhelming at its worst. People with schizophrenia experience even greater difficulty, in part because of impediments such as short attention spans, slow processing, and cognitive disorganization compounded by the complexity of their illness.

Clients with schizophrenia often require extensive practice in the skill areas of communication, assertiveness, and conflict management. In addition, they require education on the importance of being an active participant in their own health care. Many of these clients also require intensive education on their psychiatric symptoms and how medication affects those symptoms as well as instruction regarding any other medical illness or symptoms they may experience. Finally, because many clients have had at least some negative experiences with the medical community, it is important to help them cope with any fears related to speaking out on their own behalf.

SKILL: Making a Doctor's Appointment on the Phone

RATIONALE: Most people, at some time or another, need to see a doctor. Often it is up to the person who is not feeling well to make the appointment. We have found that making appointments goes more smoothly if people follow the steps presented here.

STEPS OF THE SKILL:

1. Identify yourself or give your name.
2. Tell the person that you would like to make an appointment to see the doctor.
3. Listen to the person's response. Be ready to provide any information that he or she may ask for.
4. Repeat back the time and date of the appointment given to you and then thank the person for his or her help.

SCENES TO USE IN ROLE PLAYS:

1. You need to make an appointment because you have been feeling sick for more than a week and do not seem to be getting any better.
2. You realize that you need to make an appointment for your annual physical.
3. You think that your medication isn't working, so you call your doctor for an appointment.
4. You notice that you are experiencing some early warning signs of relapse and make an appointment to see your doctor.
5. You are experiencing side effects from your medication and want to make an extra appointment to see your psychiatrist.

SPECIAL CONSIDERATIONS WHEN TEACHING THIS SKILL:

1. Group leaders should help clients identify the information they are likely to be asked for when making a doctor's appointment (e.g., the nature of the problem, insurance information, etc.).
2. Group leaders should also remind clients that they may need to be specific but brief when describing why they want an appointment. Clients should also be reminded that it is important that they speak in a slow and clear manner so that they can be understood. In addition, clients should be warned of the likelihood that the receptionist may put them "on hold" for a while and that they will have to be understanding about this.

SKILL: Asking Questions about Medications

RATIONALE: It is important to understand why a doctor has prescribed a certain medication for us and how to take that medication properly. It is equally important to feel that the medication is being helpful. When people have questions about the medications they are taking, they need to seek out someone who is knowledgeable and talk to that person about their concerns.

STEPS OF THE SKILL:

1. Choose a person to speak to, such as a case manager, a nurse, a doctor, or a family member.
2. Ask the person your question about medication. Be specific.
3. If you do not understand the person's answer, ask more questions.
4. Thank the person for his or her help.

SCENES TO USE IN ROLE PLAYS:

1. You are having trouble sleeping and are wondering if it is related to the new medication you are taking.
2. Your doctor has suggested that you begin taking a new medication, but you have concerns about its possible side effects.
3. You want to stop taking your medication because you are feeling better.
4. You don't think that the current dose of medication you are taking is helpful and want to increase it.
5. You want to know whether you can have a beer if you take the medication that has been prescribed.

SPECIAL CONSIDERATIONS WHEN TEACHING THIS SKILL:

1. It will be useful for group leaders to discuss with clients the importance of writing down any questions they may have (so they do not forget) before speaking to a specific person about their medication concerns.
2. Group leaders should also emphasize the importance of clients understanding the answers they receive. Clients should be encouraged to ask more questions or even ask another person their question if they do not understand the answer they have received.

SKILL: Asking Questions about Health-Related Concerns

RATIONALE: Talking to others about our health can sometimes feel uncomfortable or scary. This may especially be true if we need to speak with a doctor or a nurse. It is important that we understand what is going on with our health, however. Asking questions of someone who is knowledgeable will enable us to better take care of ourselves.

STEPS OF THE SKILL:

1. Choose a person to speak to, such as a case manager, a nurse, or a doctor.
2. Ask the person your question.
3. If you do not feel comfortable with the person's answer or if you do not understand, ask more questions.
4. Thank the person for his or her help.

SCENES TO USE IN ROLE PLAYS:

1. You ask a staff member at the community residence about what to expect at your upcoming physical examination.
2. Your doctor just changed your medication dose, and you want to know how it will affect you.
3. You are having trouble sleeping and ask your doctor if he or she can prescribe any medication to help.
4. Recently you have noticed that you have gained some weight, and you want to do something about it. You ask your nurse about the best ways to lose weight.
5. You haven't been feeling well lately and want to see a doctor. You ask your case manager to make an appointment for you.

SPECIAL CONSIDERATIONS WHEN TEACHING THIS SKILL:

1. Before beginning to practice this skill, it may be useful for group leaders to spend some time helping members identify different people they might want to ask questions about health-related issues. This list may include people such as doctors, nurses, case managers, therapists, and family members.
2. It may also be of use to have the group generate a list of different health care providers, such as psychiatrists, dentists, physical therapists, gynecologists, and so forth, and then discuss what aspect of health they specifically focus on.

<u>SKILL</u>: Complaining about Medication Side Effects

<u>RATIONALE</u>: Most people, at one time or another, have been on medication. Some people take medication only occasionally, like antibiotics for an infection, whereas others take them for more chronic conditions such as diabetes, depression, or schizophrenia. Unfortunately, not every medication is perfect. Each medication comes with side effects, some more severe than others, and everyone responds to medication differently. A medication that causes little to no side effects in one person may cause severe side effects in another. It is therefore important to let your health provider or other people in your life (e.g., family, support staff) know when you are experiencing them.

<u>STEPS OF THE SKILL</u>:

1. Choose a person to speak to, such as a staff member, a nurse, a doctor, or a family member
2. Tell the person you are concerned that you may be experiencing side effects from your medication
3. Describe the symptoms you are experiencing. <u>Remember to be specific</u>.
4. If you are speaking to a medical person, ask for advice about how to handle the symptoms. If you are speaking to a nonmedical person, ask for help in setting up a medical appointment.

<u>SCENES TO USE IN ROLE PLAYS</u>:

1. You have noticed that you have gained some weight since beginning your medication and want to talk to the doctor about it.
2. You recently have had your medication dosage increased and are noticing that you are having a hard time waking up in the morning. You wonder if this is a side effect of the dosage increase.
3. You are worried that your hand tremors are related to your medication.
4. You have been feeling down and have no desire to do anything. A staff member suggests you talk to your doctor to see if whether these feelings are related to your medication.
5. You want to stop taking your medication because you believe it has too many side effects.

<u>SPECIAL CONSIDERATIONS WHEN TEACHING THIS SKILL</u>:

1. Mastering this skill assumes that clients know what medications they are taking, why they are taking them, how they will feel when taking them, and the potential side effects, both common and rare. Therefore, it is extremely helpful if group leaders know what medications their clients are taking and then teach the clients about them. If a group leader is not familiar with a medication, he or she can contact the local pharmacy or talk to a doctor for information. It may also be helpful to consult books written for lay people about psychiatric medications. One book that has useful information is *Integrated Treatment for Dual Disorders* (Mueser, Noordsy, et al., 2003).
2. Group leaders may also find it helpful to "normalize" medication side effects by discussing the side effects of nonpsychiatric and over-the-counter medications. In addition, it is important that group leaders emphasize how important it is to tell a doctor about possible side effects because in most cases, the side effects can be managed or eliminated by changing the dose of medication or trying a new medication.

<u>SKILL</u>: Requesting a Change in Your Medication Dosage

<u>RATIONALE</u>: There are many reasons people may want a change in their dosage of medication. Some of these reasons include experiencing uncomfortable side effects, feeling that your medication is no longer helpful because your symptoms haven't improved, or that you no longer need your medication because you are feeling better. Whatever your reason for wanting a change in your medication dosage, it is important to speak to your doctor about your concerns. Keep in mind that changing the dosage of your medication without the guidance of a medical professional can be dangerous. The following steps have been found to be useful to facilitate a discussion with you doctor.

<u>STEPS OF THE SKILL</u>:

1. Choose an appropriate person to speak to (e.g., a nurse or doctor).
2. Explain why you want a change in your medication dosage.
3. Discuss the advantages and disadvantages of changing your medication dosage.
4. Ask questions if you do not understand what is being said.
5. If you disagree with the advice, suggest a compromise.

<u>SCENES TO USE IN ROLE PLAYS</u>:

1. You have been feeling well for the past few months and want to stop taking your medication
2. You have recently been discharged from the hospital and feel worse than before you went in. You want to know if there has been a change in your medication dosage.
3. You have noticed that it has been hard for you to concentrate on the job and wonder if you need an increase in your medication dosage.
4. You feel that your current dosage of medication is no longer working.
5. A family member notices that you have been more irritable lately and you wonder whether it is related to your medication.

<u>SPECIAL CONSIDERATIONS WHEN TEACHING THIS SKILL</u>:

1. Group leaders should remind clients that making a request to change their medication dosage does not guarantee that their doctor will agree. Therefore, a review of the skill Compromise and Negotiation may be useful.
2. It is important that before seeing their doctor, clients have specific reasons for wanting a change in their medication dosage. As it may helpful for clients to have with them a list of the specific reasons for medication dosage change, group leaders should explore possible reasons (e.g., unpleasant side effects) during the group.

SKILL: Asking about a New Medication You Have Heard About

RATIONALE: New medications are being developed for different illnesses at a faster pace than ever. In addition, advertisers trying to sell these new medications are finding ways to make more people aware of them. You can find these advertisements on television, in magazines, on pamphlets in the waiting rooms of health facilities, and even on writing pens. You may also hear about new medications from friends and family members. It is therefore very important to talk to your doctor about any new medications you believe might benefit you. We have found that talking with your doctor may be easier if you use the following steps.

STEPS OF THE SKILL:

1. Tell your doctor that you have heard about a new medication called _____.
2. Ask your doctor if he or she thinks that this medication may be helpful for you.
3. Discuss the pros and cons of changing to a new medication.
4. Listen carefully to what the doctor says.
5. Let the doctor know what you think.

SCENES TO USE IN ROLE PLAYS:

1. You saw a commercial on television promoting a new medication and wonder whether it is right for you.
2. You are waiting to see your doctor and notice pamphlets in the waiting room describing new medications.
3. A friend tells you that the new medication he is taking makes him feel great. He tells you it has just come out on the market and that you should try it.
4. You are reading a magazine and notice a full-page advertisement describing a new medication that is supposed to make you feel better. The advertisement says to discuss this with your doctor to see if it is right for you.
5. You have read in the newspaper that the local university will pay people to test a promising new medication. You need the money but want to talk to your doctor before making any decisions.

SPECIAL CONSIDERATIONS WHEN TEACHING THIS SKILL:

1. Group leaders can open a discussion about whether or not a new medication is necessarily a better medication.
2. Group leaders should encourage clients to have a list of questions prepared before seeing the doctor. Clients can generate possible questions during the group.

SKILL: Reporting Pain and Other Physical Symptoms

RATIONALE: It is very important to report pain and/or other physical symptoms to people you trust. This is especially true if you are worried about what the symptoms may be related to. Some people find it difficult or embarrassing to talk about these issues with others; however, that is not a good reason to avoid telling someone.

STEPS OF THE SKILL:

1. Choose an appropriate person to speak to.
2. Tell the person that you are not feeling well.
3. Describe the symptoms (e.g., pain, dizziness) to that person.
4. Listen to that person's response and ask for help if you need it.

SCENES TO USE IN ROLE PLAYS:

1. You twisted your ankle a few weeks ago, and it is still causing you pain. You wonder if you should tell someone about it.
2. You have been experiencing blurred vision when you read. You don't want to bother anyone because you think it's no big deal.
3. You recently underwent gall bladder surgery and wonder if the pain you are feeling in your stomach is something that you should be worried about.
4. You have noticed that you experience dizziness every time you stand up and are worried that there might be something seriously wrong. You feel afraid to mention it to anyone.
5. You had sex with your boyfriend recently and are now not feeling well. You are worried that you might be pregnant but are embarrassed to talk to anyone about it.

SPECIAL CONSIDERATIONS WHEN TEACHING THIS SKILL:

1. This may be a good time to have a general discussion about the importance of taking care of health issues early so as to lessen the risk of complications related to these health issues. Group leaders can also elicit from the clients the advantages of reporting symptoms to others and list them on a flipchart.
2. Not all clients will feel comfortable discussing pain and other physical symptoms with others; they may need to identify one support person whom they trust and then practice with that person.

VOCATIONAL/WORK SKILLS

Most clients with schizophrenia do not work, and among those who do, difficulties at the workplace are common. Despite low rates of employment in people with schizophrenia and other severe mental illnesses, most of these people want to work. The work clients most prefer are regular competitive jobs, paying competitive wages, in integrated community settings, working alongside others who do not have a psychiatric disability. The vocational skills included in this section are designed to help clients get and keep jobs, as well as to negotiate social situations at the workplace.

A variety of work-related social situations require training. Some clients benefit from job interviewing skills, especially if they plan to obtain a job without the direct assistance of a supported employment counselor. At the workplace, effective social skills are required for interacting with coworkers, customers (when applicable), and supervisors. The social skills required for these situations overlap with many other social skills covered in this book, including conversational skills, assertiveness skills, and conflict resolution skills, so that competence in these skills will facilitate workplace adjustment. Because many of the social situations for which clients need skills training are unique to the job, social skills training to improve functioning at the workplace is usually most effective when provided after a client has obtained work in his or her area of interest. Providing skills training after clients have obtained work is also helpful, because their motivation to keep a job and the social situations that are the focus of skills training have high personal relevance.

SKILL: Interviewing for a Job

RATIONALE: Making a good first impression is important when trying to get hired for a job. Having an interview for a job provides a person with that opportunity. We have found that interviews are more likely to go smoothly when people have an idea about what will be asked of them and when they keep the following steps in mind.

STEPS OF THE SKILL:

1. Make eye contact with the interviewer.
2. Shake the interviewer's hand and introduce yourself. Remember to use a confident voice tone.
3. Tell the interviewer why you are interested in the job.
4. Answer any job-related questions the interviewer asks you.
5. Thank the interviewer for his or her time.

SCENES TO USE IN ROLE PLAYS:

1. You are interviewing for a volunteer position at your local library.
2. You are interviewing for a position at the vocational training program.
3. You are interviewing for a job at the supermarket.
4. You are interviewing for a job at a landscaping business.

SPECIAL CONSIDERATIONS WHEN TEACHING THE SKILL:

1. Group leaders should review with clients the most common questions asked during an interview. It will be important for clients to have ready answers for such questions as "What past experience or skills do you have that qualify you for this job?" What makes you interested in this job?" and "What do you consider your strengths to be?"
2. Group leaders need to spend time discussing the importance of making a good first impression when going on an interview. It is useful to discuss grooming, hygiene, and appropriate dress for a particular job.
3. Clients should be frequently reminded that maintaining eye contact and speaking in a firm, confident manner are very important and will help them make a good first impression.

SKILL: Asking for Feedback about Job Performance

<u>RATIONALE</u>: Most people want feedback on their job performance at some point during their work careers. However, asking for that feedback may feel awkward or scary. We have found that people feel less awkward when they keep certain steps in mind.

<u>STEPS OF THE SKILL</u>:

1. Identify an area of your job that you would like some feedback about.
2. Request feedback from the appropriate person. Say something like "I am interested in knowing how you think I am doing with _____; I would like to talk to you about it when you have a chance."
3. Listen carefully to the person's response, especially any suggestions that he or she may make.
4. If you do not understand the suggestions, ask the person to clarify them.
5. Thank the person for his or her time.

<u>SCENES TO USE IN ROLE PLAYS</u>:

1. You have been at your new job for about a month and are wondering how your boss thinks you are doing.
2. You have been working on a project with a coworker and ask for his or her feedback on how things are going on your part of the project.
3. You have been feeling unsure about the progress you have made on a new project and ask your supervisor for some feedback.
4. You have been given additional responsibilities at work and ask for feedback about how you are doing.
5. Recently your supervisor commented that you have been working too slowly. Since then you have tried to speed up your productivity and are wondering if you are now working at an acceptable pace.

<u>SPECIAL CONSIDERATIONS WHEN TEACHING THIS SKILL</u>:

1. Some clients have little experience with working at a job as an adult and may not be able to readily identify what things people ask for regarding feedback. It will be helpful if group leaders spend some time helping clients identify appropriate things one might seek feedback about.
2. Group leaders may need to remind clients that they will often have to make an appointment or wait some time before a supervisor has an opportunity to speak to them. It is important that the clients anticipate this so that they are able to respond without getting angry or upset.
3. It is also important that group leaders discuss with clients the importance of listening to a supervisor's feedback *without* interrupting or getting defensive.

SKILL: Responding to Criticism from a Supervisor

<u>RATIONALE</u>: Receiving criticism from a supervisor can be an upsetting experience. Most people have been on the receiving end of criticism at work at some point or another. Knowing how to respond to that criticism can help make the experience more tolerable and even turn it into something productive.

<u>STEPS OF THE SKILL</u>:

1. Without interrupting or getting angry, listen carefully to what is being said to you.
2. Repeat back what your supervisor said.
3. Ask your supervisor what you can do to improve the situation.
4. If you do not understand what was said, continue to ask questions until it becomes clear.

<u>SCENES TO USE IN ROLE PLAYS</u>:

1. You have arrived late to work on several occasions, and your supervisor confronts you about it.
2. Your supervisor tells you that you are working too slowly.
3. Your boss tells you that he or she is unhappy with the quality of your work.
4. Your boss tells you that the way you dress does not meet the office dress code standards.
5. Your supervisor tells you that he or she is unhappy with how messy you keep your work space.

<u>SPECIAL CONSIDERATIONS WHEN TEACHING THIS SKILL</u>:

1. Group leaders should remind clients that no one likes to be the recipient of criticism. However, it is important to remain calm and listen carefully to what is being said so that you can remedy the situation.
2. Because receiving criticism is an upsetting event, group leaders may want to review with the clients ways to manage angry or upsetting feelings.

SKILL: Following Verbal Instructions

RATIONALE: Being able to follow instructions is a skill that is required in almost all settings, such as at school, at home, or on the job. It is especially important to be able to follow verbal instructions on the job, where having an accurate understanding of a particular assignment is essential to the overall functioning of the workplace.

STEPS OF THE SKILL:

1. Listen carefully to the person giving instructions.
2. If you are confused about what was said, ask the person to repeat the instructions.
3. Repeat back the instructions to the person.
4. Ask more questions if you still do not understand.

SCENES TO USE IN ROLE PLAYS:

1. Your job coach has just given you instructions about the best route to take to your job.
2. It is your first day on the job, and your supervisor instructs you to go to the orientation given for new employees. It is a large building, and you are not sure how to find the room.
3. You have just been asked to take on more responsibilities at work and are confused about what is expected of you.
4. Your supervisor has asked you and a coworker to work on a project together. The supervisor has split the project responsibilities between the two of you; however, it is still not clear to you what you need to be doing.
5. Your vocational counselor has given you a rather complicated homework assignment. You realize that you need some clarification about it.

SPECIAL CONSIDERATIONS WHEN TEACHING THIS SKILL:

1. Many clients have trouble following instructions as a result of their symptoms and cognitive deficits. Therefore, it will be helpful to begin the role plays using simple instructions and then work up to harder ones. In addition, simple instructions should be given to clients who are very symptomatic or have severe cognitive deficits.
2. It may also be helpful for group leaders to help clients come up with strategies for remembering instructions, such as writing them down on a sheet of paper.

SKILL: Joining Ongoing Conversations at Work

RATIONALE: There will be times at work when you may want to join a conversation that is in progress with some coworkers, such as during lunch or a break. Learning how to join a conversation without being rude or creating an awkward situation can be accomplished by simply following a few steps.

STEPS OF THE SKILL:

1. Wait for a break or a pause in the flow of the conversation.
2. Say something like "Mind if I join you?"
3. Say things related to the conversation topic.

SCENES TO USE IN ROLE PLAYS:

1. You are on your lunch break and see some people whom you would like to join who are eating their lunch and talking.
2. You are on a break and see some coworkers gathered around the vending machines. You decide to join them.
3. There has been a temporary power outage at work, and you find yourself with nothing to do. You hear two people talking about the outage and are curious to find out what they know.

SPECIAL CONSIDERATIONS WHEN TEACHING THIS SKILL:

1. This skill requires that clients be able to make judgments about when it is appropriate to join a conversation. Some clients will have difficulty recognizing when there is a break or pause in the flow of the conversation. Therefore, it may be helpful to spend some time, before beginning the role plays, having clients observe the group leaders talking and seeing if they are able to identify when the conversation flow has been broken.
2. This skill also requires that clients make judgments about when it is not OK to join a conversation. For instance, it may not be appropriate if the people talking look upset, angry, or serious. It would be helpful for the group leaders to spend some time reviewing how people identify different affects.

SKILL: Solving Problems

<u>RATIONALE</u>: All of us experience problems at one time or another. Problems can be big or small and can occur in any setting. Learning a systematic way of dealing with problems is an important skill needed to function in the world, as well as to maintain and excel in our jobs.

<u>STEPS OF THE SKILL</u>:

1. Define the problem.
2. Use brainstorming to generate a list of possible solutions.
3. Identify the advantages and disadvantages of each solution.
4. Select the best solution or combination of solutions.
5. Plan how to carry out the best solution.
6. Follow up the plan at a later time.

<u>SCENES TO USE IN ROLE PLAYS</u>:

1. You have been put on probation at work because you frequently show up late in the morning.
2. You have been offered a job that you would like to take, but the hours conflict with your weekly therapy appointment.
3. You have a job as a maintenance worker in a cafeteria. Your supervisor tells you that you are working too slowly and asks you to figure out a way to improve your productivity.

<u>SPECIAL CONSIDERATIONS WHEN TEACHING THIS SKILL</u>:

1. Because this skill is somewhat more complicated and takes longer to practice than the other skills, it is taught using a somewhat different format. Instead of having each group member complete a role play individually, group leaders should present a scenario to the entire group and then assist them through the steps of the skill together. Teaching the skill in this format has two functions: (a) It keeps all clients interested and involved, and (b) it provides the clients with experience in working together toward a common goal (which requires that they put to use some other skills that they have learned).
2. Step 2 requires group members to generate a list of possible solutions. During this step, group leaders need to emphasize the importance of writing down all ideas without judging whether they are good or bad. This technique is called *brainstorming*.
3. The Problem Solving and Goal Achievement Worksheet in Appendix A is helpful in teaching this skill.

COPING SKILLS FOR DRUG AND ALCOHOL USE

Problems with drug and alcohol use are very common among people with schizophrenia and other severe mental illnesses, with about 50% of all such individuals developing a substance use problem over their lifetimes. The high susceptibility of people with schizophrenia to substance abuse is partly due to their biological vulnerability, which makes them highly sensitive (or "supersensitive") to the effects of even small quantities of drugs and alcohol. Additional reasons for the high rate of substance abuse include efforts to self-medicate unpleasant symptoms and feelings, the desire to "feel normal" and fit in with others, boredom, and the desire to have something to do and to look forward to. Because substance use often takes place in a social setting, the ability of clients to resist offers to use substances is crucial to their developing a sober lifestyle.

Teaching substance refusal skills is a natural extension of assertiveness skills training, and experience with these skills pays off for clients in many situations involving substance use. Conflict resolution skills may also be helpful to clients in managing substance use situations, as these skills can be useful in resolving disagreements about how to spend time with friends. Although substance refusal skills are crucial for helping clients recover from drug and alcohol problems, it is important not to assume that all clients with these problems are motivated to stop using substances. Thus, the use of motivational interviewing techniques to instill and strengthen motivation to address substance use problems is crucial for most clients with such problems. The combination of motivational interviewing and social skills training can be a potent treatment package that can help many individuals recover from their substance use problems.

SKILL: Offering an Alternative to Using Drugs and Alcohol

RATIONALE: Because so many people use drugs and alcohol, each of you is likely to be pressured by someone to get high or drink. When faced with these situations, it is sometimes difficult to say "No." This can be really hard when the person is someone whom you know well, such as a family member or a friend. Sometimes you just want to spend time with the person, but all he or she wants to do is get high or drink. It is at these times that suggesting or finding an alternative activity can provide a way for you to spend time with the person *without* using drugs or alcohol. The following steps have been found to be helpful when refusing someone's request to get high or drunk.

STEPS OF THE SKILL:

1. Look at the person. Make eye contact.
2. Use a firm voice and tell the person that you don't want to use drugs or alcohol.
3. Give the person a reason why you do not want to use.
4. Suggest another activity. If the person has drugs or alcohol with him or her, leave the situation.

SCENES TO USE IN ROLE PLAYS:

1. You run into an old friend who tells you that there is going to be a party that will be attended by many people you have not seen in a while. You know that it is likely that drugs and alcohol will be present.
2. You are attending a relative's birthday party, and the host wants you to join in a toast and hands you a glass of wine.
3. A friend wants you to go to a bar to have a beer. You agree to go but order a soda instead. After you leave the bar, your friend suggests that you smoke a joint with him.
4. You are taking a walk when a person you know asks you if you want to buy some drugs.
5. You go to a movie with a new friend you met at work. Before the movie starts, your friend tells you'll enjoy the movie more if you are high and asks if you want to light up a joint.

SPECIAL CONSIDERATIONS WHEN TEACHING THIS SKILL: It is important to make sure that clients have identified for themselves reasons for refusing as well as alternative suggestions. Therefore, group leaders should spend a session helping group members brainstorm one or two reasons for refusing drugs and/or alcohol. These reasons should be written on a large flipchart by the group leaders. Another list should be generated containing alternatives to drug and/or alcohol use. These lists can help clients identify reasons and alternative suggestions that are tailored to their unique situations. Remember, the more meaningful the reasons for refusal and alternative suggestions, the greater the likelihood that they will be used outside the group. In addition, it is important to emphasize that sometimes people who ask clients to use will have drugs or alcohol with them, and when this happens, providing an alternative will be ineffective because it is clear that the person plans to use the drugs or alcohol; therefore, it is best to just leave the situation.

SKILL: Requesting That a Family Member or Friend Stop Asking You to Use Drugs and Alcohol

RATIONALE: Sometimes when you say no to drugs or alcohol, people can give you a hard time. They keep pressuring you, or they make you feel bad. Often it is someone you know, such as a family member or a friend, who is pressuring you to use drugs with him or her. The following steps have been found to be helpful when you need to say no under pressure.

STEPS OF THE SKILL:

1. Look at the person. Make eye contact.
2. Use a firm voice and tell the person that you don't want to use drugs or alcohol.
3. Give the person a reason why you do not want to use.
4. Request that the person not ask you to use drugs or alcohol.

SCENES TO USE IN ROLE PLAYS:

1. You are approached by a friend at the day program, who tells you he's going out back to get high and wants you to join him. You don't want to lose him as a friend.
2. You are stocking shelves at the local convenience store, when you see an old high school friend and say hello. He asks you to join him and a few other guys you used to hang out with for a drink after you get off work. You used to be close friends, and he won't take no for an answer.
3. You are attending your parents' 50th wedding anniversary and are handed a glass of champagne for the toast that is about to be given in your parents' honor. You are seated at your parents' table and are worried that they will be offended if you refuse.
4. You have just completed a rigorous job training program, and your family wants to take you out to dinner to celebrate. You know alcohol will be served and that your family believes one drink won't hurt you.
5. You are hanging out with some cousins after a holiday dinner and want to reconnect with them. They insist that you smoke a joint with them. You don't want them to know you have a drug problem.

SPECIAL CONSIDERATIONS WHEN TEACHING THIS SKILL: Group leaders should have clients list ways others may pressure them to use. Be sure the list includes examples that would lead the person refusing to be concerned that refusal will lead to a loss of respect from someone they care about. For example, a friend might say, "So I'm not good enough for you now?" or "Do you think you're better than me?" It is also very important to help each client identify a few personalized reasons why they can't use drugs or alcohol. It may also be helpful for clients to identify possible situations in which they may be pressured to use. When practicing the skill, group leaders should be persistent and make at least three attempts to persuade the person to use before stopping. For specific examples demonstrating how to be persistent during a role play, see Chapter 9, "Working with Clients Who Abuse Drugs and Alcohol."

SKILL: Responding to a Stranger or a Drug Dealer

RATIONALE: There are times when you may be approached by a drug dealer pressuring you to buy drugs or a stranger who wants you to use. When you are faced with these situations, the skills we have learned for refusing drugs from a friend or family member usually do not apply. Often it is not necessary to provide a reason for refusal, if you feel as though you are in danger, you can make up a reason, such as you are broke, and then leave immediately. The steps provided here offer some guidance on how to handle these difficult situations.

STEPS OF THE SKILL:

1. Decide whether to make eye contact.
2. Tell the person that you don't want to use drugs or alcohol. Be brief.
3. *If appropriate*, give the person a reason why you do not want to use.
4. Leave the situation.

SCENES TO USE IN ROLE PLAYS:

1. A dealer you used to buy from approaches you and asks why you haven't been around. He wants to know if you are buying from someone else.
2. You have recently been discharged from rehab and have been out of circulation for a while. A guy with whom you used to get high sees you and thinks you have been avoiding him. To prove you have not been avoiding him, he wants you to get high with him.
3. A person who appears to be high approaches you on the street and believes he knows you. He says that you owe him and demands that you repay him by buying some drugs.
4. You have just gotten off work and are greeted by two guys who work for the local drug dealer. They know you have cash and are pressuring you to buy from them.
5. You are riding the bus home when you notice a person staring at you. When you get off at your stop, he follows and catches up to you. You recognize the person as someone you used to get high with. He offers you some drugs.

SPECIAL CONSIDERATIONS WHEN TEACHING THIS SKILL: Although the steps of the skill are listed, it is important for group leaders to tailor the steps to each client. For example, some will not feel comfortable making eye contact with a drug dealer. Others will want to leave the situation without saying anything, and some may feel that they need to explain why they don't want to use this one time (such as needing to be clean for a urine test), believing that the dealer might leave them alone if he or she thinks that they will be back another day. It is also important to discuss how to assess the level of danger in any situation and then modify the steps accordingly. For example, if a group member believes that he or she is in a dangerous situation, it may be best to bypass some of the steps and remove him- or herself from the situation immediately.

Appendix A

Materials Useful to Group Leaders

SOCIAL SKILLS ORIENTATION FOR PROFESSIONALS

What Are Social Skills?

Social skills are the specific behaviors people use when interacting with others that enable individuals to be effective at achieving their personal goals. Situations such as having a casual conversation, making friends, expressing feelings, or obtaining something from another person all require the use of social skills.

What Are Some Examples of Social Skills?

Good social skills include both *what* is said during a social interaction and *how* it is said. When communicating with another person, the verbal content of the message, that is, the person's choice of words or phrases, is important. *How* that message is communicated can be just as important. For example, appropriate facial expressions, body language, eye contact, and a good, firm voice tone all help to communicate the message. Social skills training aims at improving both what people say during interactions and how they say it.

Why Are Social Skills Important?

People with psychiatric illnesses usually experience many problems in their relationships with others, including treatment providers, family members, and other clients. These problems result in difficulties in community adjustment and an impoverished quality of life. For many clients, poor social functioning is related to inadequate social skills. For example, clients may have difficulty starting a conversation, speak in a low monotone voice, or fail to establish eye contact. Helping clients to improve their social skills can enhance their social functioning in the community.

What Are the Causes of Social Skills Deficits?

There are many possible causes of skill deficits in people with psychiatric illnesses. Some clients become ill before they have been able to fully develop their social skills. Others may have grown up in an environment in which they did not have good role models. Still others may have learned good social skills but later lost them as they developed their illness and withdrew from other people. Clients who have spent long periods of time in hospitals where there were few expectations placed on their behavior may be out of practice and need help relearning skills and knowing when to use them. Any combination of these possibilities can contribute to deficits in social skills.

Are All Problems in Social Functioning Due to Deficits in Social Skills?

No, social dysfunction can arise from other problems as well. Medication side effects can cause problems in social functioning. In addition, if the social environment in which a client resides is not conducive and supportive to appropriate and assertive social behavior, social dysfunction will result.

(continued)

What Is Social Skills Training?

Social skills training is a set of psychotherapeutic techniques based on social learning theory that has been developed to teach social skills to individuals. Social skills training uses the same methods that were developed more than 25 years ago for assertiveness training. Social skills training involves several steps. The first step is to provide a rationale or help the client to understand why it is important to learn the skill. The second step is to demonstrate (model) the skill in a role play. The third step is to engage the client in a role play, and the fourth step involves providing feedback to the client and suggestions for improvement. Fifth, the client is encouraged to practice on his or her own.

How Often Should Social Skills Training Be Conducted?

As often as possible! It is preferable to have the social skills group meet at least two times per week, but clients can be reminded to practice the skills often, even on a daily basis. The more opportunities clients have to practice social skills, the better they get and the more natural the skills become.

What Types of Social Skills Can Be Taught?

A wide variety of skills can be taught, depending on the client's needs. Some of the most common skills include initiating and maintaining conversations, making requests of other people, expressing feelings, resolving conflicts, making friends, and being assertive.

How Can Staff Members Help Clients to Learn These Skills?

Staff members are as important to the success of social skills training as the group leaders are themselves. Staff members can help clients by knowing what skills are being taught, demonstrating these skills in their own interactions with clients (and each other), prompting and encouraging clients to use the skills in specific situations, and giving them positive feedback when they demonstrate good social skills. Furthermore, staff members can help clients learn better skills by engaging them in brief role plays conducted *outside* the regular group sessions. This additional practice may help some clients to become more familiar and comfortable with the skills, enabling them to use them on their own. In summary, staff members play a *vital* role in assisting clients to improve their social skills and are an extended part of the social skills training team.

SOCIAL SKILLS ORIENTATION FOR CLIENTS

What Is Social Skills Training?

Social skills training teaches people how they can better communicate their feelings, thoughts, and needs to others. It also teaches them how they can better respond to other people's feelings, thoughts, and needs. Social skills help people to get what they want more often and help them to avoid doing things that they do not want to do.

How Is Social Skills Training Different from Other Groups?

Social skills training is different from other forms of therapy groups. Group members do not sit around and talk about their problems. Instead, members spend group time trying out ways to actually solve their problems. They do this by practicing different skills during the group and then trying out these skills in real-life situations.

What Is Expected of Group Members?

Group members must be willing to keep an open mind. They must be willing to try new techniques designed to communicate with one other. Group members will learn about new skills and discuss how to use them in their lives. When they are ready, they will practice the skills in group and in real-life situations.

How Do Group Members Learn and Practice a New Skill?

Group members practice a new skill through role playing, initially with the group leaders and then with each other. Role playing is similar to rehearsing for a play but is more relaxed and fun. Group members are first given a handout that has the skill being taught broken down into a few easy steps. Next they watch the group leaders role play the skill with each other. (Role playing is acting in a pretend situation.) When members are feeling comfortable, they get to role play the skill. They will also be asked to do "homework," whereby they will practice the skill outside the group. Nobody is ever forced to role play or to do homework if he or she does not feel comfortable.

How Can Social Skills Training Help Me?

Social skills can help you communicate better with your friends, relatives, and employers. They can help you talk to people you are interested in dating. You can focus on skills that will allow you to become more independent. Social skills training can help you improve the skills you need to achieve almost any goal you choose. Before the first session, each group member meets with a group leader. The leader helps the group member identify his or her own personal goals to work on in group.

PROBLEM SOLVING AND GOAL ACHIEVEMENT WORKSHEET

Step 1: Define the problem or goal.

Talk about the problem or goal, listen carefully, ask questions, get everybody's opinion. Then write down *exactly* what the problem or goal is:

_____

Step 2: Use brainstorming to make a list of possible solutions.

Write down *all* ideas, even bad ones. Get everybody to come up with at least one possible solution. List the solutions *without discussion* at this stage.

1. _____
2. _____
3. _____
4. _____
5. _____
6. _____

Step 3: Identify the advantages and disadvantages of each solution.

Quickly go down the list of possible solutions and discuss the *main* advantages and disadvantages of each one.

Step 4: Select the best solution or combination of solutions.

Choose the solution that can be carried out most easily to solve the problem.

Step 5: Plan how to carry out the best solution.

List the resources needed and major obstacles to overcome. Assign tasks and set a timetable.

Step 1. _____
Step 2. _____
Step 3. _____
Step 4. _____

Step 6. Set a date for follow up: _____

First focus on what you have accomplished. *Praise all efforts.* Then review whether the plan was successful and revise it as necessary.

_____

Adapted by permission from Mueser and Gingerich (in press). Reprinted in *Social Skills Training for Schizophrenia* (2nd ed.) by Alan S. Bellack, Kim T. Mueser, Susan Gingerich, and Julie Agresta. Permission to photocopy this form is granted to purchasers of this book for personal use only (see copyright page for details).

SOCIAL SKILLS GROUP FORMAT

Instructions: This format is to be used for each skill group held. Group leaders should remind themselves of these 10 steps before the start of each group.

1. Establish a rationale for the skill.
___ Elicit reasons for learning the skill from group members.
___ Acknowledge all contributions made by group members.
___ Provide any additional rationales not mentioned.

2. Discuss the steps of the skill.
___ Discuss the reasons for each step.
___ Check group members for their understanding of the reasons.

3. Model the skill using a role play and review the role play with the group members.
___ Explain that you will demonstrate the skill in a role play.
___ Use two group leaders to model the skill.
___ Keep the role play brief and to the point.
___ Discuss whether each step of the skill was used in the role play.
___ Ask group members to evaluate the effectiveness of the role play.

4. Engage a group member in a role play using the same situation modeled.
___ Start with a member who is more skilled or is likely to be cooperative.
___ Request that the member try the skill in a role play with one of the leaders.
___ Ask the client questions to check his or her understanding of the goal of the role play.
___ Instruct the remaining group members to observe the client. Consider assigning each member a specific step, or part of a step, to observe.

5. Provide positive feedback.
___ Elicit positive feedback first from group members who have been assigned a specific step to observe.
___ Encourage feedback that is *specific*.
___ Cut off any negative feedback or criticism.
___ Praise all efforts.

6. Provide corrective feedback (suggestions for improvement).
___ Elicit suggestions for ways the client could perform the skill better.
___ Limit feedback to one or two suggestions.
___ Strive to communicate the suggestions in a positive, upbeat manner.

(continued)

7. **Engage the group member in another role play using the same situation.**
   ___ Request that the client change *one* behavior during the role play.
   ___ Check the client's understanding of the suggestions.
   ___ Focus on behaviors that are salient and changeable.

8. **Provide additional feedback.**
   ___ First focus on the behavior that was to be changed.
   ___ Consider using other behavior-shaping strategies to improve client skills, such as coaching, prompting, and supplemental modeling.
   ___ Be generous but *specific* when providing feedback.

9. **Engage other group members in role plays and provide feedback, as in Steps 4 through 8.**

10. **Assign homework that will be reviewed at the beginning of the next session.**
   ___ Give an assignment to practice the skill—use homework record sheets.
   ___ Ask group members to identify situations in which they could use the skill.
   ___ When possible, tailor the assignment to each client's skill level and personal goals.

SOCIAL SKILLS GROUP LEADER SELF-RATING CHECKLIST

Group Leader: _____   Date: _____

Instructions to group leader: Complete this checklist after conducting a session. For each item, check off whether you performed this skill "not at all," "partially," or "fully." It is helpful to complete this checklist every 3 months.

General structuring and positive engagement skills	Not at all	Partially	Fully
Created a warm, welcoming atmosphere.			
Spoke clearly, using a voice neither overloud nor oversoft.			
Established an agenda and maintained the structure of the session.			
Provided ample positive feedback for participation.			
Redirected group members who interrupted or strayed from the topic, using a kind but firm manner.			
Asked group members for examples of personal experiences in which skills could be or were used.			
Used a shaping approach to help members gradually learn new social skills by reinforcing small steps toward the targeted skill.			
Encouraged each group member to be actively involved in the session. (Members can be active in different ways, such as reading the steps of the skill out loud, providing a rationale, providing feedback for role plays, participating in role plays, contributing examples of personal experience.)			

(continued)

Steps of social skills training	Not at all	Partially	Fully
Reviewed homework from the previous group session.			
Established a rationale for using the skill.			
Discussed the steps of the skill with group members.			
Modeled the skill in a role play.			
Reviewed the modeled role play with group members.			
Engaged all group members in a role play of the skill.			
Provided or elicited behaviorally specific positive feedback for each group member's role play.			
Provided or elicited behaviorally specific suggestions for improvement for each group member's role play.			
Assigned specific homework to practice the skill outside the group.			

SOCIAL SKILLS GROUP OBSERVATION CHECKLIST

Group Leader(s): _____ Date: _____

Observer: _____

Instructions to observer: Complete this checklist after observing the group leader(s) conduct a session. For each item, check off whether the group leader(s) performed this skill "not at all," "partially," or "fully." It is helpful to complete this checklist every 3 months.

General structuring and positive engagement skills	Not at all	Partially	Fully
Created a warm, welcoming atmosphere.			
Spoke clearly, using a voice neither overloud nor oversoft.			
Established an agenda and maintained the structure of the session.			
Provided ample positive feedback for participation.			
Redirected group members who interrupted or strayed from the topic, using a kind but firm manner.			
Asked group members for examples of personal experiences in which skills could be or were used.			
Used a shaping approach to help members gradually learn new social skills by reinforcing small steps toward the targeted skill.			
Encouraged each group member to be actively involved in the session. (Members can be active in different ways, such as reading the steps of the skill out loud, providing a rationale, providing feedback for role plays, participating in role plays, contributing examples of personal experience.)			

(continued)

Steps of social skills training	Not at all	Partially	Fully
Reviewed homework from the previous group session.			
Established a rationale for using the skill.			
Discussed the steps of the skill with group members.			
Modeled the skill in a role play.			
Reviewed the modeled role play with group members.			
Engaged all group members in a role play of the skill.			
Provided or elicited behaviorally specific positive feedback for each group member's role play.			
Provided or elicited behaviorally specific suggestions for improvement for each group member's role play.			
Assigned specific homework to practice the skill outside the group.			

Instructions: A copy of these rules (poster size) should be posted in the room where the group is held so that they can be referred to as needed.

1. Stay on the Group Topic.

2. Only One Person May Speak at a Time.

3. No Name-Calling or Cursing.

4. No Criticizing or Making Fun of Each Other.

5. No Eating or Drinking during Group.

GUIDELINES FOR GIVING CONSTRUCTIVE FEEDBACK

1. Be alert to group members using the skill, even if it is only for a brief moment.

2. Start by giving praise. Find the positive behavior to highlight. A good way to begin is "I really like the way you _____."

3. Be specific about what the group member did well. For example, "I like the way you looked at me when you were talking."

4. *Avoid* critical comments and terms such as *wrong* or *bad*.

5. Make suggestions for improvement in only one area at a time. Some group members may not be able to accept any suggestions at first; for them, stick to praise for what was done well.

GUIDELINES FOR COMMUNICATING WITH CLIENTS
WHO ARE EXPERIENCING SYMPTOMS

1. Speak slowly and clearly.

2. Make only a few statements at a time.

3. Periodically ask if the client understands what you are saying.

4. Ask the client to repeat back what you have just said.

5. If the client is not able to follow what you are saying, repeat the information using fewer words and sentences.

6. Ask the client to repeat back what you have just said.

FACTS ABOUT HIV AND GUIDELINES FOR SAFER SEX

Facts about HIV (the Virus That Causes AIDS)

1. HIV is transmitted through the exchange of certain body fluids (semen, vaginal discharges, and blood infected with the HIV virus).

2. HIV cannot be spread through casual contact such as shaking hands, hugging, sneezing, or sharing bathrooms and kitchens.

3. HIV cannot be spread through insect bites or by donating blood.

4. People infected with HIV usually look and feel healthy.

5. AIDS is caused by HIV infection.

6. There is no vaccine or cure for HIV and AIDS at this time.

Guidelines for Safer Sex Practices

The following guidelines should be used by everyone. *Anyone* who is sexually active and has not been in an *exclusively* monogamous sexual relationship since 1978 is at risk of contracting the HIV virus. Anyone who engages in unsafe sex practices with a partner who has been exposed to the HIV virus is also at risk of contracting AIDS. For example, people may have been exposed unknowingly to the virus through blood transfusions or intravenous drug use. It is important to note that following these guidelines will not guarantee safety from infection. However, strict adherence to them can greatly reduce the chances of infection.

1. Have sex only with a partner who is not infected, who has sex only with you, and who does not use needles or syringes.

2. Always use (or have your partner use) a latex condom and a spermicide if you do not know for sure that your sexual partner is uninfected. Use a new condom each time you engage in sexual intercourse; never use the same condom more than once.

3. Use a water-based lubricant with your condom to add safety. Do not use oil-based jelly, baby oil, or any other substance that is not water-based because it can cause the condom to break.

4. Avoid the exchange of blood, semen, and vaginal secretions during sexual activity.

From *Social Skills Training for Schizophrenia* (2nd ed.) by Alan S. Bellack, Kim T. Mueser, Susan Gingerich, and Julie Agresta. Copyright 2004 by The Guilford Press. Permission to photocopy this form is granted to purchasers of this book for personal use only (see copyright page for details).

SUPPLEMENTAL READING LIST

Books

Bellack, A. S. (1989) *A clinical guide for the treatment of schizophrenia*. New York: Plenum Press.

Bellack, A. S. (2003). Psychosocial rehabilitation. In A. Tasman, J. Lieberman, & J. Kay (Eds.), *Psychiatry* (2nd ed.). London: Wiley.

Douglas, M., & Mueser, K. (1990). Teaching conflict resolution skills to the chronically mentally ill. *Behavior Modification, 14*(4), 519–547.

Drake, R. E., & Bellack, A. S. (in press). Psychiatric rehabilitation. In B. J.Sadock & V. A. Sadock (Eds.), *Kaplan & Sadock's Comprehensive textbook of psychiatry*. Baltimore: Lippincott, Williams & Wilkins.

Hirsch, S. R., & Weinberger, D. (Eds.). (2003). *Schizophrenia* (2nd Edition). Oxford, England: Blackwell Scientific.

Lieberman, J., & Murray, R. M. (Eds.). (2001). *Comprehensive care of schizophrenia*. London: Martin Dunitz.

Mueser, K., & Gingerich, S. (in press). *Coping with schizophrenia: A guide for families* (2nd ed.). New York: Guilford Press.

Mueser, K. T., & Tarrier, N. (Eds.). (1998). *Handbook of social functioning in schizophrenia*. Needham Heights, MA: Allyn & Bacon.

Pratt, S., & Mueser, K. T. (2002). Social skills training for schizophrenia. In S. G. Hofmann & M. Tomson (Eds.), *Treating chronic and severe mental disorders: A handbook of empirically supported interventions* (pp, 18–52). New York: Guilford Press.

Sharma, T., & Harvey, P. (2000*). Cognition in schizophrenia*. Oxford, England: Oxford University Press.

Spaulding, W. D., Sullivan, M. E., & Poland, J. S. (2003). *Treatment and rehabilitation of severe mental illness*. New York: Guilford Press.

Torrey, F. (2001). *Surviving schizozophrenia: A manual for families, consumers, and providers* (4th ed.). New York: HarperCollins.

Videotapes

Monkey See Productions. (2002). *Living with schizophrenia*. New York: Guilford Press.

Wheeler Communications. (1996). *I'm still here: The truth about schizophrenia*. Honeoye, NY: Wheeler Communications Group.

RESOURCES FOR PACKAGED ACTIVITIES
AND GAMES RELATED TO SOCIAL SKILLS

Center for Psychiatric Rehabilitation, University of Chicago: 708-614-4770, *www.ucpsychrehab.org*.

Childswork/Childsplay: 1-800-962-1141, *www.childswork.com*.

Eldersong: 1-800-397-0533, *www.eldersong.com*.

National Research and Training Center on Psychiatric Disability, University of Illinois at Chicago: 312-422-8180, *www.psych.uic.edu/uicnrtc*

Sea Bay World Wide Games: 1-800-568-0188, *www.seabaygame.com*.

Shake Loose a Memory: *www.shakelooseamemory.com*.

Wellness Reproductions: 1-800-669-9208, *www.wellness-resources.com*

Appendix B

Materials Related to Assessment

SOCIAL FUNCTIONING INTERVIEW

Name: _____   Date: _____

Clinician: _____

Role Functioning, Present and Past

Daily routine at home
- Where are you currently living?
- With whom do you live?
- Can you describe a typical day at home for me?
- What do you do to stay busy?
- Are there times when you are not doing anything and may be bored?
- What kind of living situation have you enjoyed most?

Education and work activities
- Are you taking classes or studying subjects on your own?
- Do you work part-time or full-time?
- Do you volunteer?
- Are you participating in a vocational rehabilitation program?
- What kinds of jobs did you have in the past?
- What kinds of careers interest you now? What careers interested you in the past?

Leisure activities
- What do you like to do with your spare time?
- What are your hobbies?
- What sports do you like to watch or participate in?
- Do you like to read? Do you like to write and/or keep a journal?
- Do you listen to music or play an instrument?
- Do you watch videos or TV shows?
- Do you like to draw or look at art?
- What hobbies and activities did you used to enjoy?

Relationships
- With whom do you spend time regularly? Family? Friends? Classmates? Coworkers? Spouse/ significant other? Roommates? Children?
- Do you have someone whom you feel close to, whom you can talk to about things that are important to you?
- Is there anyone whom you would like to spend more time with?
- Do you want to have more close relationships?

Spiritual supports
- Is spirituality important to you?
- What do you find comforting spiritually?
- Are you involved in a formal religion?
- Do you meditate?
- Do you look to nature or the arts for spirituality?

(continued)

Health
- What do you do to take care of your health?
- How would you describe your diet?
- Do you get some exercise?
- What is your sleep routine?

Social Situations That Are Problematic

Sometimes there are specific social situations that people feel they don't handle as well as they would like. Which of the following kinds of situations are difficult for you? Describe each situation as specifically as possible, providing one example if possible. What happens in the situation? What do you do/what does the other person do?

Starting and holding conversations

Managing conflicts, avoiding arguments

Asserting yourself, standing up for yourself

Living with other people

Having good relationships (friends, family, spouse or significant others, children)

Talking with doctors and other members of the treatment team

Working or volunteering

(continued)

Personal Goals Identified during the Interview

Short-term goals (within the next 6 months)

1. _____
2. _____

Long-term goals (within the next year)

1. _____
2. _____

Social Skill Strengths and Weaknesses Observed by the Clinician during the Interview

Strengths

1. _____
2. _____
3. _____
4. _____

Weaknesses

1. _____
2. _____
3. _____
4. _____

SOCIAL ADAPTIVE FUNCTIONING EVALUATION (SAFE)

Resident Name: _____   Evaluation Date: _____

Staff Name: _____

Instructions: Complete for the *typical* behavior **during the past month**. Circle one response for each item. When considering a rating for a particular behavior, it is important to compare the resident's ability with that of a person in a nonpsychiatric population. Group leaders should complete this scale once every 3 months.

0. No impairment
1. Mild impairment
2. Moderate impairment
3. Severe impairment
4. Extreme impairment

1. Bathing and Grooming	0	1	2	3	4
2. Clothing and Dressing	0	1	2	3	4
3. Eating, Feeding, and Diet	0	1	2	3	4
4. Money Management	0	1	2	3	4
5. Neatness and Maintenance	0	1	2	3	4
6. Orientation/Mobility	0	1	2	3	4
7. Reading/Writing	0	1	2	3	4
8. Impulse Control	0	1	2	3	4
9. Respect for Property	0	1	2	3	4
10. Telephone Skills	0	1	2	3	4
11. Conversational Skill	0	1	2	3	4
12. Instrumental Social Skill	0	1	2	3	4
13. Respect and Concern for Others	0	1	2	3	4
14. Social Appropriateness/Politeness	0	1	2	3	4
15. Social Engagement	0	1	2	3	4
16. Friendship	0	1	2	3	4
17. Recreation/Leisure (Nonsocial)	0	1	2	3	4
18. Participation in House Social Activities	0	1	2	3	4
19. Cooperation with Treatment	0	1	2	3	4

TOTAL _____

(continued)

1.   Bathing and grooming

0. No impairment. The person bathes and grooms him- or herself without prompting and assistance. He or she appears to be aware of and takes pride in his or her appearance.

1. Mild impairment. The person can perform most bathing and grooming tasks. *Occasionally*, he or she needs to be reminded to cut fingernails, shave, bathe, or comb his or her hair but, when prompted, corrects these problems.

2. Moderate impairment. The person can perform less complex grooming tasks (combing hair, showering) but may need assistance in performing more complex aspects of grooming (shaving, cutting fingernails). He or she regularly requires reminding to maintain grooming.

3. Severe impairment. The person does not initiate any activities of grooming. He or she is willing to be bathed and groomed but needs extensive assistance to perform the basic grooming tasks (showering, combing hair). He or she may insist on an unusual and eccentric style of hair arrangement or makeup.

4. Extreme impairment. The person is uncooperative and/or actively resists grooming and bathing, creating a health hazard.

2. Clothing and dressing

0. No impairment. The person is able to dress him- or herself without help; he or she dresses appropriate for the season from among his or her possessions, and, if given funds or the opportunity, is able to purchase or appropriately select clothing.

1. Mild impairment. The person dresses him- or herself without prompting or assistance, but sometimes appears sloppy (e.g., soiled or torn clothing, shirttails exposed, buttons or zippers open, shoelaces untied).

2. Moderate impairment. The person needs some prompting or assistance to dress him- or herself. He or she sometimes may dress in odd combinations of clothes (pants are on inside-out; wears multiple layers of clothing) or in seasonally inappropriate clothing (heavy coat in summer). The person may not realize when his or her clothes need to be cleaned.

3. Severe impairment. The person needs extensive assistance in dressing but does not resist this assistance. He or she may often dress in odd combinations or seasonally inappropriate clothing. He or she may disrobe without realizing that the situation is inappropriate.

4. Extreme impairment. The person refuses to wear clothes or is so unresponsive that dressing is ineffective, and therefore spends most of the time in pajamas or robe.

(continued)

3. Eating, feeding, and diet

0. No impairment. The person is able to feed him- or herself without assistance and has specific food preferences. If given funds or opportunity, the person would be able to choose his or her own diet, buy additional food items, or prepare a simple and adequately nutritious meal.

1. Mild impairment. The person can use eating utensils and supplement the meals provided by the residence with food purchased at neighborhood stores. He or she is somewhat sloppy in eating habits and table manners and might choose an unusual diet if unsupervised (e.g., only sweets or only potato chips).

2. Moderate impairment. The person occasionally eats spontaneously but needs constant prompting in order to finish the meal. Use of eating utensils is poor, and use of hands instead of utensils is not unusual. He or she cannot independently care for all dietary needs.

3. Severe impairment. The person accepts food but needs to be supervised while eating. The person may occasionally refuse food, eat excessively, or eat nonnutritive, hazardous substances.

4. Extreme impairment. The person swallows food when fed, but supplements are necessary in order to survive (high-caloric, high-protein supplements or intragastric feeding). If unsupervised, the person may be at risk of choking.

4. Money management

0. No impairment. The person is able to manage his or her own money without assistance. The person knows how much money he or she has, can count money, is capable of budgeting, and spends it accordingly.

1. Mild impairment. The person is able to manage his or her own money with some assistance. He or she may need some help in budgeting his or her money but is able to spend budgeted money without significant assistance.

2. Moderate impairment. The person needs considerable assistance with budgeting, counting, and spending money. If unsupervised, he or she may spend money impulsively or give large sums away. However, he or she is capable of performing some or most of these activities *with the help of staff* prompting or monitoring (e.g., purchasing an item).

3. Severe impairment. Most aspects of money management need to be performed or closely supervised by staff members. The person is not capable of performing even the simplest of tasks involving money without assistance, but he or she wishes to have money or values what it can purchase.

4. Extreme impairment. The person is unwilling to participate in any aspects of money management and is uninterested in money and buying things. The person's money is completely managed by others.

(continued)

5. Neatness and maintenance activities

0. No impairment. The person keeps his or her room neat and helps staff in maintenance activities in the house.

1. Mild impairment. The person requires some prompting to keep his or her room neat. He or she sometimes helps out with maintenance in the house when asked by staff.

2. Moderate impairment. The person needs extensive prompting or actual assistance to keep his or her room clean.

3. Severe impairment. The person can only minimally participate in any household maintenance tasks. He or she can do some simple activities when prompted (e.g., picking up clothes from the floor), but otherwise staff must maintain his or her room.

4. Extreme impairment. The person does not assist in any household maintenance tasks.

6. Orientation/mobility

0. No impairment. Person is able to leave the house on his or her own and return at the appropriate and agreed-upon time.

1. Mild impairment. The person knows his or her way around the neighborhood and can leave the house unaccompanied, but he or she is sometimes late when arriving at destinations.

2. Moderate impairment. The person can usually leave the house unaccompanied, but he or she sometimes fails to arrive at a destination or fails to return on time. The person may know some parts of the neighborhood.

3. Severe impairment. The person can leave the house only when escorted and would otherwise fail to arrive at his or her destination. The person knows few parts of the neighborhood.

4. Extreme impairment. The person does not leave the house and shows no incentive to leave.

7. Reading/writing

0. No impairment. The person writes letters and reads (e.g., newspapers, books).

1. Mild impairment. The person writes a little (e.g., a simple note, occasional brief letter) and reads a little (e.g., a brief newspaper article) on his or her own. The person needs help with correctly addressing and mailing a letter.

2. Moderate impairment. The person reads and/or writes some if prompted, but rarely does so on his or her own initiative. The person cannot read beyond simple sentences.

(continued)

3. Severe impairment. The person signs his or her name, or reads simple signs, but not more, even if prompted.

4. Extreme impairment. The person is essentially illiterate; he or she does not read or write at all, even if prompted, and does not sign his or her name.

8. Impulse control

0. No impairment. The person waits as necessary in order to have his or her needs met.

1. Mild impairment. Occasionally, the person is impatient (e.g., repeats the same demand, is excessively emphatic when making a request). His or her impulses can be controlled with simple reminders.

2. Moderate impairment. The person is sometimes intrusive if his or her needs are not met immediately. He or she may have loud outbursts but is not violent. Verbal commands or brief periods of time in a quiet room are adequate to maintain control of his or her impulses.

3. Severe impairment. The person often has problems with outbursts that require seclusion (e.g., at least once every week or two). Certain topics of conversation or certain situations are avoided to prevent these outbursts.

4. Extreme impairment. The person is prone to violent outbursts that require seclusion (e.g., several times per week) and is avoided by other clients and staff members.

9. Respect for property

0. No impairment. The person follows social rules regarding respect for others' property and adequately maintains his or her own property.

1. Mild impairment. The person maintains his or her property and respects the property of others, but sometimes needs reminders to obey these social rules.

2. Moderate impairment. The person understands the difference between his or her property and that of others. He or she may occasionally take others' property but is willing to return it when requested. The person sometimes may not notice or protest when someone takes his or her property.

3. Severe impairment. The person has a limited understanding of the distinction between his or her property and that of others and often disobeys social rules regarding property (e.g., regularly takes others' property or gives his or her own away). The person responds to prompts to follow conventional rules regarding property (e.g., giving others' property back when instructed to).

4. Extreme impairment. The person does not follow social rules in regard to respecting others' property or maintaining his or her own and does not respond to prompts to follow these rules.

(continued)

10. Telephone skills

0. No impairment. The person uses the telephone appropriately, including the use of directory assistance.

1. Mild impairment. The person dials most telephone numbers without assistance but needs help in using directory assistance.

2. Moderate impairment. The person uses the telephone but consistently needs assistance in dialing.

3. Severe impairment. The person needs extensive assistance with using the telephone (e.g., dialing, speaking into the receiver, speaking loudly enough, knowing when to hang up).

4. Extreme impairment. The person refuses or is incapable of using the telephone, even when extensive assistance is offered.

11. Conversation skill

0. No impairment. The person converses with others in a socially appropriate, skilled manner (e.g., choice of topic, level of self-disclosure, good eye contact, and voice loudness).

1. Mild impairment. The person has fairly good skills when conversing with others. His or her choice of conversational topic or self-disclosure may occasionally be inappropriate, or his or her nonverbal skills (eye contact, interpersonal distance) or paralinguistic skills (voice tone, loudness) may need some improvement. Feedback is successful in getting the person to alter his or her behavior.

2. Moderate impairment. The person has some ability to engage in conversations with others (e.g., can talk for several minutes with another person), but often demonstrates poor skills (e.g., choice of topic, nonverbal, and paralinguistic skills). Feedback produces only small improvements in these skills.

3. Severe impairment. The person has great difficulty sustaining any conversation for more than a very brief period (e.g., 30 seconds to 1 minute). People have difficulty following the person's conversations, which may revolve around delusions or lead nowhere in particular. The person appears not to listen to others but can briefly engage other people in conversations. Feedback is ineffective at improving the person's ability to converse.

4. Extreme impairment. The person is incapable of engaging in even very brief conversations, even when prompted. The person is mute, speaks in a garbled fashion, has severely disordered syntax, or is so preoccupied with delusions that even brief conversations are impossible.

(continued)

12. Instrumental social skills

0. No impairment. The person understands the house rules and the roles of staff members and is able to ask for specific services from appropriate staff members in a socially skillful manner. The person regularly attains the instrumental (tangible) goals of his or her interactions.

1. Mild impairment. The person is often able to achieve the instrumental goals of his or her interactions. The person may occasionally ask an inappropriate person for something. Social skill problems may occasionally limit the person's ability to achieve instrumental goals (e.g., the person demands something rather than requests it; he or she stands inappropriately close to the other person; he or she speaks in a low voice tone).

2. Moderate impairment. The person sometimes achieves the instrumental goals of his or her interactions with others, but his or her success is often hampered by poor social skills (e.g., lack of specificity, prominent deficits in nonverbal and paralinguistic skills). The person may misperceive social roles (e.g., asking the cook for a change in medication). Despite these limitations, the person tries regularly to obtain instrumental goals.

3. Severe impairment. The person rarely attains instrumental goals of social interactions because of poor social skills and misperception of social roles. The person approaches others occasionally to achieve instrumental goals.

4. Extreme impairment. The person never approaches others to achieve instrumental goals.

13. Respect and concern for others

0. No impairment. The person shows appropriate respect and concern for others' feelings in his or her interactions, even during emotionally charged conflicts.

1. Mild impairment. The person occasionally shows inappropriate disregard for others' feelings (e.g., during a conflict). When prompted, the person can demonstrate more appropriate respect.

2. Moderate impairment. The person sometimes appears unaware of how others may feel about what he or she says (e.g., insulting others).

3. Severe impairment. The person sometimes makes crude and inappropriate comments. He or she makes lewd sexual comments or crude racial slurs without regard to how these remarks are perceived by his or her audience.

4. Extreme impairment. The person frequently makes crude and inappropriate comments without regard to how they are perceived by others.

(continued)

14. Social appropriateness/politeness

0. No impairment. The person's interactions with others are well mannered and polite. Even in emotionally charged situations, he or she usually conducts him- or herself in a thoughtful and considerate fashion.

1. Mild impairment. The person is sometimes socially awkward but is usually polite. He or she may occasionally be impolite (e.g., asking an intrusive question, not responding to a greeting) but responds when given feedback about such behaviors.

2. Moderate impairment. The person often fails to demonstrate common polite behaviors (e.g., making greetings, getting out of someone's way, responding to simple requests such as turning down the radio) and is sometimes socially inappropriate. When the person is given feedback about his or her behavior, some small improvements are possible.

3. Severe impairment. The person is almost never polite and is often socially inappropriate. Attempts to correct his or her behavior are largely unsuccessful.

4. Extreme impairment. The person is socially inappropriate nearly all the time. His or her behavior and speech are characterized by unacceptable social conduct.

15. Social engagement

0. No impairment. The person both initiates social interactions with others on a regular basis (e.g., several times per day) and is responsive to interactions initiated by others. Social interactions are not limited to very brief periods but may extend to longer periods of time (e.g., more than 15 minutes).

1. Mild impairment. The person both initiates social interactions with others and is responsive to others, but interactions tend to be shorter or occur less frequently.

2. Moderate impairment. The person regularly participates in social interactions, but he or she usually reciprocates social interactions, rather than initiates them.

3. Severe impairment. The person usually avoids social contacts. He or she rarely initiates social interactions, and when others initiate an interaction, he or she is only minimally responsive. Most interactions are quite brief.

4. Extreme impairment. The person actively refuses to interact with others and may leave the room when someone enters. He or she may react with fear or aggression if forced to interact.

(continued)

16. Friendships

0. No impairment. The person has friendly relationships with others inside and outside the house. At least one of these friendships goes beyond acquaintance, and the nature of the friendship is close, stable, long-lasting, and mutually rewarding.

1. Mild impairment. The person has several acquaintances but has difficulties in forming and maintaining close, stable friendships. The person may interact preferentially with staff members instead of peers. Or he or she may have friendships that are based on abnormal content or motivation. For example, the person exploits or is being exploited sexually or financially, or the relationship is based on inappropriate or unusual attractions.

2. Moderate impairment. The person may seek out and spend time with one other person, but without meaningful interaction (e.g., sitting silently). The person may seek out a staff member with whom he or she attempts to be friendly.

3. Severe impairment. The person has one or two acquaintances with whom he or she maintains some contact, but these relationships are maintained solely on the initiative of the other person.

4. Extreme impairment. The person has no contacts with either peers or staff members.

17. Recreation/leisure (nonsocial)

0. No impairment. The person has well-developed, specific interests or hobbies (e.g., knitting, running, reading, crossword puzzles) in which he or she participates *more than once* a week.

1. Mild impairment. The person has definite interests or hobbies, to which he or she devotes regular, but less than frequent, time (once a week or less).

2. Moderate impairment. The person has some specific interests, but involvement in activity is irregular (once or twice a month).

3. Severe impairment. The person has some superficial interests (favorite TV program or magazine; follows a sports team) in which he or she engages.

4. Extreme impairment. The person has no superficial interests or hobbies. He or she may spend his or her free time involved in nondiscriminating TV viewing or sitting around smoking cigarettes.

(continued)

18. Participation in house social activities

0. No impairment. The person takes appropriate and selective advantage of social activities offered by the house staff and appears to enjoy them.

1. Mild impairment. The person often participates in social activities organized by the house staff, but occasional prompting is needed.

2. Moderate impairment. The person participates in some social activities organized by the house staff, but he or she often needs to be prompted and occasionally leaves before the activity is completed.

3. Severe impairment. The person passively and reluctantly participates in occasional social activities organized by the house staff, but rarely or never of his or her own accord.

4. Extreme impairment. The person refuses to participate in social activities organized by the house staff.

19. Cooperation with treatment

0. No impairment. The person fully cooperates with the treatment plan and implementation. He or she understands the benefits and the risks of the treatment and is an active participant in his or her treatment (e.g., requests a specific medication). The person is able to accurately report adverse effects from medication or intercurrent medical illnesses.

1. Mild impairment. The person is fully compliant with treatment and other suggestions or reasonable requests, but he or she does not actively participate in the treatment plan and occasionally overemphasizes or underemphasizes adverse effects of medication or intercurrent medical illnesses.

2. Moderate impairment. The person is compliant with most suggestions but occasionally refuses treatment or other reasonable requests. He or she may often complain of medical problems that have no physiological explanation.

3. Severe impairment. The person is only selectively compliant with treatment suggestions. Medical illnesses or psychotic symptoms may be exacerbated because of noncompliance with medication or other suggestions.

4. Extreme impairment. The person refuses to comply with treatment to the extent that severe health problems result. He or she may need to be restrained or medicated by force or through court intervention.

SOCIAL SKILLS CHECKLIST

Name: _____   Date: _____

Clinician's name: _____

Check Rating Period: Initial ___; 3 months ___; 6 months ___; 12 months ___; other time period ___

Directions: Complete this checklist to provide an assessment of the person's social behavior and functioning over the past month. For some behaviors, it may be necessary to ask for additional information from others who have more frequent contact with the person and are aware of a wide variety of his or her interactions and activities. Depending on the setting, this may be a counselor, nurse, therapist, psychiatric aide, "primary staff member," case manager, or a significant other (such as a family member). When possible, the same clinician should complete this form at each rating period.

Social skill	Not at all or rarely	Some of the time	Often or most of the time	Data not available
Looks at the other person while talking.				
Maintains appropriate social distance (approximately an arm's length away).				
Makes other people feel comfortable (e.g., greets others, listens to others, says positive or supportive things to others).				
Initiates conversations.				
Maintains conversation.				
Expresses positive feelings to others.				
Can resolve conflicts without arguments.				
Has social contact with other people.				
Maintains at least one close relationship (with friend, family, boyfriend/girlfriend, staff member).				
Speaks up for self assertively and politely.				
Asks for help assertively and politely.				
Communicates with members of the treatment team by asking questions and/or expressing concerns.				

OBSERVATION OF ROLE-PLAY TESTS

EXAMPLES OF SITUATIONS THAT CAN BE USED IN ROLE-PLAY TESTS

The staff member gives these instructions to the person participating in the role-play test: "The purpose of this procedure is to find out how you react to situations that might typically occur on a day-to-day basis. Each situation will require you to interact with another person. I will explain what the situation is to you. I would like you to imagine that you are in that situation. After I have described the situation, I will say something. Each time I say something, I would like you to respond as you would if I were talking to you in the real situation. Remember to listen carefully to the situation I describe to you. Again, in each situation, respond as if it were actually occurring."

The following role-play scenes contain descriptions of specific situations and statements or questions for the staff member to make to the person participating in the role play. The staff member must allow time for the person to respond to each question or statement. Some role plays include alternatives for the staff member, depending on the response of the person participating in the role play. For example, in the role play for Making Requests, there is one set of statements if the person is able to make a request and another set of statements if the person just engages in conversation.

NOTE: The staff member should *not* read aloud the name of the skill that the situation is meant to assess (Expressing Positive Feelings, Making Requests, Expressing Unpleasant Feelings, etc.).

Expressing positive feelings

Situation: You get on a crowded bus with two heavy packages. An acquaintance of yours, who is sitting down, sees you and offers to give you his seat, saying:

1. "Hi, _____, why don't you take my seat?"
2. "That package looks really heavy."
3. "Seems like the buses get more crowded every day."

Making Request

Situation: You've received a letter from the Internal Revenue Service (IRS) about your taxes. You've read the letter carefully, but you don't understand what the letter is about. You think your counselor at the mental health center would understand the letter. You know she is in the office this afternoon, and you stop by to see her about it. She says:

1. "Hi, _____."

If the person makes the request:

2. "I'd like to help you. But I'm really busy at the moment. Could you come back later?"
3. "It could take me a long time."

If the person does not make the request:

2. "It's good to see you today."
3. "I'm glad you stopped by."

(continued)

Making Complaints

Situation: You are in a restaurant and have just finished your meal. The waiter brings your check, and you notice he has overcharged you by two dollars. He says:

1. "Thank you. Please come again."

If the person brings up the mistake in the bill:

2. "No, I don't think so."
3. "I usually don't make mistakes."

If the person does not bring up the mistake in the bill:

2. "It's been a pleasure to serve you."
3. "You can pay on your way out."

Compromise and Negotiation

Situation: You and your friend have decided to do something together on Friday evening. Your friend wants to rent a horror movie. You really dislike horror movies, and you try never to watch them. She says:

1. "I'm really in the mood to see a horror movie. Let's rent _____, the horror movie that just came out on video."
2. "I'm in the mood for a movie, so I thought we'd see that one."
3. "OK, let's do that."

Starting a Conversation with a New or Unfamiliar Person

Situation: You are sitting in the lounge waiting for your group to begin. You notice a stranger sitting across the room. This person looks at you and says:

1. "Hi."
2. "This is my first day here."
3. "Thanks for talking to me."

Responding to Complaints

Situation: You have broken a vase belonging to your roommate. It was an unavoidable accident, but you are blamed for breaking it. Your roommate says:

1. "Did you break my vase?"
2. "How can you be so clumsy?"
3. "You can't be trusted around any of my things."

(continued)

310

Asking Questions about Health-Related Concerns

Situation: You are at the doctor's office for a physical checkup. He gives you an examination and checks your heart and blood pressure. He tells you his findings. But he uses medical terms that you don't understand. He turns and starts to leave, saying,

1. "That's all. You can get dressed and leave now."

If the person asks for clarification:

2. "I can explain what I meant in more simple language. _____."
3. "Thank you for letting me know that I wasn't being clear."

If the person does not ask for clarification:

2. "OK. You can see my secretary about a follow-up appointment."
3. "Have a nice day."

Refusing Requests

Situation: You are having lunch with a friend, when she asks to borrow five dollars until payday. You are short on money and were planning to spend it on something for yourself. Your friend says:

1. "Please lend me the money. I'll pay you back next week."

If the person says he or she cannot lend the money:

2. "But I really need the money."
3. "I don't know what I'll do if I don't have the money."

If the person agrees to lend the money:

2. "Thanks. You are a real friend."
3. "I knew I could count on you."

Expressing Unpleasant Feelings

Situation: You have a friend who is always late. He promised to pick you up at 4:00 P.M. to go shopping. He finally shows up at 4:45. You are bothered by this and decide to tell him. He says:

1. "Hi. I'm here."

If the person expresses negative feeling:

2. "I got held up in traffic."
3. "I can't help it if there are a lot of cars on the road at this time of day."

If the person does not express negative feelings,:

2. "You look like you're ready to do some serious shopping."
3. "I think we're going to find some good things on sale today."

(continued)

311

Expressing Positive Feelings

Situation: You are in the hospital recovering from minor surgery. A relative comes in to visit you. She says:

1. "I just wanted to stop in to say hello."
2. "How are you feeling?"
3. "We'll have to get together after you get out of the hospital."

EXAMPLES OF BEHAVIORS RATED AS "OCCUR/NONOCCUR" IN A ROLE PLAY TEST

Behaviors That Can Be Rated in Most Role Plays

Gaze

Definition: Looks at the other person while speaking and listening, without staring.

Example: Eye contact is maintained intermittently, interspersed by gazing in the direction of the partner.

Appropriate volume

Definition: Voice volume is neither too soft nor too loud; can easily be heard by the other person.

Facial expressiveness

Definition: Smiles, frowns, and other facial gestures are congruent with verbal content.

Example: Smiles when telling or hearing something amusing, frowns when hearing or telling something upsetting or aggravating, lifts eyebrows when confused or asking a question.

Speaking with inflections

Definition: Voice tone is not monotonic, and inflection is used to communicate emphasis and emotion.

Timely responses

Definition: Response latency should generally be brief, and mediators such as "Let me think about that" and "Hmm" are employed when a response must be contemplated.

Example: Speech rate is at a normative conversational level. There are no long pauses or total silences in response to what another person is saying.

(continued)

Behaviors That Can Be Rated in Specific Role Plays

Verbal expression of positive feelings

Definition: Verbal content expressing positive feelings (e.g., appreciation, admiration, approval, or gratitude for some aspect of another person's behavior or manner).

Example: "Thank you for giving up your bus seat so that I can sit down. I really appreciate it." "You are very kind to visit me in the hospital. It makes me feel good to see you."

Nonverbal expression of positive feelings

Definition: Positive affective displays with or without specific content.

Example: Laughs, makes affectionate physical gestures, smiles.

Verbal expression of negative feelings

Definition: Verbal content expressing negative feelings (e.g., dissatisfaction, upset feelings, disapproval, or displeasure in regard to the other person's behavior).

Example: "It upsets me when you are late. I would really appreciate it if you could call me if you are going to be late."

Nonverbal expression of negative feelings

Definition: Negative affect or affective tone with or without explicit verbal content.

Example: Uses a firm tone, does not laugh or giggle.

Making a request

Definition: Specifies what the request entails. Tells the other person that his or her help would be appreciated.

Example: "I would appreciate it if you could help me understand this letter I have received. It uses terms that I don't understand. I would feel more confident if you could take a look at it."

Making a complaint

Definition: Explains what the situation is that is prompting the complaint. Suggests how the problem could be corrected.

Example: "I think the addition is incorrect on my bill. I would appreciate it if you could add it up again."

(continued)

Compromise and negotiation

Definition: Explains one's own viewpoint, acknowledges the other person's viewpoint. Suggests a compromise or agreeable alternative.

Example: "I don't want to see a horror film. But I know we both like comedies. Could we see a comedy tonight?"

Initiating conversation

Definition: Introduces oneself (or greets the other person by name if he or she is an acquaintance). Makes small talk.

Example: "Hi. My name is Xavier. I haven't seen you here before. How do you like it so far?"

Refusing a request

Definition: Tells the person he or she cannot do what has been requested.

Example: "I'm sorry, I can't lend you money today. I don't have any to spare."

EXAMPLES OF 5-POINT SCALES THAT CAN BE USED TO RATE ROLE-PLAY TESTS

Overall Social Skill

Overall Social Skill (OSS) is a general measure of a person's social competence. It subsumes other social skill variables, including verbal, nonverbal, and paralinguistic (voice tone, loudness, etc.) elements. The person with good social skill is easy to understand, responds smoothly (e.g., no lengthy pauses or talking over another person), and does not engage in disconcerting behavior. He or she seems comfortable or confident in the particular situation, even if it is difficult. Emotional expressiveness is appropriate and not excessive. When appropriate, the person is task oriented, but he or she appears to be sensitive to social cues from a partner and is able to modify his or her behavior when necessary.

OSS is scored on a 5-point scale:

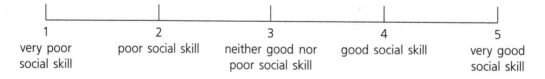

1	2	3	4	5
very poor social skill	poor social skill	neither good nor poor social skill	good social skill	very good social skill

(continued)

Apparent Discomfort

Apparent Discomfort (AD) reflects a person's general level of anxiety, nervousness, tension, or discomfort in a particular situation. Discomfort is reflected in verbal content, paralinguistic aspects of communication (e;.g., speech dysfluencies, stuttering, tremulousness of voice), and nonverbal behavior (motoric tension, nervous gestures, body sway or trembling, foot tapping). Nonverbal manifestations of discomfort may be difficult to distinguish from akathisia; if in doubt, get confirmation from other sources, such as the medical record.

AD is scored on a 5-point scale:

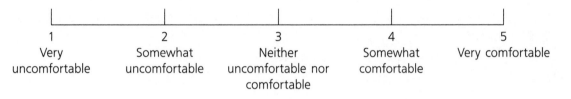

1	2	3	4	5
Very uncomfortable	Somewhat uncomfortable	Neither uncomfortable nor comfortable	Somewhat comfortable	Very comfortable

SOCIAL SKILLS GOALS SELF-RATING SCALE

Name: _____   Date: _____

Check Rating Period: Initial ___; 3 months ___; 6 months ___; 12 months ___; other time period ___

The following is a list of goals that you set before or while participating in social skills training. On a scale of 1 to 5, please rate how close you are to achieving each goal.

Goals	How close am I to achieving this goal?				
	1 = no progress toward achieving this goal 2 = a little progress toward achieving this goal 3 = moderately close to achieving this goal 4 = very close to achieving this goal 5 = this goal has been achieved				
	1	2	3	4	5
	1	2	3	4	5
	1	2	3	4	5
	1	2	3	4	5
	1	2	3	4	5
	1	2	3	4	5
	1	2	3	4	5
	1	2	3	4	5
	1	2	3	4	5

SOCIAL SKILLS GOALS CLINICIAN RATING SCALE

Name: _____   Date: _____

Clinician: _____

Check Rating Period: Initial ___; 3 months ___; 6 months ___; 12 months ___; other time period ___

Clinician: Please list all goals set at initial meeting as initial goals. All goals that are modified should be listed in the lower section under "Modified/New Goals." Any goals set in subsequent meetings are also recorded in the "Modified/New Goals" section. Dates of goal outcomes should be placed in the selected boxes.

Initial Goals

Goals	Date set	Not achieved	Partially achieved	Fully achieved	Modified (see below)
1.					
2.					
3.					
4.					

Modified/New Goals

Goals	Modified from goal #	Date set	Not achieved	Partially achieved	Fully achieved	Modified
5.						
6.						
7.						
8.						

SOCIAL SKILLS TRAINING GROUP PROGRESS NOTE

Group Member: _____   Clinician: _____

Group Member's Goal(s): _____

_____

Dates of sessions	Skill taught	Number of role plays	Atten- tive- ness*	Coopera- tion**	Perfor- mance ***	Homework com- plete?****	Homework assigned?

*To rate attentiveness:

1 = attentive 1–20% of the time; may at times know what is being discussed, but usually is self-absorbed or preoccupied.

2 = attentive 20–40% of the time; fades in and out of awareness, but on average is following the group less than half the time.

3 = attentive 40–60% of the time; about half the time the person is following what is going on in the group and the other half is distracted or acting bored.

4 = attentive 60–80% of the time; most of the time knows what is going on, although there may be a few lapses in attention.

5 = attentive 80–100% of the time; gives relevant and specific answers to questions.

(continued)

**To rate cooperation:

1 = only minimally willing to participate; openly defiant and disruptive; considerable time is taken to encourage client to participate.

2 = rather reluctant to participate, but shows some definite efforts; may answer questions when called upon, but refuses to role play.

3 = willing to do what is asked with no resistance; answers questions and engages in role pays, but does not volunteer.

4 = actively participates, at least partly without prompting; may start off hesitantly, but warms up quickly and displays some enthusiasm.

5 = easy to engage in discussions and role plays; enthusiastic and volunteers to be involved in group activities; may spontaneously give supportive feedback to others.

***To rate performance of the skill:

1 = requires tremendous amount of assistance to perform the skill; shows little or no ability to rehearse the skill without extensive therapist coaching.

2 = requires considerable coaching and/or redirection, but is able to demonstrate some skill spontaneously; on average can follow only two steps of the skill.

3 = needs some help or redirection, but on average can follow at least three steps of the skill.

4 = needs little corrective feedback following role plays; follows at least three steps and needs help only in "fine-tuning" role plays.

5 = no assistance necessary to follow all steps of the skill; may perform the role play in a creative, inventive way.

****To rate homework completion

1 = did not complete any of the homework assignment.

2 = partially completed the homework assignment.

3 = fully completed the homework assignment.

SOCIAL SKILLS HOMEWORK RECORD

Name: _____ Date Assigned: _____

Staff or Family Member Assisting with Homework (optional): _____

Date Assignment Is Due: _____

Skill Being Practiced: _____

Brief description of assignment:

_____

_____

_____

Date practiced: _____ Time: _____ Location: _____

Briefly describe what took place:

_____

_____

_____

How effective were you at using the skill during the homework? Please check one:

___ 1. not at all effective

___ 2. a little effective

___ 3. moderately effective

___ 4. very effective

___ 5. highly effective

Additional comments:

_____

_____

_____

SOCIAL SKILLS EFFECTIVENESS SELF-RATING SCALE

Name: _____   Date: _____

Clinician: _____

Check Rating Period: Initial ___; 3 months ___; 6 months ___; 12 months ___; other time period ___

Skill	An example of a situation in which I might need to use this skill	How effective am I at dealing with situations that require the use of this skill? 1 = not at all effective 2 = a little effective 3 = moderately effective 4 = very effective 5 = highly effective
		1 2 3 4 5
		1 2 3 4 5
		1 2 3 4 5
		1 2 3 4 5
		1 2 3 4 5
		1 2 3 4 5
		1 2 3 4 5

References

Andreasen, N. C. (1982). Negative symptoms in schizophrenia: Definition and reliability. *Archives of General Psychiatry, 39*, 784–788.

Bandura, A. (1969). *Principles of behavior modification*. New York: Holt, Rinehart & Winston.

Becker, D. R., & Drake, R. E. (2003). *A working life for people with severe mental illness*. New York: Oxford University Press.

Becker, D. R., Drake, R. E., Bond, G. R., Xie, H., Dain, B. J., & Harrison, K. (1998). Job terminations among persons with severe mental illness participating in supported employment. *Community Mental Health Journal, 34*, 71–82.

Bellack, A. S. (in press). Social skills for severe mental illness. *Psychiatric Rehabilitation Journal*.

Bellack, A. S., Bennett, M. E., & Gearon, J. S. (2000). *Behavioral treatment for substance abuse in schizophrenia*. Unpublished treatment manual. Baltimore, MD.

Bellack, A. S., Blanchard, J. J., & Mueser, K. T. (1996). Cue availability and affect perception in schizophrenia. *Schizophrenia Bulletin, 22*, 535–544.

Bellack, A. S., & DiClemente, C. C. (1999). Treating substance abuse among patients with schizophrenia. *Psychiatric Services, 50*, 75–80.

Bellack, A. S., & Hersen, M. (Eds.). (1979). *Research and practice in social skills training*. New York: Plenum.

Bellack, A. S., & Morrison, R. L. (1982). Interpersonal dysfunction. In A. S. Bellack, M. Hersen, & A. E. Kazdin (Eds.), *Interpersonal handbook of behavior modification and therapy* (pp. 717–748). New York: Plenum Press.

Bellack, A. S., Morrison, R. L., Mueser, K. T., Wade, J. H., & Sayers, S. L. (1990). Role play for assessing the social competence of psychiatric patients. *Psychological Assessment: A Journal of Consulting and Clinical Psychology, 2*, 248–255.

Bellack, A. S., & Mueser, K. T. (1993). Psychological treatment for schizophrenia. *Schizophrenia Bulletin, 19*, 317–336.

Bellack, A. S., Mueser, K. T., Wade, J., Sayers, S. L., & Morrison, R. L. (1992). The ability of schizophrenics to perceive and cope with negative affect. British *Journal of Psychiatry, 160*, 473–480.

Bellack, A. S., & Thomas-Lohrman, S. (2003). *Maryland Assessment of Social Competence*. Unpublished assessment manual. Baltimore, MD.

Benton, M. K., & Schroeder, H. E. (1990). Social skills training with schizophrenics: A meta-analytic evaluation. *Journal of Consulting and Clinical Psychology, 58*, 741–747.

Birchwood, M., Smith, J., Cochrane, R., Wetton, S., & Copestake, S. (1990). The Social Functioning Scale: The development and validation of a new scale of social adjustment for use in family intervention programmes with schizophrenic patients. *British Journal of Psychiatry, 157*, 853–859.

Bond, G. R., Becker, D. R., Drake, R. E., Rapp, C. A., Meisler, N., Lehman, A. F., Bell, M. D., & Blyler, C. R. (2001). Implementing supported employment as an evidence-based practice. *Psychiatric Services, 52,* 313–322.

Bond, G. R., Drake, R. E., Mueser, K. T., & Latimer, E. (2001). Assertive community treatment for people with severe mental illness: Critical ingredients and impact on clients. *Disease Management and Health Outcomes, 9,* 141–159.

Buztlaff, R. L., & Hooley, J. M. (1998). Expressed emotion and psychiatric relapse: A meta-analysis. *Archives of General Psychiatry, 55,* 547–552.

Carey, K. B. (1996) Substance use reduction in the context of outpatient psychiatric treatment: A collaborative, motivational, harm reduction approach. *Community Mental Health Journal, 32,* 291–306.

Center for Psychiatric Rehabilitation of the University of Chicago. (1998). *Street smarts: Skills for surviving in an urban setting.* Chicago: University of Chicago.

Childswork/Childsplay. (1995). *Everyone has feelings!* [poster]. Plainview, NY: Authors.

Childswork/Childsplay. (1998). *Face it!* [card game]. Plainview, NY: Authors.

Corrigan, P. (1995). Wanted: Champions of psychiatric rehabilitation. *American Psychologist, 50,* 514–521.

Corrigan, P., & Lundin, R. (2001). *Don't call me nuts: Coping with the stigma of mental illness.* Chicago: Recovery Press.

Corrigan, P. W. (1991). Social skills training in adult psychiatric populations: A meta-analysis. *Journal of Behavior Therapy and Experimental Psychiatry, 22,* 203–210.

Daniels, L. (1998). A group cognitive-behavioral and process-oriented approach to treating the social impairment and negative symptoms associated with chronic mental illness. *Journal of Psychotherapy Practice and Research, 7,* 167–176.

Davidson, L. (2003). *Living outside mental illness: Qualitative studies of recovery in schizophrenia.* New York: New York University Press.

Davis, M., Eshelman, E., & McKay, M. (1995). *The relaxation and stress reduction workbook* (4th ed.). Oakland, CA: New Harbinger.

Dezan, N. (1995). *Yesterdays.* Mt. Airy, MD: Eldersong.

Dezan, N. (1996). *You be the judge.* Mt. Airy, MD: Eldersong.

Dilk, M. N., & Bond, G. R. (1996). Meta-analytic evaluation of skills training research for individuals with severe mental illness. *Journal of Consulting and Clinical Psychology, 64,* 1337–1346.

Dixon, L., Haas, G., Weiden, P. J., Sweeney, J., & Frances, A. J. (1991). Drug abuse in schizophrenic patients: Clinical correlates and reasons for use. *American Journal of Psychiatry, 148,* 224–230.

Dixon, L., McFarlane, W., Lefley, H., Lucksted, A., Cohen, C., Falloon, I., Mueser, K. T., Miklowitz, D., Solomon, P., & Sondheimer, D. (2001). Evidence-based practices for services to family members of people with psychiatric disabilities. *Psychiatric Services, 52,* 903–910.

Donahoe, C. P. J., & Driesenga, S. A. (1988). A review of social skills training with chronic mental patients. In M. Hersen, R. M. Eisler, & P. M. Miller (Eds.), *Progress in behavior modification* (Vol. 24, pp. 131–164). Newbury Park, CA: Sage.

Drake, R. E., Essock, S. M., Shaner, A., Carey, K. B., Minkoff, K., Kola, L., Lynde, D., Osher, F. C., Clark, R. E., & Rickards, L. (2001). Implementing dual diagnosis services for clients with severe mental illness. *Psychiatric Services, 52,* 469–476

Eckman, T. A., Wirshing, W. C., Marder, S. R., Liberman, R. P., Johnston-Cronk, K., Zimmermann, K., & Mintz, J. (1992). Technique for training schizophrenic patients in illness self-management: A controlled trial. *American Journal of Psychiatry, 149,* 1549–1555.

Falloon, I. R. H., Boyd, J. L., & McGill C. W. (1984). *Family care of schizophrenia.* New York: Guilford Press.

Falloon, I. R. H., Laporta, M., Fadden, G., & Graham-Hole, V. (1993). *Managing stress in families: Cognitive and behavioural strategies for enhancing coping skills.* London: Routledge.

Freeman, S. (1989 and 1999). *Penny ante* (Version 1 and Version 2). Hillsborough, NC: Activities and Approaches.

Furman, W., Gleller, M., Simon, S. J., & Kelly, J. A. (1979). The use of a behavioral rehearsal procedure for teaching job-interviewing skills to psychiatric patients. *Behavior Therapy, 10,* 157–167.

Gingerich, S., & Bellack, A. S. (1995). Research-based family interventions for the treatment of schizophrenia. *The Clinical Psychologist, 48,* 24–27.

Glynn, S. M., Marder, S. R., Liberman, R. P., Blair, K., Wirshing, W. C., Wirshing, D. A., Ross, D., & Mintz, J. (2002). Supplementing clinic-based skills training with manual-based community support sessions: Effects on social adjustment of patients with schizophrenia. *American Journal of Psychiatry, 159,* 829–837.

Gould, R. A., Mueser, K. T., Bolton, E., Mays, V., & Goff, D. (2001). Cognitive therapy for psychosis in schizophrenia: A preliminary meta-analysis. *Schizophrenia Research, 48,* 335–342.

Green, M. F., Kern, R. S., Braff, D. L., Mintz, J. (2000). Neurocognitive deficits and functional outcome in schizophrenia: Are we measuring the "right stuff"? *Schizophrenia Bulletin, 26,* 119–136.

Halford, W. K., & Hayes, R. (1991). Psychological rehabilitation of chronic schizophrenic patients: Recent findings on social skills and family psychoeducation. *Clinical Psychology Review, 23,* 23–44.

Harvey, P. D., Davidson, M., Mueser, K. T., Parrella, M., White, L., & Powchik, P. (1997). Social-Adaptive Functioning Evaluation (SAFE): A rating scale for geriatric psychiatric patients. *Schizophrenia Bulletin, 23,* 131–145.

Heinssen, R. K., Liberman, R. P., & Kopelowicz, A. (2000). Psychosocial skills training for schizophrenia: Lessons from the laboratory. *Schizophrenia Bulletin, 26,* 21–46.

Hersen, M., & Bellack, A. S. (1976). A multiple-baseline analysis of social-skills training in chronic schizophrenics. *Journal of Applied Behavior Analysis, 9,* 239–245.

Hersen, M., & Bellack, A. S. (1976). Social skills training for chronic psychiatric patients: Rationale, research findings and future directions. *Comprehensive Psychiatry, 17,* 559–580.

Hersen, M., Bellack, A. S., & Turner, S. M. (1978). Assessment of assertiveness in female psychiatric patients: Motoric and physiological measures. *Journal of Behavior Therapy and Experimental Psychiatry, 9,* 11–16.

Jeste, D. V., Alexopoulus, G. S., Bartels, S. J., Cummings, J. L., Gallo, J. L., Gottlieb, G. L., Hailpain, M. C., Palmer, B. W., Patterson, T. L., Reynolds, C. F., & Lebowitz, B. D. (1999). Consensus statement on the upcoming crisis in geriatric mental health: Research agenda for the next decade. *Archives of General Psychiatry, 556,* 848–858.

Jonikas, J., & Cook, J. (1993). *Safe, secure, and street-smart: Empowering women with mental illness to achieve greater independence in the community.* Chicago: National Research and Training Center on Psychiatric Disability. University of Illinois at Chicago.

Katz, M. M., & Lyerly, S. B. (1963). Methods for measuring adjustment and social behavior in the community: 1. Rationale, description, descriminative validity and scale development. *Psychological Reports, 13,* 503–535.

Keefe, R. S., & Harvey, P. D. (1994). *Understanding schizophrenia.* New York: Free Press.

Kopelowicz, A., Corrigan, P. W., Schade, M., & Liberman, R. P. (1998). Social skills training. In K. T. Mueser & N. Tarrier (Eds.), *Handbook of social functioning in schizophrenia* (pp. 307–326). Boston: Allyn & Bacon.

Kopelowicz, A., Wallace, C. J., & Zarate, R. (1998). Teaching psychiatric inpatients to re-enter the community: A brief method of improving the continuity of care. *Psychiatric Services, 49,* 1313–1316.

Lecomte, T., Cyr, M., Lesage, A., Wilde, J., Leclerc, C., & Ricard, N. (1999). Efficacy of a self-esteem module in the empowerment of individuals with schizophrenia. *Journal of Nervous and Mental Disease, 187*(7), 406–413.

Lehman, A. F., & Steinwachs, D. M. (1998). Patterns of usual care for schizophrenia: Initial results from the Schizophrenia Patient Outcomes Research Team (PORT) client survey. *Schizophrenia Bulletin, 24,* 11–20.

Liberman, R. P., Blair, K. E., Glynn, S. M., Marder, S. R., W., W., & Wirshing, D. A. (2001). Generalization of skills training to the natural environment. In H. D. Brenner, W. Boker, & R. Genner (Eds.), *The treatment of schizophrenia: Status and emerging trends* (pp. 104–120). Seattle, WA: Hogrefe & Huber.

Liberman, R. P., Lillie, F., Falloon, I. R. H., Harpin, R. E., Hutchinson, W., & Stoute, B. (1984). Social skills training with relapsing schizophrenics: An experimental analysis. *Behavior Modification, 8,* 155–179.

Liberman, R. P., Mueser, K. T., Wallace, C. J., Jacobs, H. E., Eckman, T., & Massel, H. K. (1986). Training skills in the psychiatrically disabled: Learning coping and competence. *Schizophrenia Bulletin, 12,* 631–647.

Liberman, R. P., Wallace, C. J., Blackwell, G., Kopelowicz, A., Vaccaro, J. V., & Mintz, J. (1998). Skills training versus psychosocial occupational therapy for persons with persistent schizophrenia. *American Journal of Psychiatry, 155,* 1087–1091.

Marder, S. R., Wirshing, W. C., Mintz, J., McKenzie, J., Johnston, K., Eckman, T. A., & Johnston-Cronk, K. (1996). Two-year outcome for social skills training and group psychotherapy for outpatients with schizophrenia. *American Journal of Psychiatry, 153,* 1585–1592.

Marsh, D. T. (1998). *Serious mental illness and the family: The practitioner's guide.* New York: Wiley.

Martin, G., & Pear, J. (1996). *Behavior modification: What it is and how to do it* (5th ed.). Upper Saddle River, NJ: Prentice-Hall.

Matousek, N., Edwards, J., Jackson, H. J., Rudd, R. P., & McMurry, N. E. (1992). Social skills training and negative symptoms. *Behavior Modification, 16,* 39–63.

McFarlane, W. R. (2002). *Multifamily groups in the treatment of severe psychiatric disorders.* New York: Guilford Press.

McKay, M., & Fanning, P. (1987). *Progressive relaxation and breathing* [audiocassette]. Oakland, CA: New Harbinger.

Miller, W. R., & Rollnick, S. (2002). *Motivational interviewing* (2nd ed.): *Preparing people for change.* New York: Guilford Press.

Morrison, R. L. (1990). Interpersonal dysfunction. In A. S. Bellack, M. Hersen, & A. E. Kazdin (Eds.), *International handbook of behavior modification and therapy* (3rd ed., pp. 503–522). New York: Plenum Press.

Mueser, K. T. (1998). Social skill and problem solving. In A. S. Bellack & M. Hersen (Eds.), *Comprehensive clinical psychology* (Vol. 6, pp. 183–201). New York: Pergamon Press.

Mueser, K. T., Bellack, A. S., Douglas, M. S., & Morrison, R. L. (1991). Prevalence and stability of social skills deficits in schizophrenia. *Schizophrenia Research, 5,* 167–176.

Mueser, K. T., Bellack, A. S., Douglas, M. S., & Wade, J. H. (1991). Prediction of social skill acquisition in schizophrenic and major affective disorder patients from memory and symptomatology. *Psychiatry Research, 37,* 281–296.

Mueser, K. T., Doonan, R., Penn, D. L., Blanchard, J. J., Bellack, A. S., Nishith, P., & deLeon, J. (1996). Emotion recognition and social competence in chronic schizophrenia. *Journal of Abnormal Psychology, 105,* 271 275.

Mueser, K. T., Foy, D. W., & Carter, M. J. (1986). Social skills training for job maintenance in a psychiatric patient. *Journal of Counseling Psychology, 33,* 360–362.

Mueser, K. T., & Gingerich, S. L. (in press). *Coping with schizophrenia: A guide for families* (2nd ed.). New York: Guilford Press.

Mueser, K. T., & Glynn, S. M. (1999). *Behavioral family therapy for psychiatric disorders* (2nd ed.). Oakland, CA: New Harbinger.

Mueser, K. T., Noordsy, D. L., Drake, R. E., & Fox, L. (2003). *Integrated treatment for dual disorders: A guide to effective practice.* New York: Guilford Press.

Mueser, K. T., Torrey, W. C., Lynde, D., Singer, P., & Drake, R. E. (2003). Implementing evidence-based practices for people with severe mental illness. *Behavior Modification, 27,* 387–411.

Mueser, K. T., Yarnold, P. R., & Bellack, A. S. (1992). Diagnostic and demographic correlates of substance abuse in schizophrenia and major affective disorder. *Acta Psychiatrica Scandinavica, 85,* 48–55.

Patterson, T. L., McKibbin, C., Taylor, M., Goldman, S., Davila-Fraga, W., Bucardo, J., & Jeste, D. V. (2003). Functional Adaption Skills Training (FAST): A pilot psychosocial intervention study in middle-aged and older patients with chronic psychotic disorders. *American Journal of Geriatric Psychiatry, 11,* 17–23.

Penn, D. L., Corrigan, P. W., Bentall, R. P., Racenstein, J. M., & Newman, L. (1997). Social cognition in schizophrenia. *Psychological Bulletin, 121,* 114–132.

Pilling, S., Bebbington, P., Kuipers, E., Garety, P., Geddes, J. R., Martindale, B., Orbach, G., & Morgan, C. (2002). Psychological treatments in schizophrenia: II. Meta-analyses of randomized controlled trials of social skills training and cognitive remediation. *Psychological Medicine, 32,* 783–791.

Pope, H. G., Ionescu-Pioggia, M., Aizley, H. G., & Varma, D. K. (1990). Drug use and life style among college undergraduates in 1989: A comparison with 1969 and 1978. *American Journal of Psychiatry, 147,* 998–1001.

Pratt, S., Bartels, S., Mueser, K., & Haddad, S. (2003). *Psychosocial rehabilitation in older adults with SMI: A review of the research literature and suggestions for development of rehabilitative approaches.* Manuscript submitted for publication.

Prochaska, J. O., & DiClemente, C. C. (1992). Stages of change in the modification of problem behaviors. In M. Hersen, R. M. Eisler, & P. M. Miller (Eds.), *Progress in behavior modification* (Vol. 28). Sycamore, Illinois: Sycamore Publishing Company.

Prochaska, J. O., DiClemente, C. C., & Norcross, J. C. (1992). In search of how people change: Applications to addictive disorders. *American Psychologist, 47,* 1102–1114.

Rosen, A., Hadzi-Pavlovic, D., & Parker, G. (1989). The Life Skills Profile: A measure assessing function and disability in schizophrenia. *Schizophrenia Bulletin, 15,* 325–337.

Schooler, N., Hogarty, G., & Weissman, M. (1979). Social Adjustment Scale II (SAS-II). In W. A. Hargreaves, C. C. Atkisson, & J. E. Sorenson (Eds.), *Resource materials for community mental health program evaluations* (pp. 290–303). Rockville, MD: National Institutes of Mental Health. DHEW Publication No. (ADM) 79–328.

Scott, J. E., & Lehman, A. F. (1998). Social functioning in the community. In K. T. Mueser & N. Tarrier (Eds.), *Handbook of social functioning in schizophrenia* (pp. 1–19). Boston: Allyn & Bacon

Shelley, P., & Wheeler, J. (2000). *Shake loose more memories.* Carnation, WA: Shake Loose a Memory.

Skinner, B. F. (1938). *The behavior of organisms: An experimental analysis.* New York: Appleton-Century-Crofts.

Skinner, B. F. (1953). *Science and human behavior.* New York: Macmillan.

Smith, T. E., Bellack, A. S., & Liberman, R. P. (1996). Social skills training for schizophrenia: Review and future directions. *Clinical Psychology Review, 16,* 599–617.

Smith, T. E., Hull, J. W., Romanelli, S., Fertuck, E., & Weiss, K. A. (1999). Symptoms and neurocognition as rate limiters in skills training for psychotic patients. *American Journal of Psychiatry, 156,* 1817–1818.

Tauber, R., Wallace, C. J., & Lecomte, T. (2000). Enlisting indigenous community supporters in skills training programs for persons with severe mental illness. *Psychiatric Services, 51,* 1428–1432.

Torrey, E. F. (2001). *Surviving schizophrenia: A manual for families, consumers and providers* (4th ed.). New York: HarperTrade.

Tsang, H. W. (2001). Applying social skills training in the context of vocational rehabilitation for people with schizophrenia. *Journal of Nervous and Mental Disease, 189,* 90–98.

Tsang, H. W., & Pearson, V. (2001). Work-related social skills training for people with schizophrenia in Hong Kong. *Schizophrenia Bulletin, 27,* 139–148.

Wallace, C. J. (1998). Social skills training in psychiatric rehabilitation: Recent findings. *International Review of Psychiatry, 10,* 9–19.

Wallace, C. J. (2003). *Final report to the National Institutes of Mental Health on Project 1RO1MH57029: A clinical pilot of the workplace fundamentals module.* Los Angeles: University of California at Los Angeles.

Wallace, C. J., Liberman, R. P., Tauber, R., & Wallace, J. (2000). The Independent Living Skills Survey: A comprehensive measure of the community functioning of severely and persistently mentally ill individuals. *Schizophrenia Bulletin, 26,* 631–658

Wallace, C. J., Tauber, R., & Wilde, J. (1999). Teaching fundamental workplace skills to persons with serious mental illness. *Psychiatric Services, 50,* 1147–1153.

Wellness Reproductions, L.C.C. (2003). *Emotions plus* [poster]. Plainview, NJ: Author.

Wheeler, J., & Shelley, P. (1996). *Shake loose a memory.* Carnation, WA: Shake Loose a Memory.

Wheeler, J., & Shelley, P. (1997). *Shake out the truth.* Carnation, WA: Shake Loose a Memory.

Wykes, T, & Sturt, E. (1986). The measurement of social behaviour in psychiatric patients: An assessment of the reliability and validity of the Social Behavior Schedule. *British Journal of Psychiatry, 148,* 1–11.

Index

Note: Page numbers in **bold** indicate skill sheets.